Washington DC
1987

BC

Predicting fertility : demographic
studies of birth expectations

Predicting Fertility

Predicting Fertility

Demographic Studies of Birth Expectations

Edited by

Gerry E. Hendershot
Paul J. Placek
National Center for
Health Statistics

LexingtonBooks
D.C. Heath and Company
Lexington, Massachusetts
Toronto

Library of Congress Cataloging in Publication Data

Main entry under title:

Predicting fertility.

Includes bibliographical references and index.
1. Fertility, Human—Addresses, essays, lectures. 2. Family size—
Addresses, essays, lectures. 3. Population forecasting—Addresses, essays,
lectures. I. Hendershot, Gerry E. II. Placek, Paul J., 1945-
III. Title: Birth expectations.
HB901.P73   304.6'3   79-9686
ISBN 0-669-03618-8

Published simultaneously in Canada

Printed in the United States of America

International Standard Book Number: 0-669-03618-8

Library of Congress Catalog Card Number: 79-9686

Contents

Preface

Four decades ago, the now classic Indianapolis Study introduced the notion of studying the social-psychological motivations behind women's fertility orientations. Two decades ago, the authors of the monographs from the 1955–1960 Growth of American Families Surveys were confident that women's birth expectations were valid and reliable predictors of future fertility, at least in the aggregate. Measurement of these orientations continued in the 1965 and 1970 National Fertility Surveys, but the authors of the reports of those studies were less optimistic that birth expectations were accurate enough for precise fertility predictions. With the availability of the longitudinal data on fertility orientations from the 1975 National Fertility Survey, new evaluations of birth expectations were undertaken. In the meantime, the National Survey of Family Growth, now the nation's continuing national-fertility survey, has made measurement of fertility orientations (especially birth expectations) an important part of data collection and analysis. Also, questions about birth expectations were asked in the 1964–1966, 1967–1969, and 1972 National Natality Surveys, and are being asked in the 1980 National Natality Survey and 1980 National Fetal Mortality Survey. Furthermore, the Current Population Survey has been measuring birth expectations since the 1971 annual June supplement, and the World Fertility Surveys have routinely included questions on fertility orientations.

Thus predicting fertility through birth expectations is not only a matter of historical interest but is also a salient area of investigation for current and future fertility surveys. Given the considerable interest expressed in this topic by the professional community, the time seems to be right for assessing our knowledge about fertility orientations. The purpose of this book, therefore, is to assemble a significant part of the accumulated methodological, conceptual, and theoretical knowledge about birth expectations.

This book includes a wide range of demographic studies of birth expectations and will be useful as basic background reading for anyone interested in contemporary demography. It is our intention that this book be useful also to people in fields other than demography. Educational planners doing school-enrollment projections, economists utilizing future population size as a relevant variable, market researchers anticipating demands for their products, agricultural experts planning ahead for needed food output, business and military persons doing manpower projections, health planners anticipating future client loads and facility needs, medical-care providers anticipating the need for certain specialties, and health practitioners in the family-planning field all have an interest in understanding the extent to which birth expectations are useful in projecting future fertility.

We acknowledge with gratitude the contributions made by the authors of the various chapters. They worked under rigid deadlines, and their cooperative spirit made this project a pleasure. We appreciate the latitude and encouragement provided by our branch chiefs and division director—Robert Heuser, chief of the Natality Statistics Branch; William Pratt, chief of the Family Growth Branch; and John Patterson, director of the Division of Vital Statistics. However, the conclusions are strictly those of the authors. No official support or endorsement by the Division of Vital Statistics is intended or should be inferred. Also, Kenneth C.W. Kammeyer of the University of Maryland reviewed the first draft and provided valuable suggestions, most of which we incorporated. Very special words of appreciation go to Rebecca Paytash Placek, who typed most of the manuscript, and, with Tabetha Penn Hendershot, assisted in the statistical verification.

Part I
Historical Development and Current Issues

1 Introduction

Paul J. Placek and
Gerry E. Hendershot

Why Predict Fertility?

It is useful to be able to predict the size and composition of population in the future for many reasons, including economic forecasting, evaluations of the quality of life, school-enrollment projections, and assessments of our ability to prosper given finite resources. Since many countries have low and fairly constant mortality rates, and international migration is negligible, the primary determinant of future population trends is fertility. It therefore follows that predicting fertility is the crux of population forecasting.

Future Fertility: Fate versus Control

Drawing on the framework introduced to demography by Back (1967), the notions of *fate* and *control* are useful in conceptualizing the prediction of fertility through women's birth expectations. Typically, fertility-survey questions on birth expectations ask: "Do you expect to have more children? (If definitely or probably yes): How many more children do you think you will probably have?" Respondents who reply, "As many as God sends," or, "I'll probably have more, but I don't know how many more will come along," regard future childbearing as a matter predestined by God or fate. Respondents who reply, "I definitely plan to have one more child in about two years," regard their future fertility as a matter under their firm control.

The concept of fate is an important variable in understanding human fertility in many societies where fertility is relatively high and is a concomitant of the expression of sexual needs. People may not want to control fertility, may have only hopes and fears about future fertility, may drift along toward higher fertility through nondecisions about contraceptive use, or may not have enough reasons to avoid subsequent births. Women may not know that fertility control is technically possible or ethically allowable. They may not have sufficient motivation or a planning orientation, the appropriate psychological makeup, or a social environment that permits decision making.

Control is an equally critical factor in understanding fertility, particularly since women's ability to forecast their own future fertility has improved in recent decades. Women can now better manipulate demo-

3

graphic events that were previously beyond their personal control, such as contraceptive use, abortion, the choice of a marriage partner, work during marriage, or the right to divorce an unsuitable husband. Thus in modern society we increasingly move toward control of fertility.

The traditional methods of demography often submerge the individual choices that influence fertility. Trends, rates, and the influence of macrochanges on these rates are used in making statements about future fertility, without much regard for individual decisions. The perspective is that women are merely passive recipients in the grip of social, economic, and biological forces. While social frameworks and group contexts must be taken into consideration, the role of individual decision making may have become more salient as control over the environment allows more prerogatives over "demographic fate." Thus, the social-psychological approach suggested by the concept of birth expectations may become increasingly useful in demographic studies that predict future fertility.

Birth Expectations and Other Approaches to Population Forecasting

Alternative approaches used in forecasting fertility involve conceptual frameworks other than the social-psychological intentions implied in birth expectations. For example, Easterlin (1978) asserts that age-structure differences resulting from the relative sizes of birth cohorts is the engine of social and economic change in post–World War II America. In large cohorts there is a glut of young people in the labor market, job competition is intense, and the family-formation process is inhibited; young people are less willing to marry and have children. In small cohorts there are relatively fewer young adults competing for jobs, the family-formation process is encouraged, and optimistic couples increase their childbearing aspirations. Easterlin's model is cyclical; every two decades a substantial shift occurs in the relative supply of younger and older workers. Therefore, Easterlin projects a rise in the birth rate in the 1980s owing to the smaller cohorts born in the 1960s. Swings in the age-cohort pendulum exert a powerful leverage on social and economic change and thereby affect fertility aspirations.

A different rationale for the projection of future fertility is provided by Westoff (1978). Amassing a list of normative changes in women's roles as well as of shifts in marital and familial patterns, Westoff concludes that a continuation of current low-fertility patterns lies ahead. Through the development of modern contraceptive technology we have almost achieved the perfect-contraceptive society. Factors associated with postponed marriage, more women working, cohabitation, high divorce rates, a declining remarriage rate, and increased out-of-wedlock childbearing attenuate rather than encourage high fertility, especially in the early, more fecund years of adulthood. Predicting that fertility in the United States and other developed countries will fall to very low levels, probably below replacement, Westoff asserts that Easterlin's forecast is based on only two repetitions of a cyclical pattern in the United States and ignores these recent changes in marriage and the family.

Still another economic model of fertility behavior is presented by William Butz and Michael Ward (1979), who use family income and opportunity costs of women's time during economic growth and recession to predict variation in fertility rates. However, neither Easterlin's cohort-size theory, Westoff's focus on broad sociocultural change, nor the Butz-Ward wage and fertility model regard women's birth expectations as the ultimate determinants of future fertility.

A possible limitation of these approaches is that the individual decisions culminating in a birth are neglected. With these macro approaches, one must implicitly assume that changing economic fortunes and social forces are being perceived by individual women, interpreted in some fairly uniform way, and acted on in terms of expected (and completed) fertility. Are cohort size and broad social changes types of fate, which predetermine future fertility, or are they factors taken into account by individuals attempting to exercise control in achieving a desired level of fertility?

This discussion of conceptual frameworks raises some of the questions that pervade the contemporary study of fertility. Diverse points of view on cause and effect, on relevant variables, and on appropriate methodology presently characterize demographic studies of birth expectations. This book reflects that diversity and ultimately attempts to reconcile some of the major differences of opinion expressed by the contributors.

Organization and Content

This book is divided into four parts. Part I describes the historical development of the study of fertility orientations and identifies current issues; part II provides a sampling of the various methodologies and applications utilized in quantifying fertility orientations; part III describes substantive trends and patterns in birth expectations; and part IV identifies common elements in the various approaches (to the extent that this is possible) and recommends approaches that should be taken in future studies. The editors have added a short note to introduce each chapter and to point out the chapter's relationship to other chapters and to several general issues throughout the book. Also, a list of publications not referred to elsewhere is provided for the benefit of those readers who wish to read still more about birth expectations (see appendix A). Finally, a section on survey questions is provided so that the reader may compare the wide variety of questions used to measure fertility orientations (see appendix B).

In part I Oakley describes in chapter 2 how an inadequate demographic-data base provided the incentive for inventing better predictive measures of fertility. She traces the evolution of specific questions that have been employed and discusses the use that is eventually made of the resulting data. Oakley outlines the controversies that have emerged and suggests that their resolution may be possible through the study of "uncertainty," a promising but relatively unexplored area of fertility orientations. The degree of certainty in expectations may be the critical factor in their accurately predicting fertility intentions.

Part II contains various methodologies and applications used to study fertility orientations, and discusses the issues that have evoked controversy. Long and Wetrogan in chapter 3 review the four basic ways in which birth expectations have been used in making population projections:

1.   Questions on total births expected can be used to project completed cohort fertility.
2.   Births expected by cohorts of young adult women can be used to project completed fertility for females not yet of childbearing age.
3.   Questions on births expected in the very near future can be used to predict short-term fertility.
4.   Knowledge of birth expectations can be used as an ex post facto rationalization for fertility assumptions made from other analyses.

Using a variety of sources of expectations data, the strengths and limitations of the four basic uses are evaluated; and the authors conclude that the use of birth-expectations questions has not yet fulfilled its promise of shifting the burden of responsibility for making accurate fertility projections from the forecaster to the mother.

In chapter 4 Westoff evaluates how accurately data on fertility preferences predict actual subsequent fertility using evidence from four longitudinal studies—the Kelly Study of Engaged Couples, the Princeton Fertility Study, the Detroit Study, and the National Fertility Study (NFS). Westoff asserts that fertility preferences reflect, rather than anticipate, changes in conditions that lead to fluctuations in fertility rates, and thus are no better than conventional period indexes of fertility. He concludes that women's departures from their initial fertility predictions increase with time but that compensating mechanisms obviate these changes in the aggregate. Hendershot and Placek, in chapter 5, examine the aggregate validity, stability, and reliability of birth expectations using the 1972 National Natality Survey (NNS) and the 1973 and 1976 National Surveys of Family Growth (NSFG). Intersurvey reliability is investigated by comparing birth expectations of women with births in 1972 as measured by the NNS and the 1973 NSFG. Temporal stability is investigated by comparing birth expectations of women in the populations that were measured by the NSFG in 1973 and 1976. Finally, predictive validity is investigated by comparing birth expectations in the 1973 NSFG with the actual fertility of women from the same populations as reported in the 1976 NSFG. It was found that women bore 30 percent more children than they expected, suggesting that women's expectations may have remained unchanged but that they also had births that were mistimed and unwanted.

Lee's model for forecasting fertility from birth-expectations data, discussed in chapter 6, provides a conceptual and mathematical framework for predicting fertility when target levels of completed fertility are changing. He shows how turning points in period fertility rates may precede by several years the turning points in desired completed fertility, and how the amplitude of fluctuations in period fertility rates may be much greater than those in reproductive goals. He suggests a two-step procedure: first, forecasting future trends in cohort goals taking contraceptive failure rates into account, and second, combining these forecasted trends with base-period data on children ever born to obtain duration-specific future fertility rates. The mathematics of this approach, which Lee describes as "aiming at a moving target," are lucidly presented.

In chapter 7 Ryder documents changes in the intentions aspect of women's fertility orientations, using the 1970 and 1975 NFS studies—specifically, intended parity, ideal parity, and desired parity. He considers the face validity of the questions producing these three indicators as well as their empirical interconnections. In noting the decline in parity orientations for all three measures, marriage-cohort, period, and marital-duration effects are specified for Catholics and non-Catholics. Ryder also grapples with causes and effects between intended and ideal parity and between intended and desired parity. He recommends abandoning the ideal- and desired-family-size concepts since they do not predict reproductive intentions.

Using 1975 Sri Lanka Fertility Survey data, Pullum (chapter 8) proposes and compares three different strategies for determining the extent to which stated fertility preferences can be used to predict mean completed fertility if women could implement their preferences throughout their family-building careers. The marital-duration strategy uses recently married women's face-value completed-family-size preferences. The second strategy consists of a rationalization model, which adjusts for the fact that women predict what they in fact already have in order to avoid the feeling that they may have failed in achieving their fertility goals. The synthetic-cohort strategy utilizes information about the wantedness status of the latest pregnancy and parity-progression ratios in constructing a synthetic family-building cohort model. Adding religion and region as specifying variables, the three procedures are evaluated for their relative utility in accomplishing a variety of predictive tasks.

Part III on trends and patterns in birth expectations begins with Moore's review (chapter 9) of empirical findings from the 1967 Survey of Economic Opportunity and 1971 through 1979 Current Population Surveys (CPS), both conducted by the Bureau of the Census. He tracks the decrease in family-size norms and transition to lower average parity, and gives special attention to the recency of investigating fertility expectations of single women in the CPS. He concludes that completed cohort fertility can be projected utilizing birth-expectations data, particularly if adjustments are made to allow for the confounding effects of the exclusion of single women from the surveys, recent sharp declines in fertility, reduction in average parity, and the nuances observed for women in certain racial and educational groups. He asserts that while individual-level predictions are not precise, compensating errors balance each other to produce accuracy in the aggregate.

In chapter 10 Masnick uses both completed cohort-fertility data for women born since 1940 and CPS birth-expectations data to complete the fertility histories of younger women who have not yet completed their childbearing. Using an innovative technique, he relates the proportions of each cohort's completed family size, which are at varying levels, to the mean family size for the cohort. He concludes that the youngest cohorts, for whom childbearing is not yet completed, have favored the two-child norm yet have simultaneously postponed births; they are therefore unlikely to "catch up," and Masnick's 1981, 1986, and 1991 projections forecast very low fertility.

In chapter 11 O'Connell examines interstate variations in birth expectation using previously unpublished 1977–1978 CPS data and new estimates of total fertility rates for states for intercensal years. He examines the extent to which there has been a convergence of state total fertility rates over time to a complete cohort fertility rate equivalent to the prevailing average number of lifetime births expected by women 18 to 29 years of age. He concludes that there has not been much evidence of a convergence in state total fertility rates from 1940 to 1977, but that birth-expectations data for women 18 to 29 years old for the period 1977–1978 indicate a uniform expected family size of two children per women across the United States.

Hirsch, Seltzer, and Zelnik, in chapter 12, explore desired-family-size preferences of teenaged women in the 1971 and 1976 National Surveys of Young Women (NSYW). Average desired family size declined from 2.68 in 1971 to 2.52 in 1976; the authors quantify declining family-size desires by race, age, marital status, education, family stability, number of siblings, religion, religiosity, premarital sex activity, and parity. Finally the investigators explore ten reasons that young women gave for wanting a particular number of children (optimum number, population explosion, sex distribution, parental management abilities, finances, and so on).

Blake and Del Pinal bring a unique perspective to the study of predicting fertility by examining attitudes toward childlessnesss in chapter 13. (The 1978 CPS found that 18 percent of single women aged 18 to 24 stated their intention to remain childless.) Using the results of five questions commissioned from a 1978 national survey, five issues are examined—the direct costs of children, opportunity costs (lost and gained), economic perceptions, long-term noneconomic returns for the parents, and children as interaction goods. These issues are examined in relation to a set of other attitudinal predictors about housework, childrearing responsibilities, and working mothers.

Finally, in chapter 14 Cho and Kantrow review Korea, Malaysia, Nepal, Pakistan, Thailand, Fiji, Indonesia, and Sri Lanka World Fertility Survey (WFS) findings on fertility orientations. In these less-developed countries at vastly different stages of social, economic, and family-planning-program development, women have more children than they say they want. The authors assert that total fertility would be significantly reduced if actual family size conformed to desired family size; women in these countries had typically achieved their desired family size by age 30. However, because women in these countries may rationalize for their fertility behavior already completed or may give "courtesy responses" in survey interviews, their measured family-size desires might not be an adequate guide to their future fertility. Cho and Kantrow broaden our notions of the term *rationality* as it is used in understanding fertility orientations, providing us with much-needed cross-cultural perspective.

Given the wide sampling of substantive approaches in analysis, concepts, and methodological applications, the considerable task of part IV is to synthesize. In chapter 15 Campbell evaluates the relative predictability of short-term and long-term expectations and specifically recommends certain research activity for demographers. He states that research on short-term expectations should include:

1. continued comparisons between expectations and subsequent fertility;
2. more emphasis on subgroups, as well as longitudinal analyses of predicted fertility;
3. a focus on five-year rather than shorter intervals;
4. comparisons of expected and actual fertility for all women, not just for currently married women;
5. the development of alternative methods for forecasting short-term fertility.

Campbell also recommends six areas of research needed on long-term birth expectations:

1. The expectations of young women should be verified, separating those who were and were not included in the study samples.
2. Birth expectations should be published by the census bureau for birth cohorts of women, rather than for standard age groups only.
3. There should be greater utilization of cross-cultural data to conduct the proposed research.
4. Continued comparisons should be made between women's birth expectations, cumulative fertility, and the level of age-specific fertility required for them to realize their expectations.
5. The stability and validity of expected births at given orders needs more study.
6. Alternative methods of forecasting completed fertility must be developed, including models that better quantify social and economic factors.

Chapter 16, finally, attempts a synthetic exposition of the diverse material presented by the contributors. The aim is to reconcile conflicting conceptual models and their attendant conclusions, as well as to suggest some new testable hypotheses. An innovative framework is provided that incorporates the macro demographic, economic, and social perspectives with the micro social-psychological approach implied in the concept of birth expectations.

It is hoped that this current appraisal of demographic studies of birth expectations will yield empirically grounded new beginnings and conceptual clarity in future studies of predicting fertility.

References

Back, Kurt W. "New Frontiers in Demography and Social Psychology." *Demography* 4 (1967): 90–97.

Butz, William P., and Ward, Michael P. "The Emergence of Countercyclical U.S. Fertility." *American Economic Review* 69(1979):318–328.

Easterlin, Richard A. "What Will 1984 Be Like? Socioeconomic Implications of Recent Twists in Age Structure." *Demography* 15 (1978): 397–432.

Westoff, Charles F. "Some Speculations on the Future of Marriage and Fertility." *Family Planning Perspectives* 10 (1978): 79–83.

2 Reflections on the Development of Measures of Childbearing Expectations

Deborah Oakley

In this chapter Deborah Oakley describes the historical circumstances that led to the first attempts to measure birth expectations. She traces the subsequent development of various techniques used to measure expectations in demographic studies, several of which are considered in part II, "Methods and Issues."—*Eds.*

The first modern sample fertility survey was conducted in the late 1930s in Indianapolis, Indiana. It was designed to determine whether the births reported had been planned or unplanned and what social, psychological, and economic factors affected fertility. The measures used in analysis were the number of children ever born (CEB) and the planning status of each birth as derived from detailed pregnancy and contraceptive histories. The survey also included a question: "If you could begin your married life over again, and the size of your family could be determined only by your liking for children, how many would you have?" (Reed 1947). This question was wisely bypassed in analyses of predicting fertility since it had numerous deficiencies, including a hypothetical context purposely unrelated to either past or future reality.

Rather, the contribution of various social, economic, and psychological factors to past fertility was measured by means of scaling and factor analysis (Borgatta and Westoff 1954) and applied to predicting fertility as if past relationships would necessarily apply to future reproductive decisions. Unfortunately, the variables included in the study could account for only a minor part of the variance in CEB, not an adequate base for predicting future fertility.

Thus by the end of World War II demographers interested in national fertility trends were dependent for their data on vital statistics, decennial census returns, isolated surveys such as the one in Indianapolis, and small-scale studies. The national birth-registration system did not include all states until 1933, when Texas joined; and as late as 1942 President Franklin Roosevelt had lamented that there was "great confusion in vital records" (U.S. Department of Health, Education, and Welfare 1950, p. 11). New

11

census data came only at ten-year intervals, with delays in producing and distributing its limited fertility data. And most small-scale studies of fertility were confined to special clinic or hospital populations (for example, Stix 1935; Wiehl and Berry 1937; Wiehl 1938). The only substantial fertility study up to that time was the Indianapolis survey, which demonstrated the possibility of gathering data about personal factors including pregnancy and contraceptive histories (Whelpton and Kiser 1946–1958). However, even this pioneering effort did not produce results that could be translated into quantitative fertility indexes. With the results of the Indianapolis study as their best source of information, demographers had no sound theoretical base on which to construct a new predictive measure.

The best measures then available for assessing fertility trends were age-specific birth rates, which dealt only with the past; and the synthetic measure, the total fertility rate (TFR), which had validity for predicting fertility only if there were no intercohort changes in fertility behavior. Since the central professional and public-policy question for demographers was precisely whether there were such changes in process, neither the birth rates nor the TFR were useful as predictors.

Given the inadequate measures, theories, and data about fertility, the prolonged postwar increase in the birth rate challenged demographers. Their predictions of the trend in the birth rate proved to be inaccurate, and their projections of the future population were embarrassingly discrepant from reality. Better measures as well as better data and theories were clearly called for. The measurement of childbearing expectations was one part of the development of better measures; and as the empirical data accumulated, interpretations of expectations data inevitably became entangled in the attempt to develop better theories as well.

Early in the postwar period Whelpton recognized the importance of tracing cohort as well as period fertility patterns and prepared the cohort-fertility measures that have now become standard in fertility analysis (Whelpton 1954; Whelpton and Campbell 1960). With this refinement in the techniques of fertility analysis came the ability to disaggregate overall change into components resulting from changes in average completed fertility and changes in timing. Parity distributions by cohort, including the proportions ever bearing children, could also be compared across age groups. Cohort-fertility tables showed that only 8 percent of the increase in births among women aged 30 to 34 in 1958 as compared to women of that same age in 1942 could be attributed to fifth and higher-order births. Twenty-one percent of the increase was caused by an increase in the number of women having any births at all, and another 59 percent could be attributed to progression to second and third orders (Whelpton and Campbell 1960). Thus it could be shown that, in addition to changes in timing, a major factor in the postwar baby boom was an increase in the proportion of women having children. But the question still remained as to whether there was also an increase in preferred size of families.

The Indianapolis study had provided evidence of a widespread use of contraception; and it was assumed that as the planning of births increased and fertility came under voluntary control, people would become better predictors of their own childbearing.

Development of the Measurement of Expectations

Given these circumstances, Whelpton and Freedman advocated the use of a straightforward approach to a new measure: asking women themselves about their own expectations. The question, "How many children do you expect to have altogether?" was first asked in the 1954 Detroit Area Study of a sample of 427 married women under the age of 40. Response rates were adequate, and the question was shown to elicit responses that were reliable in the short term (Goldberg, Sharp, and Freedman 1959).

In 1955 the first large-scale national-sample survey of married women was conducted for the purpose of investigating women's expectations of future births.[1] These Growth of American Families (GAF) respondents were asked: "Do you expect to have another child? If it is possible for you to do so, would you say definitely yes, probably yes, probably no, or definitely no?" In addition to the categories mentioned, the category "uncertain" was provided as a possible response (Freedman, Whelpton, and Campbell 1959, p. 437). In the 1960 GAF II survey the context and question were slightly different: "You now have _____ living children (or soon will after the baby comes). Do you expect to have (more) children (after this baby)? Would you say definitely yes, probably yes, you're uncertain, probably no, or definitely no?" This was followed by: "How many children do you expect to have in all (counting those you now have)? (Whelpton, Campbell, and Patterson 1966, p. 417).

Similar questions were used in the 1955 and 1958 Detroit Area Study surveys (Goldberg, Sharp, and Freedman 1959), and in a panel study early in 1962, with a followup late in the same year. As early as 1960 Freedman had commented: "What is needed is a time series on an annual basis for the national population of expected and desired number of children" (Freedman 1962, p. 218). Questions on childbearing expectations were added to some of the multipurpose national surveys conducted by the University of Michigan's Survey Research Center, during the 1962–1964 period (Axelrod et al. 1963; Freedman, Goldberg, and Slesinger 1963, 1964), but even these nationally representative samples were thought to be too small to allow useful analysis by some sets of subgroups. A step in the direction of a larger-scale national time series was made when the 1965 National Fertility Study

(NFS), the first fertility survey ever funded by the U.S. government, included questions on expectations:

> We have now asked you questions about the number of children you would like to have and the number you intend to have, about your physical ability to have children, and questions on family planning. Taking all this into account, how many more children do you expect to have (in addition to those you already have)? [Ryder and Westoff 1971, p. 39.]

The responses allowed were "none," some number, or "don't know."

Two other approaches were taken toward incorporating expectations in time-series data. Chronologically, the first was a question on expectations in the series of National Natality Followback Surveys, which were questionnaires mailed to mothers of a sample of legitimate live births in the years 1964–1966 and repeated in 1967, 1968, 1969, and 1972. In the first survey the question was: "After each birth, some couples feel that their families are completed, while others expect more children. In your case, do you expect to have more children?" In 1972 the question was changed to: "Do you expect to have more children?" In all years response categories were the same: "definitely yes," "probably yes," "probably no," and "definitely no." The total number expected was also obtained.

In 1965 the U.S. National Committee on Vital and Health Statistics recommended the Current Population Survey (CPS) as the ideal vehicle for a continuing national survey of expectations of nonmothers as well as those of the mothers surveyed by the National Natality Surveys (NNS) (National Center for Health Statistics 1965, p. 20). A question on expectations was introduced into the Survey of Economic Opportunity conducted by the Bureau of the Census in 1967 and later adopted as routine, annually repeated questions in the CPS. Over the years the question changed from the 1967 version, which asked: "Do you expect to have one or more (additional) children?" with response categories of "yes," "no," and "uncertain" (U.S. Bureau of the Census 1971, p. 6) to: "Looking ahead, do you expect to have any (more) children?" with the same response categories (U.S. Bureau of the Census 1979, p. 81).

Questions on expectations were also included in the 1973 and 1976 National Surveys of Family Growth (NSFG). Rather than emphasizing the most likely number of children only, these surveys asked for the largest and smallest number expected. In the 1976 version this read: "No one can be certain about the future, but you probably have some idea of how close you will come to the number you intend to have. What is the *largest* number of (additional) babies you expect to have?" The next question asked: "What is the *smallest* number of (additional) babies you expect to have?" (Italics were in the original.) Response categories for both questions were either the number or "don't know."

In addition to these national surveys, expectations questions have been included in small-scale and local surveys (for example, Mason 1975; Oakley and Schechtman 1979; Ory 1976).[2]

Uses and Limitations of Expectations Data

The two major uses of the data produced by expectations measures have been in the building of population projections and in the investigation of fertility differentials. Although expectations as a measure were developed to aid in projecting population, more recently they have been used in studies of fertility differentials and as an aid in understanding whether there is stability in family-size norms as circumstances change. For instance, in 1978 the U.S. National Committee on Vital and Health Statistics supported collection of longitudinal panel data on expectations and other variables "to allow an estimation of the effects of number and timing failures on subsequent family size desires and expectations" (National Center for Health Statistics 1978, p. 14). As Ryder has pointed out in chapter 7, from a theoretical point of view it is difficult to justify the use of expectations in the study of fertility differentials since they represent unspecified and probably changing mixes of normative and reality factors. In this chapter, therefore, attention will be devoted to the history of the use of expectations data in population projections.

"The primary purpose of the 1955 and 1960 studies of Growth of American Families was to provide information needed in order to improve population projections for the United States" (Whelpton, Campbell, and Patterson 1966, p. 371). The intent of these studies was to supplement the then newly constructed measures of past cohort fertility, as developed by Whelpton, by melding with them the expectations, by cohort, of women surveyed about their future births. As the U.S. National Committee on Vital and Health Statistics Subcommittee on Fertility Measures, chaired by Kiser,[3] said in 1965 about the accumulation of data from various surveys:

> Data on the number of children expected as well as other kinds of fertility data made available through the surveys should be sensitive to changes in cohort births, probably more sensitive than a continued refinement of conventional data (using period measures). For example, 1955–57 age-specific birth rates for all women imply a total fertility of about 3.7 children per woman. Yet there is nothing in the survey data collected from married women to suggest that any national cohort will reach that level. [National Center for Health Statistics 1965, p. 19]

Combining cohort expectations with past cohort fertility was a conceptual improvement over dependence on either period rates or the artificial TFR.[4]

However, the accuracy of expectations in comparison with actual completed fertility depended on the proportion in the cohort that were represented in the cohorts sampled. Elaborate adjustments to take these factors into account (for example, Freedman, Whelpton, and Campbell 1959, appendixes F and G; Whelpton, Campbell, and Patterson 1966, chapter 10) highlighted the limited contribution of expectations as compared to other sources of data and judgment.[5]

As for the proportion of the cohorts from which the samples were drawn, the early samples were confined to currently married women living with their husbands or with husbands temporarily absent for military service. Among these women GAF I surveyed only those who were white and aged 18 to 39. GAF II included a small subsample of black women. In the 1967 Survey of Economic Opportunity, the sample included a more representative and adequate sample of black women, and the age range was extended to ages 14 to 39 years. In the NNS only births known or inferred to be legitimate were sampled, but the age of the mother was not restricted. The NFS in 1965 and 1970 surveyed ever-married women, while the 1973 and 1976 NSFG studies surveyed women who were ever-married or single with children. A sample of all women was finally obtained in the 1976 CPS, which was a sample of never- as well as ever-married women, independent of whether the woman already was a mother or not.[6] To the extent that other women's fertility diverged from that of the particular population sampled, the projected expectations would be discrepant with later reality. Adjustments made for the fertility of women not represented in the sample had to be made on the basis of assumptions that were more arbitrary than empirical. O'Connell and Moore subsequently showed that this criticism was stronger in theory than in reality, since for 1976 the effect of later additions on cohorts of married women's expectations was minor, less than 0.1 child for the period 1971–1976. This was true because, while fertility expectations of later-married women were decidedly lower than those of women married at the time of the first interview, their relative contribution to cohort fertility was very small compared to the contribution of the women married by the earlier date (O'Connell and Moore 1977). However, the higher the proportion of the cohort that delays marriage, the greater their proportionate contribution to total cohort fertility. The impact of this change probably differs by cohort and would depend on the differential in their expectations as compared to expectations of the earlier-marrying cohort members.

Another problem with extrapolating from expectations data for projection purposes was that cohorts younger than those surveyed would not have been questioned at all. One analysis concluded that by the end of a five-year period, births to women in the age groups younger than those surveyed would constitute the majority of total births (Ryder and Westoff 1971, p. 48; see also Siegel and Akers 1969, p. 102).

There was also the problem of timing of cohort fertility throughout a cohort's reproductive years, a piece of information required to convert cohort data into the period rates used in component projections. Despite their interest in the potential of expectations data for projections, the U.S. National Committee on Vital and Health Statistics noted:

> There has been considerable controversy as to whether or not the basic assumptions regarding cohort fertility [in projections] should be based on extrapolation of past trends or on the expressed expectations of women as derived from a survey such as the Growth of American Families Study. Although the results of the survey should certainly be taken into account, its usefulness is somewhat limited, since the survey cannot cover women not yet of childbearing age and in a very few years it will be they who will be bearing most of the children. Even if survey results are used to establish the level of completed fertility, it may be desirable to use past [cohorts'] experience to determine the timing of births. . . . [National Center for Health Statistics 1965, p. 22]

In the government publications issued by the census bureau's projections branch since the introduction of expectations data, the cohort-fertility assumptions for cohorts then in the reproductive ages did bracket the figures provided by various surveys, but the assumptions continued to modify the data. For instance, for 1967 census-bureau projections:

> the GAF figure was used only as the pivotal value for four other values of the terminal level of completed fertility, derived essentially by historical analysis. Second, the variations by age [cohort] were not used; on the other hand the variations by age were not so great as to make it unreasonable to use a single value for all ages. The use of a single value also takes advantage of counter-balancing errors within cohorts and between cohorts. [Siegel and Akers 1969, p. 111]

Moreover, past timing patterns followed by cohorts already having completed the reproductive years uniformly provided the timing patterns, despite the fact that comparisons of the aggregate five-year expectations data in the 1955 GAF were highly accurate when compared with actual fertility experienced during the intervening five years by the 1960 GAF II sample (Whelpton, Campbell, and Patterson 1966).[7]

One further practical matter concerning sample coverage of the total cohort deserves mention. Even among those interviewed there were some whose expectations were not reported because they expressed uncertainty in various ways. In GAF I, 9 percent were uncertain whether they expected more births (Freedman, Whelpton, and Campbell 1959). In GAF II the comparable figure was 4 percent (Whelpton, Campbell, and Patterson 1966, p. 420). In the 1965 NFS, only 3 percent were categorized as uncertain, but the question itself contained no response categories at all and interviewers were instructed to probe for a number if they received a nonnumerical response (Ryder and Westoff 1971, p. 39). In the 1967 Survey of Economic Opportunity, the percentage classified as not reporting on birth expectations was 19.7, of which 12 percent were recorded as uncertain, an additional 7 percent gave no answer of any kind, and 1 percent were considered to have given inconsistent answers (U.S. Bureau of the Census 1971, pp. 6, 22). The similar figure for the first CPS using this question, in 1971, was 18.4 percent (U.S. Bureau of the Census 1974, p. 135); in 1974, the figure was 20.6 percent (of which 8.8 percent were "uncertain"). In 1975 the tabulations were switched from currently married to ever-married women, and the percentage recorded as not reporting was 17.2. In the 1976 CPS 11 percent were uncertain about expectations, and altogether 15.5 percent of ever-married respondents were recorded as not reporting. (U.S. Bureau of the Census 1975, 1976, 1979, appendix A; Maurice Moore, personal communication.)

The treatment of respondents who are uncertain or not reporting is particularly important when high rates of uncertainty are recorded and when subgroups have differential reporting rates. As shown in columns 1 and 2 of table 2-1, the highest rates for nonreporting for two years in the CPS seem to be at the very beginning and at the middle of the reproductive years.

In analysis of results from the various surveys, those who are uncertain or are otherwise classified as not stating an expectation have been allocated in some surveys, while in others they have been ignored. In GAF I the 9 percent uncertain were assigned an additional number of children, either the "maximum number that they said they would have altogether if they bear additional children" or an arbitrary 0.5 additional births if they had not given any maximum (Freedman, Whelpton, and Campbell 1959, p. 220). In GAF II the 4 percent of white women who were uncertain were treated as unknowns and assigned an expectations number according to the GAF I expectations of women of the same age, religion, parity, and contraceptive use. In the NFS studies they were excluded from analysis, as they were in the Survey of Economic Opportunity and the CPS analyses. In the NNS, however, respondents who, because of uncertainty or other reasons, did not respond to the expectations question have had responses imputed to them according to various characteristics.

Through these various approaches those who express uncertainty have either been excluded from analysis entirely or have been included according to various assumptions. According to their proportion of the cohort sampled and the differentials in fertility expectations, these decisions would have an impact on the quality of expectations data produced by the surveys. While excluding the low percentage uncertain in the 1965 NFS, Ryder and Westoff (1971, p. 40) reported that the uncertain women had current parity that was 15 percent higher than for other respondents. For the CPS, differentials in fertility by reporting status on expectations depended on age, but

Table 2–1
Reporting on Expectations by Age and on Numbers of Children Ever Born for Those Reporting and Not Reporting on Expectations, 1967 and 1971

| Ages | Percentage Not Reporting | | Children Ever Born per 1,000 Wives | | | | | |
	1967 (1)	1971 (2)	1967 Reporting (3)	1967 Not Reporting (4)	Ratio (4) ÷ (3) (5)	1971 Reporting (6)	1971 Not Reporting (7)	Ratio (7) ÷ (6) (8)
Total 14–39 years	19.7	18.4	2,425	2,414	0.99	2,132	2,012	0.94
14–17	22.4	32.4	—	—	—	412	468	1.14
18–19	19.8	16.0	731	1,717	2.35	571	634	1.11
20–21	20.4	16.7	969	1,989	2.05	771	833	1.08
22–24	19.0	18.2	1,366	2,100	1.54	1,123	1,127	1.00
25–29	23.4	20.0	2,312	2,246	0.97	1,950	1,824	0.94
30–34	21.0	19.1	3,049	2,889	0.95	2,804	2,576	0.92
35–39	15.0	16.3	3,214	2,887	0.90	3,218	3,151	0.98

Sources: 1967: U.S. Bureau of the Census, "Previous and Prospective Fertility: 1967," *Current Population Reports*, series P-20, no. 211 (1971), table 6; (1971); ibid., "Fertility Histories and Birth Expectations of American Women: June 1971," *Current Population Reports*, series P-20, no. 263 (1974), table 63.

the magnitude of the differences seems to have differed in various years. As shown in columns 3 through 8 of table 2–1, the number of children ever born was greater among those not reporting if the women were under 25 years of age, but the reverse was true for those over age 25; and the effect was larger for four out of six age groups in 1967 than in 1971.

In 1967 the number of children ever born for those not reporting expectations exceeded the number of children ever born for those reporting among whites, but the reverse was true among the black women surveyed. In 1971 births to those reporting expectations were 7 percent higher among whites and 4 percent higher among blacks as compared to their respective racial groups not reporting expectations. Among women with some college education, those not reporting had just 2 percent more children ever born as compared with those reporting, but among women who were not high-school graduates the relationship was reversed, with fertility of those not reporting only 88 percent of those reporting expectations (U.S. Bureau of the Census 1974, table 63).

These differentials are important in the interpretation of the utility of expectations data, particularly for population projections. If some arbitrary number of additional children, such as the 0.5 additional births assigned in the GAF I analysis, is used without regard to age or any other characteristic of the women, the degree to which their expectations are accurately represented within their cohort is questionable. And if they are excluded from consideration altogether, their expectations are as absent from consideration as those excluded from the sampled population or the younger cohorts.

Criticisms

In addition to criticisms of the practical matters of sample coverage and representativeness of those actually making childbearing decisions in future years, there have also been numerous criticisms of the meaning and validity of expectations data. In essence, critics pointed out that what people say is not necessarily what they will do. Ryder and Westoff have been particularly harsh in their criticism, calling the contribution of expectations data to improving fertility forecasts not only small, but also an "untrustworthy addition to our stock of projections procedures" (1971, p. 48). As the issues evolved, two sets of arguments were put forward to support this point of view.

The first kind of argument attacking the validity of expectations data has come from two separate and quite different sources. They both suggest that answers to expectations questions do not relay accurately preferences that help determine or shape future behavior. Blake (1974) has charged that expectations are fleeting expressions that are not indicative of long-term trends. In particular, Blake has argued that there is a complex of factors associated with the desire for children, some of which were artificially suppressed among American women by the publicity associated with the movement for zero population growth. Blake has therefore argued that expectations data should be interpreted in the context of other measures, particularly the number of children respondents consider ideal.

Coombs, Freedman, Goldberg, and others have argued similarly that there are underlying preferences that are not entirely reflected in single answers to questions such as those on expectations. The measures that have been proposed and tested to investigate underlying preferences have been shown to produce results that are good predictors of future fertility (Coombs 1974, 1979), except among women with no children (Coombs 1974). The measure, now familiar to fertility researchers, is a series of paired comparisons ranking successive sets of alternative numbers of children.

The second kind of argument about the validity of expectations as a measure is that preferences play a less important role than do indirect or structural factors. This argument suggests that childbearing is affected by life circumstances that may intervene to change or affect childbearing intentions or expectations. The primary circumstance that changes, often independent of childbearing expectations, is exposure to risk as determined by age at first intercourse, age at marriage, and marital dissolution. The importance of changes in exposure to risk has been pointed out in an analysis of unwanted childbearing (Ryder and Westoff 1972), and Zelnik and Kantner (1977) have made a similar point about teenagers. Taking cognizance of these changing life circumstances, as well as using a developmental approach to value formation, Namboodiri (1974), Beckman (1975), Ory (1976), and others have documented the sequencing of some people's childbearing decision-making process, which has also been shown to be more elaborate for some people than for others (see, especially, Ory 1976).

Despite the extensive debate that has been focused on expectations as a measure during the past twenty-five years, criticism has not been directed toward the measure itself. Although the measure has evolved over the years, and its placement within the interview or questionnaire has differed, no serious attention has been directed toward measuring the effects of these varying procedures.

A New Question: Uncertainty

It has been little understood that the chances of expectations data being reliable predictors of actual fertility could be affected by the interpretation of the responses. In the 1955 GAF study, the response options included both "definitely" and "probably" answers and "uncertain." The trend in later studies was to omit the "uncertain" category but maintain the differentiation between definiteness and some uncertainty, as indicated by "probably" yes or no. In analysis, those who have answered "probably yes" have been combined with the "definitely yes" category and similarly with the groups expecting probably and definitely not to have a child or another child. In calculating the numbers of children expected, and in uses of expectations as a dependent variable in analytic studies, the "probably" responses have been treated as if they were "definitely" responses. That is, the number stated (or if a range, the center of their range), is given equal weight in calculating the total number expected, regardless of whether the response was "probably" or "definitely" yes. Similarly, those who said they probably expect no (more) children have been added into the cumulative expectations with zero expected, just as are those who say they definitely want none (or no more) children.

The potential impact of these assumptions is indicated by table 2-2, showing data for the NNS. For 1964-1966 (before the dramatic fertility decline of the early 1970s), a higher proportion of mothers expecting no more children were definite about their expectations. In other words, some uncertainty was expressed by a much higher proportion of those expecting than those not expecting a child. If this uncertainty had been traced with more careful attention, the fertility trends might have been more accurately predicted, particularly because those saying they were definite in their

Table 2-2
Distribution by Parity of Responses to a Question on the National Natality Survey, 1964-1966
Question: "Do you expect to have more children?"

Number of Living Children	Number Total	Total	Percentage			
			Yes		*No*	
			Definitely	*Probably*	*Probably*	*Definitely*
Total	3,480	100	25.5	28.6	17.8	28.2
1	1,026	100	59.5	32.1	2.9	5.5
2	900	100	18.4	37.0	13.7	30.9
3	621	100	9.9	27.9	23.3	38.8
4	393	100	5.7	15.8	34.7	43.7
5	232	100	6.4	16.7	34.8	42.1
6+	308	100	4.1	18.6	33.7	43.6

Sources: 1964-1966: National Center for Health Statistics, "Differentials in Expectations of Additional Children Among Mothers of Legitimate Live Births, U.S. 1964-1966, *Vital and Health Statistics,* series 22, no. 13 (1972), table 1.

expectations of having another child expected an average of 2.10 children, while those saying they probably would have more children expected an average of only 1.45 (National Center for Health Statistics 1972). Over the years of the NNS the four categories have received varying but approximately equal proportions of the total responses, yet no analysis has been done on these or similar data to investigate whether the different levels of certainty about expectations might have an impact on reliability.

Conclusion

The development of expectations as a measure of future fertility has been fraught with difficulties, not all of which have been adequately addressed. However, the potential for contributing otherwise unavailable information remains high. Restrictions on the samples available for surveying are being minimized. Assumptions that influence interviewing or coding techniques and analytical choices can be reexamined, and the result should be data that are more trustworthy additions to the whole range of information on which population projections are based.

Notes

1. The sample was limited to white, 18- to 39-year-old women living with their husbands or temporarily separated owing to the husbands' absence in the armed forces.

2. Questions on intentions, ideals, and desired number of children have also been asked but are not the subject of this historical assessment. Intentions have sometimes been used interchangeably with, or instead of, expectations. Ryder and Westoff (1971) demonstrated that in the 1965 NFS intentions were more reliable and elicited higher response rates than expectations questions. These findings support the idea that the two questions deal with different concepts, since there should be more uncertainty and therefore lower reliability and lower response rates associated with the infertility and contraceptive failures that should be part of expectations but not of intentions. "Our primary reason for choosing intended rather than expected parity in what follows is the greater conceptual purity of the former" (Ryder and Westoff 1971, p. 25), a reason that applies to comparisons with ideal and desired family size but not necessarily to comparisons with behavior.

3. Other members of the subcommittee were Anders Lunde, I.M. Moriyama, Donald Akers, Arthur Campbell, David Goldberg, Wilson Grabill, and Norman Ryder.

4. "Before the 1965 GAF results became available the common procedure for projecting fertility was to compute period birth rates of various types, fit straight lines or curves, and extrapolate past trends mathematically, graphically, or on a judgmental basis. In choosing among various procedures, consideration was sometimes given to the effect that changes in social and economic conditions had had on fertility in the past, and might have in the future" (Whelpton, Campbell, and Patterson 1966, p. 372).

5. In addition to making assumptions about the fertility of the people not surveyed, it was necessary to interpret the meaning of statements made by those who were surveyed. For instance: "In GAF I and GAF II those women who were classified as probably sterile, but for whom conception appeared to be neither dangerous nor likely to result in a fetal death, were assigned an additional 0.3 births if they answered that they would have another if they could." In the 1965 NFS all these women were assigned an expectation of zero additional births (Ryder and Westoff 1971, p. 40).

6. However, the sample of married women currently living with their husbands included women aged 14 to 39 years, while the sample of all other women was restricted to ages 18 to 34.

7. The authors had thought the 1965 answers stereotyped and of little value, so they did not repeat timing questions in 1960.

References

Axelrod, Morris; Freedman, Ronald; Goldberg, David; and Slesinger, Doris. "Fertility Expectations of the United States Population: A Time Series." *Population Index* 29 (1963): 25–31.

Beckman, Linda. "Couples' Decision-Making Processes Regarding Fertility." Paper presented at the Conference on Social Demography, University of Wisconsin, 1975.

Blake, Judith. "Can We Believe Recent Data on Birth Expectations in the United States?" *Demography* 11 (1974): 25–44.

Borgatta, Edgar F., and Westoff, Charles F. "Social and Psychological Factors Affecting Fertility: The Prediction of Total Fertility," *Milbank Memorial Fund Quarterly* 32 (1954): 383–419.

Coombs, Lolagene. "The Measurement of Family Size Preferences and Subsequent Fertility." *Demography* 11 (1974): 587–611.

——. "Prospective Fertility and Underlying Preferences: A Longitudinal Study in Taiwan." *Population Studies* 33 (1979): 447–455.

Freedman, Ronald. "American Studies of Family Planning and Fertility: A Review of Major Trends and Issues." In *Research in Family Planning,* edited by Clyde V. Kiser, pp. 211–227. Princeton, N.J.: Princeton University Press, 1962.

Freedman, Ronald; Goldberg, David; and Slesinger, Doris. "Current Fertility Expectations of Married Couples in the United States." *Population Index* 29 (1963): 366–391.

———. "Fertility Expectations in the United States: 1963." *Population Index* 30 (1964): 171–175.

Freedman, Ronald; Whelpton, Pascal K.; and Campbell, Arthur A. *Family Planning, Sterility and Population Growth*. New York: McGraw-Hill, 1959.

Goldberg, David; Sharp, Harry; and Freedman, Ronald. "The Stability and Reliability of Expected Family Size Data." *Milbank Memorial Fund Quarterly* 37 (1959): 369–385.

Mason, Richard. "Differences in Motivation for Childbearing among Childless Parental Couples in a Student Population." Ph.D. dissertation, Florida State University, 1975.

Namboodiri, Krishnan. "Which Couples at Given Parities Expect to Have Additional Births? An Exercise in Discriminant Analysis." *Demography* 11 (1974): 45–56.

National Center for Health Statistics. "Fertility Measurement: A Report of the United States National Committee on Vital and Health Statistics." *Vital and Health Statistics,* series 4, no. 1 (1965).

———. "Differentials in Expectations of Additional Children Among Mothers of Legitimate Live Births, U.S. 1964–1966." *Vital and Health Statistics,* series 22, no. 13 (1972).

———. "Statistics Needed for National Policies Related to Fertility: A Report of the United States National Committee on Vital and Health Statistics." *Vital and Health Statistics,* series 4, no. 18 (1978).

Oakley, Deborah, and Schechtman, Barbara. "Childlessness in the United States." Mimeographed, 1979.

O'Connell, Martin, and Moore, Maurice. "New Evidence on the Value of Birth Expectations." *Demography* 14 (1977): 255–264.

Ory, Marcia. "The Decision to Parent or Not: Normative and Structural Components." Ph.D. dissertation, Purdue University, 1976.

Reed, Robert. "The Interrelation of Marital Adjustment, Fertility Control, and Size of Family." Social and Psychological Factors Affecting Fertility, vol. 6. *Milbank Memorial Fund Quarterly* 25 (1947): 383–425.

Ryder, Norman, and Westoff, Charles. *Reproduction in the United States, 1965*. Princeton, N.J.: Princeton University Press, 1971.

———. "Wanted and Unwanted Fertility in the United States: 1965 and 1970." In *Demographic and Social Aspects of Population Growth,* edited by Charles Westoff and Robert Parke, pp. 467–487. Washington, D.C.: Commission on Population Growth and the American Future, 1972.

Siegel, Jacob, and Akers, Donald. "Some Aspects of the Use of Birth Expectations Data from Sample Surveys for Population Projections." *Demography* 6 (1969): 101–115.

Stix, Regine. "A Study of Pregnancy Wastage." *Milbank Memorial Fund Quarterly* 13 (1935): 347–365.

United States Bureau of the Census. "Previous and Prospective Fertility: 1967." *Current Population Reports,* series P-20, no. 211 (1971).

———. "Fertility Histories and Birth Expectations of American Women: June 1971." *Current Population Reports,* series P-20, no. 263 (1974).

———. "Fertility Expectations of American Women: June 1974." *Current Population Reports,* series P-20, no. 277 (1975).

———. "Fertility of American Women: June 1975." *Current Population Reports,* series P-20, no. 301 (1976).

———. "Fertility of American Women: June 1978." *Current Population Reports,* series P-20, no. 341 (1979).

United States Department of Health, Education, and Welfare. *Vital Statistics of the United States,* vol. 1. Washington, D.C.: National Vital Statistics Division, U.S. Department of Health, Education, and Welfare, 1950 (reprinted 1961).

Whelpton, Pascal. *Cohort Fertility: Native White Women in the United States.* Princeton, N.J.: Princeton University Press, 1954.

Whelpton, Pascal K., and Campbell, Arthur A. *Fertility Tables for Birth Cohorts of American Women.* Washington, D.C.: U.S. National Office of Vital Statistics, 1960.

Whelpton, Pascal K.; Campbell, Arthur A.; and Patterson, John E. *Fertility and Family Planning in the United States.* Princeton, N.J.: Princeton University Press, 1966.

Whelpton, Pascal K., and Kiser, Cylde V., eds. *Social and Psychological Factors Affecting Fertility.* New York: Milbank Memorial Fund, 1946–1958.

Wiehl, Dorothy. "A Summary of Data on Reported Incidence of Abortion." *Milbank Memorial Fund Quarterly* 16 (1938): 80–88.

Wiehl, Dorothy, and Berry, Kathleen. "Pregnancy Wastage in New York City." *Milbank Memorial Fund Quarterly* 15 (1937): 229–247.

Zelnik, Melvin, and Kantner, John. "Sexual and Contraceptive Experience of Young Unmarried Women in the United States, 1976 and 1971." *Family Planning Perspectives* 9 (1977): 55–73.

Part II
Methods and Issues

3

The Utility of Birth Expectations in Population Projections

John F. Long and
Signe I. Wetrogan

Since World War II, fertility rates in the United States and much of the developed world have experienced historically unique fluctuations from low to high and back to low. To cope with the problems engendered by these fluctuations, an unprecedented demand for population projections arose. In answering that demand, forecasters have had available since 1955 estimates of women's own birth expectations. As Long and Wetrogan show in this chapter, those expectations have been used frequently in projecting population. Sometimes they have been used simply to justify fertility projections based primarily on other considerations, sometimes to project the long-term "ultimate" level of fertility. Most often, however, they have been used to project the completed fertility of women already in their childbearing years. According to the authors they have performed very well at that task, equalling or excelling the performance of alternative projection methods.—*Eds.*

For twenty-five years birth expectations have been used in various ways to set the fertility assumptions of population projections. By now one would expect that birth expectations would have either proved their utility or been discarded. No such consensus has emerged, however. Birth expectations have been touted as a panacea for projections, decried as worthless, or temporarily accepted pending further evidence.

It is time to set the record straight. Birth expectations are no panacea. They are highly unsuitable for the critical task of population projections—setting the ultimate level of fertility fifty or seventy-five years hence. Yet they are not worthless. For certain well-defined tasks, such as completing the fertility of young cohorts of childbearing ages or determining the next five-year fertility patterns, birth expectations have been more useful than alternative atheoretical indicators of future fertility. But although birth expectations can be useful in working out these details of fertility projections, they do not replace a coherent theoretical framework of fertility behavior or the informed judgment of the forecaster.

It is easy to see why birth expectations were originally so readily accepted as a panacea for population projections. Projections of future fertility trends have always posed a major difficulty for demographers attempting to make population projections. The cohort-component model requires assumptions of the age-specific fertility rates for every year of the

29

projection. In the absence of established theory on the determinants of trends in aggregate-level fertility, demographers have been left in the unpleasant position of having to project this large matrix of yearly age-specific fertility on the basis of an atheoretical analysis of current or past trends. Efforts to project this matrix on a period basis (U.S. Bureau of the Census 1958) were widely viewed as inadequate and led researchers to look for something better.

In the mid-1950s cohort analysis of past fertility trends began to be used in preference to period-fertility measures (Whelpton 1954; Ryder 1956). Many of the advantages of fertility analysis by cohort, principally the relative stability of cohort versus period fertility, made the method attractive for fertility projections (Akers 1965, pp. 416–419). The major difficulty in applying cohort-fertility analysis to projections was the specification of completed cohort fertility. Although historical (Whelpton 1954; U.S. Bureau of the Census 1964) and mathematical-extrapolation (Ryder 1960, 1964) methods were developed to project the level at which a cohort presently in the childbearing ages might complete its fertility, a temporary fluctuation in period fertility could still be misinterpreted as a change in the cohort's completed fertility rather than a change in timing.

The advent of birth-expectations surveys promised a solution to this problem. No matter what the temporary period rates showed, surveys of women's birth expectations provided a supposedly independent estimate of the eventual completed cohort fertility. This expected completed fertility level, combined with data on the cohort's fertility to date, also implied a timing pattern for estimating the future age-specific fertility rates for the cohort.

The presence of birth expectations served as a catalyst to the production of fertility projections on a cohort basis, since birth expectations provided the independent guideline to future fertility that period-fertility analysis lacked. The Growth of the American Family (GAF) studies of 1955 and 1960 used their survey data on birth expectations to produce projections of fertility on a cohort basis (Freedman, Whelpton, and Campbell 1959; Whelpton, Campbell, and Patterson 1966). In 1963 the U.S. census bureau switched from period- to cohort-fertility analysis in its national population-projection reports—incorporating birth-expectations information to a limited extent.

While this switch to cohort-fertility projections reflected the real promise shown by birth expectations, the euphoria over the use of birth expectations in projections led to some exaggerated claims. The original GAF study asserted that birth-expectations surveys would allow a sample representative of most women in the cohorts of childbearing age to indicate their future fertility rather than relying on the judgment of the demographers, sociologists, and statisticians who made the projections (Freedman, Whelpton, and

Campbell 1959, p. 324). As birth expectations were incorporated into population-projection reports, it became clear that many decisions still required the forecaster's judgment.

Methods of Using Birth Expectations in Population Projections

Even if forecasters take the results of birth-expectations surveys at face value, they still must decide how to incorporate these expectations into the projections. This can be done in at least four basic ways:

1. Responses to the number of births expected during one's lifetime can be used to project the completed cohort fertility of cohorts now of child-bearing age.
2. The number or trend of births expected by women aged 18 to 24 can be used to project the ultimate level of completed fertility for cohorts not yet of childbearing age.
3. A question on expected births in the next five years can be used to project short-term fertility trends.
4. Birth expectations can be used as a general guideline or an ex post facto rationalization for fertility assumptions made from other methods.

Although the 1958 census-bureau projections (U.S. Bureau of the Census 1958) used a period approach to fertility, virtually all national population projections since that time have used the cohort-fertility method and have employed one or more of these methods of incorporating birth expectations (table 3-1). The 1955 and 1960 GAF studies used method 1 for completing the fertility of cohorts now in childbearing years. In addition, the 1960 GAF study used method 2 by extending the trend of birth expectations by cohort forward for the ten cohorts not yet of childbearing age in 1960. The census bureau's 1964 projection report (U.S. Bureau of the Census 1964) used the cohort approach based on historical analysis of the fertility history of previous cohorts and used the expectation data only as a general guideline to the reasonableness of the final results (method 4). The 1971 census-bureau projections (U.S. Bureau of the Census 1971) used birth expectations in a variation of methods 2 and 4. Here, birth expectations provided a guideline for selecting projection series, since the 2.6 births expected for all women estimated from the 1967 survey was about halfway between the ultimate fertility levels of the two middle series (2.78 and 2.45). In 1972 a similar rationale suggested that series B with an ultimate fertility level of 3.1 be dropped, that a new series F with an ultimate fertility level of 1.8 be added, and that series E with an ultimate fertility level of 2.1 be

Table 3–1
Summary of the Use of Birth Expectations in Population Projections Prepared since 1955

Projections Study	Base Date of Population	Birth-Expectation Survey	Expectations of Currently Married White Wives Aged 20 to 24	Equivalent Expectations For all Women [a]	Methods of Using Birth-Expectation Data [b]	Ultimate Completed Cohort Values in Projections
Freedman, Whelpton, and Campbell, 1959	1955	1955 Growth of American Families study	3.2 (ages 18–24)	2.9	1,2	2.9
U.S. Bureau of the Census, 1958	1957	Period approach to projecting fertility				I = 4.13 II = 3.76 III = 3.38 IV = 2.99
Whelpton, Campbell, and Patterson, 1966	1965	1960 Growth of American Families study [c]	3.1	2.8[c] (without adjustment) 3.1 (with adjustment)	1,2	2.8 (with adjustment)
U.S. Bureau of the Census, 1964	1963	1960 Growth of American Families study	3.1	2.8	4	A = 3.350 B = 3.100 C = 2.775 D = 2.450
U.S. Bureau of the Census, 1967	1966	1960 Growth of American Families study	3.1	2.8	4	A = 3.350 B = 3.100 C = 2.775 D = 2.450
U.S. Bureau of the Census, 1970	1969	1965 National Fertility Survey	3.1	2.8 (estimated)	4	B = 3.100 C = 2.775 D = 2.450 E = 2.110

U.S. Bureau of the Census, 1971	1970	1967 Survey of Economic Opportunity	2.8	2.6	4	B = 3.100 C = 2.775 D = 2.450 E = 2.110
U.S. Bureau of the Census, 1972	1972	1972 Current Population Survey	2.3	2.1	4	C = 2.8 D = 2.5 E = 2.1 F = 1.8
U.S. Bureau of the Census, 1975	1974	1973 Current Population Survey	2.2	1.9 (white only)	1, 4	I = 2.7 II = 2.1 III = 1.7
U.S. Bureau of the Census, 1977	1976	1974–1976 Current Population Survey	2.1	1.8 (white only)	1, 4	I = 2.7 II = 2.1 III = 1.7

[a] These values are derived from adjustments to the expectations data obtained from currently married young wives.

[b] Number refers to the corresponding method of incorporating birth-expectation data into a population-projection model described in the text.

[c] The authors of the 1960 Growth of American Families study introduced an upward adjustment to the reported birth expectations of young wives to account for the unexpected childbearing that was observed to occur in the later years of childbearing.

accepted as most likely—all on the basis of the 1971 and 1972 surveys of birth expectations.

The two most recent sets of projections done at the census bureau have returned to a limited version of method 1 for using birth expectations. The birth expectations of 18- to 24-year-olds at the time of the most recent birth-expectations surveys provide the completed fertility for these cohorts under the middle-series projection, but the ultimate fertility level for that series is 2.1, roughly equal to the level of replacement fertility (U.S. Bureau of the Census 1975, 1977).

After choosing a given method, the forecaster may decide to make additional adjustments to the birth-expectations data before using them for projections. The authors of the 1960 GAF study adjusted the expectations upward to account for unplanned births. Inasmuch as birth expectations were asked only of currently married women until 1976, most forecasters have also adjusted expectations to obtain estimates for all women. This adjustment from currently married women to ever-married women and from ever-married women to all women usually reduces the expectations in the 18- to 24-year-old age groups by about 0.3 child (table 3-1), although the 1976 and subsequent surveys have now shown a difference between expectations of currently married women and all women of only 0.1 child (O'Connell and Moore 1977). Even after adjusting birth expectations to a projected level of completed cohort fertility for all women, the forecaster still must decide on the exact timing pattern that will be followed by each cohort. The resulting matrix of age-specific fertility rates by calendar year must be further adjusted to provide a smooth transition in period fertility levels. Clearly the forecaster's judgment plays a major role in each step toward producing the final projected matrix of yearly age-specific fertility rates.

If birth expectations have not fulfilled the promise to eliminate the need for professional judgment, how well have they lived up to the other claims made for them in projecting population? Unfortunately, the tasks outlined for birth expectations were just too many—especially in the face of the most precipitous decline in fertility rates in U.S. history. Almost from the beginning of their use, their true utility in projections has been questioned (Akers 1965, pp. 418–419). From 1964 through 1976 the projection reports using birth-expectations data were almost universely too high in their fertility assumptions (U.S. Bureau of the Census 1975, p. 19). By the time of the third major nationwide study on birth expectations, its authors were already questioning their utility for forecasting (Ryder and Westoff 1967, 1971, pp. 46–47). By 1977 Westoff and Ryder had concluded that birth expectations were no better than period rates as indicators of future fertility. Were another alternative to the use of birth expectations in projections available, expectations might have been readily dropped.

In its own way, however, this conclusion that birth expectations are worthless for population projections is as wrong as the original contention that they provided all the answers. Both misconceptions stem from the failure to evaluate each of the specific methods for using birth expectations in population projections.

**Evaluation of the Utility of Birth Expectations
for Population Projections**

Evaluating the utility of birth expectations in population projections has always been difficult. There is no doubt that birth expectations do have high face validity since they have the advantage of allowing the actual women who will have the future births to indicate their future fertility. The question remains, however, whether projections based on birth expectations are more accurate than projections made on some other atheoretical basis. Unfortunately, the very advantage that expectations bring to fertility projections—information on the long-term cohort values of fertility rather than on the short-term period effects—means that many years must pass before projections made using birth expectations can be compared to actual completed cohort fertility. Most earlier evaluations of the validity of birth expectations have been limited to comparisons of actual and expected fertility during a five-year period. These comparisons have been interpreted broadly in an attempt to discuss their long-term implications (Whelpton, Campbell, and Patterson 1966; Ryder and Westoff 1967; Westoff and Ryder 1977; and O'Connell and Moore 1977). Often such interpretations have been proved wrong as assumptions made about timing have led to implied completed cohort fertility levels that did not materialize.

To make matters worse, surveys on birth expectations and the resulting projections of fertility cover a twenty-five-year period marked by changes in fertility trends from the high fertility levels of the 1950s, to the rapid declines during the 1960s and early 1970s, to the low levels of fertility of the mid-1970s. It is not at all clear whether evaluations of the utility of birth expectations obtained in one of these periods would apply to another. Even less clear is how expectations perform during a period of rapidly rising fertility such as the 1940s and early 1950s, for which no birth-expectations data exist.

Despite these problems, with twenty-five years of fertility history since the first nationwide birth-expectations data were collected, the time has come to make some specific judgments on their usefulness in projections. It is now possible to test directly how well the early birth-expectations surveys did in predicting complete cohort fertility and to make at least a preliminary evaluation of each of the four ways of using birth-expectations data for fertility projections. Even the effects of differing historical levels of fertility on the relationship between expectations and subsequent fertility levels can be handled if one is careful to refer to the particular background of fertility trends in which expectations are being measured.

This background is shown in figure 3-1, which compares the eventual completed cohort fertility of all women aged 20 to 24 in the indicated year with the estimates of their lifetime births expected from survey data and other atheoretical methods of projecting fertility. The two other measures presented here are the composite-period-fertility method represented by the total fertility rate and the completed-cohort-fertility method implied by the cumulative cohort fertility at ages 20 to 24, using the average timing patterns of the 1882-1932 cohorts. The broad historical background shows fertility declining in the 1920s, rising in the 1940s and 1950s, and declining in the 1960s and 1970s. Against this background the validity of each of the four methods of using birth expectations in population projections can be evaluated.

Validity for Completing Fertility History
of Women Currently of Childbearing Age

The original suggested use of birth expectations in projecting the completed fertility of cohorts now in the childbearing years (method 1, as previously discussed) is still the use that has the highest face validity. A general idea of the value of this method can be obtained by plotting the estimated birth expectations of all women aged 20 to 24 based on surveys from 1955 through 1977 (shown by the chain-dot line in figure 3-1) against the actual or estimated completed cohort fertility of the same cohorts when they reach ages 45 to 49 (shown by the solid curve). When possible, these estimates of birth expectations for all women aged 20 to 24 are taken from actual estimates used by previous projection studies (table 3-1). For those birth-expectations surveys that were not used in projection studies, we have subtracted the standard 0.3 child from the expectations of currently married women aged 20 to 24. For the sake of consistency in the time series of expectations, we used the same procedure for the years after 1976 even though direct responses on birth expectations of all women were available.

Comparison of these time series shows that the eventual completed fertility rates for cohorts aged 20 to 24 in 1955 were almost 0.3 child higher than the expected births of 2.9. The eventual completed cohort-fertility rates for those 20 to 24 in 1960 were within 0.1 child of their expected births. Although the completed cohort fertility of those 20 to 24 in the 1960s appears to have declined sharply, the number of births expected declined only modestly, so that the 1965 and 1967 birth expectations now appear to have been too high by 0.3 to 0.4 child. Extrapolation of the completed cohort fertility beyond the 1943–1947 cohorts (those 20 to 24 in 1967) on the basis of current data through 1977 can be quite hazardous, but it appears that the estimates of birth expectations of 1.9 to 2.1 for all women 20 to 24 extracted from the surveys of the early 1970s may prove to be only a little high. Obviously, expectations of completed cohort fertility have not declined as quickly as actual cohort fertility. As a result, projections made using the expectations data have been too high.

A fair evaluation of the utility of birth expectations in population projections looks not so much at their absolute accuracy as at their accuracy relative to alternative atheoretical methods. Two rather simplistic alternatives are illustrated in figure 3–1. A simple period approach projects completed cohort fertility for cohorts just entering the childbearing ages as equal to the total fertility rate at that date (dashed line). Another alternative is a simplified cohort method using the average timing pattern and completed cohort fertility of the 1882–1932 cohorts. If the 20- to 24-year-olds in a given year have, for example, a cumulative cohort fertility that is 10 percent above the average for 20- to 24-year-olds in the reference cohorts, the completed cohort fertility for these groups would be 10 percent above the completed fertility of the reference cohorts (dotted lines).

The relative accuracy of these three methods of projecting the eventual completed fertility of cohorts 20 to 24 depends on the level and direction of actual fertility rates (figure 3–1). In 1955, when period rates were near the peak of a twenty-year rise, a period projection of the eventual completed cohort fertility of those currently 20 to 24 (the 1931–1935 birth cohorts) would have been off by almost 0.5 child. The simplified cohort-projection method would have been around 0.3 child too high, while birth expectations were 0.3 child too low. By 1960 both the period and cohort projections of fertility were near their peaks, but it appears that the completed cohort fertility of those 20 to 24 in 1960 (the 1936–1940 birth cohorts) will be considerably lower than it was for the five earlier cohorts. Thus the period-projection alternative appears to have been more than 0.8 child too high, and the cohort-projection method appears to have been high by 1 full child. In contrast, the projection made using birth-expectations data was low by only 0.1 child. Rapid declines in period fertility in the 1960s brought the projections of eventual completed cohort fertility using period measures and birth expectations much closer. From the mid-1960s through the early 1970s, the period-fertility measure and the birth-expectations data gave almost identical results. The cohort-fertility-projection alternative gave far less accurate results for the 1960s and early 1970s as the timing of fertility changed to a notably later pattern than the average pattern of the 1882–1932 cohorts.

For the period from the middle to the end of the 1970s, it appears that total fertility rates again have diverged somewhat from data on birth

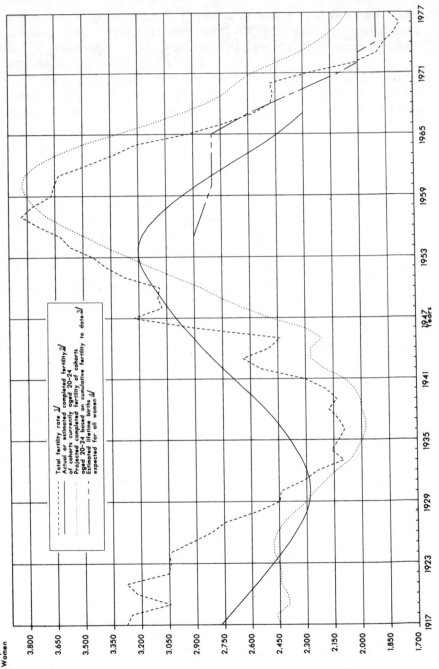

Births per
1000 Women

Legend:
Total fertility rate 1/
Actual or estimated completed fertility 2/
of cohorts currently aged 20-24
Projected completed fertility of cohorts
aged 20-24 based on cumulative fertility to date 3/
Estimated lifetime births
expected for all women 4/

[1] Sum of age-specific birth rates for the calendar year.

[2] Based on the unpublished cohort data through 1977. For the five-year cohorts who had not reached ages 45 to 49 by 1978 (the 1930–1934 and later cohorts), their remaining fertility was extrapolated on the basis of their cumulative fertility through 1977 and the fertility experience of the 1929–1933 cohorts.

[3] Based on the relationship of the cumulative fertility for cohorts aged 20 to 24 in the calendar year to the cumulative fertility to ages 20 to 24 and completed cohort rates of the cohorts aged 45 to 49 in the calendar year.

[4] Numbers of lifetime births expected for all women, based on surveys taken in selected calendar years (see table 3–1).

Figure 3–1. Birth Expectations and Fertility Trends: 1917–1977

expectations. By the early 1970s the estimate of the number of births for all women 20 to 24 had stabilized at around 1.9, while total fertility rates continued to drop, reaching 1.7 in 1976. Although it is far too early to tell whether the expectations or the period method was more accurate, there is now at least the suggestion that the birth-expectations data indicate a turn-around that would have been missed by analyzing period data alone. As previously noted, the census-bureau projections based on 1 July 1976 data (U.S. Bureau of the Census 1977) used the expectations of the 18- to 24-year-olds to complete the fertility of these cohorts, leading to a middle series that predicted an upturn in total fertility rates. The tracking report for the first three years of this projection period (U.S. Bureau of the Census 1980) reveals that such an upturn in total fertility rates has indeed occurred—an upturn that would not have been foreseen from period rates.

Only during the late 1960s and early 1970s do these data support the assertion made by Westoff and Ryder (1977, p. 449) that birth expectations are little better than period rates. In the earlier years of 1955 and 1960, period and birth-expectations data were decidedly not identical, and birth-expectations data proved considerably better than period measures in projecting completed cohort fertility of those 20 to 24 in 1960. For the most recent years, as well, birth-expectations data are showing differences from period rates.

So far this discussion has concerned only broad trends in expectations and completed fertility for the 20- to 24-year-old age group. This is the age at which birth expectations may tell us the most, since expectations are relatively well established and the bulk of fertility is still to come. But do expectations serve as well in predicting fertility for other age groups? This question can be answered by comparing the 1955 and 1960 birth expectations by five-year age groups with the actual values of completed fertility estimated for each cohort using fertility data through 1977. As table 3–2 shows, all age groups from 20 through 39 in 1955 reported expected family sizes that now seem to have been about 20 percent below their actual or currently estimated completed cohort fertility. In 1960, however, all cohorts—except the youngest—reported lifetime expectations that now appear to have been within 5 percent of their actual completed fertility. In neither study does age make a substantial difference in the ability of birth expectations to predict fertility.

Table 3–2 also compares the relative accuracy of birth expectations with the alternative period- and cohort-projection methods. The period method completes the cohort fertility rates of each five-year cohort by adding the five-year age-specific fertility rates experienced by older age groups in the 1950–1955 period (or the 1955–1960 period) to the cumulative cohort fertility attained by the cohort as of 1955 (or 1960). The cohort method multiplies the completed cohort rate of the 1906–1910 (or 1911–1915) cohort by the cumulative cohort fertility as of 1955 (or 1960) for each five-year cohort, and then divides by the cumulative cohort fertility completed as of that age by the 1906–1910 (or 1911–1915) cohort.

In 1955 these alternative methods, based on the lower average fertility of the 1950–1955 period, did better than the 1955 birth-expectation data. However, in 1960 these alternatives, based on the extremely high fertility levels of the 1955–1960 period, did much worse than the birth-expectations data. The differences between these results and those of figure 3-1 reveal more about the pitfalls of using lagged five-year data than about the differences between methods. The fairer comparison is given in figure 3-1, where current expectations are compared with current alternative period and cohort methods.

Utility of Birth-Expectations Data for Projecting the Ultimate Level of Completed Cohort Fertility

Completing the fertility history of cohorts currently of childbearing ages constitutes only a portion of the task of fertility projections. For short-run projections, completion of the fertility of cohorts now of childbearing ages may encompass most of the needed fertility projections, but longer-run projections depend heavily on assumptions about the fertility of cohorts that will not enter the childbearing ages for years to come. Within only 10 to 15 years, the age groups of highest fertility (20 to 24 and 25 to 29) will consist of persons who were not of childbearing ages at the time the projections were made. Consequently, it is no longer sufficient to have assumptions about completed cohort fertility for persons currently of childbearing ages. Given the fifty- to one-hundred-year time frame of most current national projections, the primary assumptions concern the ultimate levels of completed cohort fertility for cohorts that will not begin childbearing until many years after the projections are made. How good are birth-expectations data in dealing with this problem (previously described as method 2)?

Both expectations have been used to infer data about these ultimate levels in several ways. In the 1955 GAF study, completed cohort fertility rates for future cohorts were assumed to remain constant at the level of the youngest cohort for which expectations data were available. A similar rationale was used in several of the U.S. census bureau's projections for the late 1960s and early 1970s, in which a set of projection series was justified on the basis that the average of the middle assumptions of ultimate completed cohort fertility was close to the birth expectations of the 18- to 24-year-olds in the latest survey.

This procedure of holding the last expectation value constant for future cohorts is reasonable only under stable conditions in which fertility rates for

Table 3–2

A Comparison of Predicted Completed Cohort Fertility Using Birth Expectations, Continuation of Period Rates, and Extrapolations of Cohort Trends, Prepared in 1955 and 1960 with Cumulative or Estimated Cumulative Fertility at Age 45 to 49

Cohort	Age at Survey Date	Cumulative Fertility to Survey Date[a]	Cumulative Fertility to Age 45–49[b]	Birth Expectations[c]	Completed Cohort Fertility Projected By Various Methods					
					Percentage Difference from Cumulative Fertility at Age 45–49	Period Extrapolations[d]	Percentage Difference from Cumulative Fertility at Age 45–49	Cohort Extrapolation[e]	Percentage Difference from Cumulative Fertility at Age 45–49
Projections Based on 1955 Information									
1941–1945	10–14	—	2,524	2,867	13.6	3,263	29.3	2,284	−9.5
1936–1940	15–19	106	2,960	2,845	−4.0	3,263	10.6	3,363	14.1
1931–1935	20–24	848	3,201	2,771	−18.3	3,252	2.2	3,357	6.6
1926–1930	25–29	1,699	3,079	2,759	−23.2	3,097	1.3	3,199	8.7
1921–1925	30–34	2,182	2,856	2,753	−15.3	2,837	−2.8	2,923	9.9
1916–1920	35–39	2,335	2,573	2,530	−18.1	2,562	−4.6	2,595	9.2
1911–1915	40–44	2,312	2,353	2,339	−35.0	2,350	−7.5	2,351	−5.0
Projections Based on 1960 Information									
1946–1950	10–14	—	2,185	2,930	34.1	3,609	65.2	2,353	7.7
1941–1945	15–19	111	2,524	2,989	19.3	3,609	45.0	3,839	54.5
1936–1940	20–24	956	2,960	2,994	1.7	3,604	32.1	4,420	72.9

1931–1935	25–29	2,006	3,201	3,167	−2.9	3,496	24.7	4,165	80.7
1926–1930	30–34	2,493	3,079	3,096	2.9	3,190	18.9	3,430	59.9
1921–1925	35–39	2,639	2,856	2,860	1.8	2,879	10.6	2,925	31.8
1916–1920	40–44	2,534	2,573	2,575	5.1	2,574	2.6	2,579	15.4

[a] Robert M. Heuser, *Fertility Tables for Birth Cohorts by Color: United States, 1917–73*, DHEW Publication no. (HRA) 76–1152 (Washington, D.C.: U.S. Government Printing Office, 1976).

[b] Unpublished cohort data through 1977; and for the five-year cohorts who had not reached ages 45–49 by 1978, their remaining fertility was extrapolated on the basis of fertility through 1977 and the fertility experience of the 1929–1933 cohorts.

[c] Based on cumulative fertility to the survey date and the additional births expected from the survey date to the end of childbearing; from Ronald Freedman, Pascal K. Whelpton, and Arthur A. Campbell, *Family Planning, Sterility and Population Growth* (New York: McGraw Hill, 1959); and Pascal K. Whelpton, Arthur A. Campbell, and John E. Patterson, *Fertility and Family Planning in the United States* (Princeton, N.J. Princeton University Press, 1966).

[d] Based on cumulative fertility to the survey date and the averaged fertility of the previous five-year period.

[e] Based on the relationship of the cumulative fertility of the cohorts in childbearing in 1955 and 1960 to the cumulative and completed cohort rates of the 1906–1910 or 1911–1915 cohorts.

the distant future are expected to remain the same as current (or immediately future) fertility. As figure 3–1 shows, such a condition of stability has not existed in the more than fifty years for which we have detailed fertility data. Completed cohort fertility has gone through wide undulating cycles. Given this instability in completed cohort fertility, it is quite unlikely that a birth-expectation value that is correct for completing one cohort would also be correct for completing future cohorts. Only if fertility rates are now finally approaching a period of long-run stability would such a strategy be appropriate.

The historical cyclical pattern of completed cohort fertility also bodes poorly for the method of continuing the observed changes in expectation by cohorts into the future. This method might prove adequate as long as the trend continues but would give disastrous results at the turning points. For an example one need only look at the 1960 GAF projections, which had done so well in predicting the completion of cohorts of childbearing ages at the time of study. The 1960 study applied the past trends of rising birth expectations to cohorts not yet of childbearing age. It is now apparent that these cohorts will have much lower levels of completed cohort fertility. For the youngest cohorts in the 1960 GAF projections, the projected completed cohort fertility appears to have been far too high (table 3–2) with the 1946–1950 cohorts projected fully 34 percent above what now appears to be the best guess as to their completed cohort fertility.

For forecasters now to use birth expectations of women currently of childbearing ages to project the completed cohort fertility of future cohorts requires that the forecasters be firmly convinced that fertility will soon reach an unprecedented period of stability. If the forecasters are unprepared to make such a strong assumption, they must look for something other than birth expectations in attempting to select the ultimate levels of fertility.

Validity of Birth Expectations for Timing Information

Although the cohort-fertility method of making population projections appears to have several advantages over the period method, it does require some additional complexity. Not only must completed cohort fertility be projected, but the timing pattern for each cohort must also be determined in order to give the year-by-year projections of fertility for each age that the cohort-component method of population projection requires (Akers 1965).

As previously mentioned, some inferences about timing patterns can be made by comparing the cumulative fertility to date of a cohort with its expectations of completed fertility. The dotted line in figure 3–1 indicates the fertility that would result if the cohorts aged 20 to 24 had the same timing as the average of the 1882–1932 cohorts. If the actual timing pattern is earlier than this average pattern, a smaller proportion of the total will be born after ages 20 to 24 and the actual completed cohort fertility (solid line in figure 3–1) will be below this dotted line. Conversely, a later-than-average timing pattern would result in actual completed cohort fertility above that shown by the dotted line. Using this relationship, figure 3–1 can illustrate the changes in timing over the last fifty years. In the 1930s the implied fertility of the early ages (dotted line) was lower than the actual completed cohort fertility (solid line), indicating a late timing pattern. By the 1960s the rate of fertility implied by the rate of childbearing (dotted line) in the early ages was far above the estimated completed cohort fertility (solid line), implying an early timing pattern.

If birth expectations are a good measure of completed cohort fertility, then similar comparisons can be made between the dotted line in figure 3–1 and birth expectations (chain-dot line in figure 3–1). The resulting timing information could be used as a broad guide for projecting age-specific fertility rates, but more specific timing information requires explicit questions on timing in the birth-expectations surveys.

The use of questions on births expected during the next five years in preparing short-term population projections constitutes the third method outlined previously. Such questions were asked on the 1955 GAF study and on census-bureau surveys done in 1967 and 1972. Table 3–3 compares the expected and the actual five-year fertility for the periods 1955–1960, 1967–1972, and 1972–1977 for women who were married at the beginning of the period. The expected and actual data match very well for the 1955–1960 period, although the 1955 GAF researchers thought that the expected values seemed stereotyped and of little value (Whelpton, Campbell, and Patterson 1966, p. 15). The 1967–1972 period was one of the major declines in fertility. Although five-year expectations also fell rapidly, they were still 10 to 25 percent higher than actual five-year fertility for most age groups—and even further off for the 35- to 39-year-old age group. In 1972–1977 expected births during the five years were much closer to actual births than was the case for 1967–1972—closer, in fact, than with alternative period or cohort methods.

Although the five-year birth-expectations data have never, to our knowledge, been used in projections, the data seem to have been fairly accurate and could prove of some benefit in period projections for the very short term (Siegel and Akers 1969, p. 113). The practicality of such an approach is limited, however, since the normal time lag for the tabulation of survey results and the production of projections from these results would occupy much of the five years.

Table 3–3
Evaluation of Short-Term Birth Expectations

Age at Beginning of Period	CEB at Beginning of Period	CEB at End of Period	CEB During Period	Number Expected in Five Years at Beginning of Period	Difference Between Five-Year Expectation and Childbearing	
					Number	Percentage
1955 to 1960 Period (White Wives)[a]						
18–24	1.1	2.6	1.5	1.5	—	—
25–29	1.9	2.8	0.9	0.9	—	—
30–34	2.3	2.8	0.5	0.4	–0.1	–20.0
35–39	2.7	2.9	0.2	0.2	—	—
1967 to 1972 Period (All Wives)[b]						
14–19	0.690	1.864	1.173	1.293	+0.120	10.2
20–24	1.246	2.169	0.924	1.090	+0.166	18.0
25–29	2.312	2.836	0.524	0.579	+0.055	10.5
30–34	3.049	3.210	0.160	0.199	+0.039	24.4
35–39	3.214	3.219	0.005	0.073	+0.068	136.0
1972 to 1977 Period (All Wives)[c]						
14–19	0.577	1.631	1.054	1.051	–0.003	–0.3
20–24	0.979	1.793	0.814	0.933	+0.119	14.6
25–29	1.807	2.348	0.541	0.546	+0.005	0.9
30–34	2.749	2.933	0.184	0.148	–0.036	–19.6
35–39	3.173	3.206	0.033	0.040	+0.007	21.2

[a]Pascal K. Whelpton, Arthur A. Campbell, and John E. Patterson, *Fertility and Family Planning in the United States* (Princeton, N.J.: Princeton University Press, 1966).
[b]Signe Wetrogan, "Birth Expectations and Subsequent Fertility" (Paper presented at the Annual Meeting of the Population Association of America, New Orleans, La., 1973).
[c]Based on data from the 1972 Current Population Survey for all wives and from the 1977 Current Population Survey for wives first married prior to 1972.

**Validity of Birth Expectations as a General Guideline in
Making Fertility Assumptions for Population Projections**

The fourth method for making projections based on birth expectations is to use them only as general guidelines for, or rationalizations of, fertility assumptions obtained in other ways. It is not really possible to evaluate how effective this method has been since one is never sure how the expectations data have influenced the projection. It is likely that this influence is often subjective, coloring the forecaster's approach and ultimate choice of assumptions. This use of expectations data falls on the side of the projection effort that is referred to as an "art." No amount of searching through written methodologies will decipher its influence, yet it may well be the single major role that expectations have played in the population-projection process.

A related and less defensible use of birth expectations in population projections is as an ex post facto justification of an assumed ultimate fertility rate arrived at by some other explicit or implicit procedure. Many of the explanations of the use of expectations in the methodologies accompanying projection reports are couched as rationalizations of projections arrived at by a more subjective approach. As in the original 1955 study, it is still easier to explain assumed fertility levels by shifting the onus onto the expectations of the women who are actually going to have the births rather than the judgment of the demographers, sociologists, and statisticians who make the projections.

Conclusions

Despite conflicting evaluations of the effectiveness of birth expectations in making fertility projections, birth expectations have continued to be used for almost twenty-five years in projecting the U.S. population. Four general methods in which expectations have been or could be used are: (1) completing fertility of cohorts now of childbearing age, (2) projecting ultimate fertility levels of future cohorts, (3) determining fertility for the next five years, and (4) providing a general guideline for setting fertility assumptions. Of these four methods the most useful is the original one—completing the fertility of cohorts (especially the younger cohorts) now in the childbearing ages. While birth expectations have certainly not been infallible in this regard, they have done as well as period methods during the rapid decline in fertility from the mid-1960s to the mid-1970s and appear to have done better at the turning point of high fertility in 1960 and at what may be a plateau in the mid- to late 1970s.

Despite the relative success of birth expectations in projecting completed cohort fertility, there is no evidence that they help with the more fundamental task of establishing the ultimate fertility level. It is this level, rather than the values for completion of fertility for cohorts now in childbearing, that determines the broad outline of population trends after the initial ten or fifteen years of the projection period. Failing this task, birth expectations cannot claim to have fulfilled their promise of shifting the responsibility of making fertility projections from the forecasters to the women having children. Even if these women could foresee the approximate level of their own future fertility, they should never have been expected to indicate the fertility of future cohorts. For that task, the burden falls squarely back on the forecasters, who must use their own judgment to set ultimate levels—perhaps using data on birth expectations as one factor among many.

After twenty-five years we must once again face squarely the questions that birth-expectations data were to circumvent. These questions involve the socioeconomic determinants of fertility in the long-term historical view. Neither birth expectations nor other atheoretical methods of projecting fertility are adequate substitutes for answers to these questions. Only when forecasters are able to discover and to project these determinants can they really claim to be projecting fertility. Meanwhile, they will continue to project population based on assumptions about fertility that may include data on birth expectations as well as on historical trends, but the basic component of these projections will remain the forecasters' own judgment.

References

Akers, Donald. S. "Cohort Fertility Versus Parity Progression." *Demography* 2 (1965): 414–428.
Freedman, Ronald; Whelpton, Pascal K.; and Campbell, Arthur A. *Family Planning, Sterility and Population Growth.* New York: McGraw-Hill, 1959.
Heuser, Robert M. *Fertility Tables for Birth Cohorts by Color: United States, 1917–73.* DHEW Publication no. (HRA) 76–1152. Washington, D.C.: U.S. Government Printing Office, 1976.
Moore, Maurice, and O'Connell, Martin. "Perspectives on American Fertility." *Current Population Reports,* Special Studies, series P-23, no. 70. Washington, D.C.: U.S. Government Printing Office, 1978.
O'Connell, Martin, and Moore, Maurice J. "New Evidence on the Value of Birth Expectations." *Demography* 14 (1977): 255–264.
Ryder, Norman. "The Problems of Trend Determination During a Transition in Fertility." *Milbank Memorial Fund Quarterly* 34 (1956): 5–21.
———. "The Structure and Tempo of Current Fertility." *Demographic*

and Economic Change in Developed Countries, edited by National Bureau of Economic Research. Princeton, N.J.: Princeton University Press, 1960.

————. "The Process of Demographic Transition." Demography 1 (1964): 74–82.

Ryder, Norman B., and Westoff, Charles F. "The Trend of Expected Parity in the United States: 1955, 1960, 1965," Population Index 33 (1967): 153–168.

————. Reproduction in the United States, 1965. Princeton, N.J.: Princeton University Press, 1971.

Siegel, Jacob S. "Development and Accuracy of Projections of Population and Housing in the United States." Demography 9 (1972):51–68.

Siegel, Jacob, and Akers, Donald. "Some Aspects of the Use of Birth Expectations Data from Sample Surveys for Population Projections." Demography 6 (1969): 101–115.

United States Bureau of the Census. "Illustrative Projections of the Population of the United States by Age and Sex: 1960 to 1980." Current Population Reports, series P-25, no. 187 (1958).

————. "Projections of the Population of the United States by Age and Sex: 1964 to 1985." Current Population Reports, series P-25, no. 286 (1964).

————. "Projections of the Population of the United States by Age, Sex, and Color to 1990." Current Population Reports, series P-25, no. 381 (1967).

————. "Projections of the Population of the United States by Age and Sex: 1970 to 2020." Current Population Reports, series P-25, no. 448 (1970).

————. "Projections of the Population of the United States by Age and Sex: 1970 to 2020." Current Population Reports, series P-25, no. 470 (1971).

————. "Projections of the Population of the United States, by Age and Sex: 1972 to 2020." Current Population Reports, series P-25, no. 493 (1972).

————. "Projections of the Population of the United States: 1975 to 2050." Current Population Reports, series P-25, no. 601 (1975).

————. "Projections of the Population of the United States: 1977 to 2050." Current Population Reports, series P-25, no. 704 (1977).

————. "Fertility of American Women: June 1978." Current Population Reports, series P-20, no. 341 (1979).

————. "The 1977 Population Projections of the United States: The First Three Years." Current Population Reports, series P-25 (1980).

Westoff, Charles F., and Ryder, Norman B. "The Predictive Validity of Reproductive Intentions." Demography 14 (1977): 431–453.

Wetrogan, Signe. "Birth Expectations and Subsequent Fertility." Paper presented at the Annual Meeting of the Population Association of America, New Orleans, La., 1973.

Whelpton, Pascal K. *Cohort Fertility: Native White Women in the United States.* Princeton, N.J.: Princeton University Press, 1954.

Whelpton, Pascal K., Campbell, Arthur A.; and Patterson, John E. *Fertility and Family Planning in the United States.* Princeton, N.J.: Princeton University Press, 1966.

4

The Validity of Birth Intentions: Evidence from U.S. Longitudinal Studies

Charles F. Westoff

In chapter 3 Long and Wetrogan suggested that women's birth expectations were accurate predictors of the completed cumulative fertility of cohorts; that is, the average number of children expected by young women is quite close to the average number they bear during their lifetimes. In this chapter Charles F. Westoff reviews several longitudinal fertility studies that confirm this suggestion: The average numbers expected did in fact predict average numbers of lifetime births with an accuracy ranging from 90 to 100 percent. While that might seem to be strong endorsement of birth-expectations data, the remainder of Westoff's evidence is a stinging indictment. He argues that the aggregate-level agreement between expectations and fertility in those studies was largely fortuitous, the result of women's counterbalancing over- and underestimates of their future fertility. Because the data considered were longitudinal—that is, for the same women at two or more points in time—Westoff is able to show that many women wrongly predicted their individual fertility, even when the expectations of the group as a whole correctly predicted the group's fertility. Individual unreliability would not be so damaging to the use of expectations for predicting fertility if the errors could be counted on to counterbalance each other in the aggregate, as they seem to have done in the first three of the studies Westoff reviews. Unfortunately, Westoff shows that in a more recent study they did not balance out, and the aggregate expectation was some 15 percent below actual completed fertility. Westoff suggests that expectations do not so much predict the future as reflect current conditions, and are therefore subject to the same limitations as any other period measure of fertility.—*Eds.*

How accurately do data on fertility preferences and intentions predict actual fertility in subsequent years? Is there a large difference between the individual and the aggregate level in the predictive validity of such data? This chapter summarizes and synthesizes the evidence from several U.S. longitudinal studies. A review of the basic evidence and main conclusions of these studies is followed by an overall summary and conclusion about the usefulness of such data for predictive purposes. The importance of the longitudinal design for this purpose is that it is free from the contaminating influence of actual experience and the natural tendency to rationalize behavior that might have been unintended. In the longitudinal study, we have information on intentions before the fact of the reproductive experience we are trying to predict.

The Kelly Study of Engaged Couples

In the late 1930s the psychologist E. Lowell Kelly began a longitudinal study of marital adjustment with a sample of 300 engaged couples. Twenty years later the panel was recontacted, and a subset of 145 couples was extracted to analyze how well their fertility was predicted from their fertility preferences prior to marriage. The sample size is small; the original selection of couples was nonrandom and localized (in Connecticut); college graduates were overrepresented and Catholics underrepresented; and the 145 couples were the residue after eliminating those who had never married, had married more than once, had reported problems of sterility, had adopted any children, or had provided insufficient information. Despite these limitations, the Kelly Study data provide a unique opportunity to examine the validity of fertility preferences over a long span of marriage.

The mean number of births for the 145 couples was 2.6 (fertility was estimated to be 97 percent complete); the mean number of children reported as desired by males and females during their engagement was 2.6 and 2.8, respectively. This is a rather close correspondence (between 94 and 99 percent) in the aggregate. If such accuracy could be counted on in a larger and more general population, the usefulness of such attitudinal data for fertility forecasting would be established.

There are, however, two additional findings from the Kelly Study that discourage such a conclusion. The sample just happened to divide evenly between couples who had successfully planned all births ("planners") and couples who had experienced at least one unplanned birth ("nonplanners"). Although both groups had almost identical initial preferences (for males, 2.6 and 2.7 for planners and nonplanners respectively, and for females 2.8 and 2.9), the actual number of births differed markedly—2.2 for the planners and 3.2 for the nonplanners. Thus the similarity of the aggregate preferences and performance for the total sample is an artifact of the proportions of planners and nonplanners in the population, and there is every reason not to assume the stability of that balance.

The second finding is a very low correlation between initial preferences and performance at the individual level. The multiple correlation of male and female preferences with subsequent fertility was only 0.30. (For women alone, the correlation was 0.28.) On the one hand, it is somewhat sobering to realize that some 90 percent of the variance of completed fertility was unaccounted for by the couple's preference just before marriage. On the other hand, there are numerous reasons why the individual predictive value might be that low: The couples were not yet married, they had not yet faced the economic and domestic realities of family life, their replies may not have been thoughtful, all kinds of new and unpredictable experiences (including children themselves) could intervene to change their intentions, half the group had unplanned pregnancies, and so forth.

Nevertheless, the low predictive value of family-size preferences for eventual fertility, plus the fortuitous balance of planners and nonplanners in the sample, combine to raise serious questions about the dependability of the aggregate correspondence between preferences and actual fertility in a general population.

The Princeton Fertility Study

The questions raised by the Kelly Study and by other U.S. fertility research at the time were incorporated into the Princeton Fertility Study, which began in 1957. The design was longitudinal and involved three interviews starting at six months after the birth of the second child. The second interview took place three years later and the last interview an average of eight years after the first (the third interview was spread out over five years, beginning with the oldest women). The original sample consisted of 1,165 two-parity, native-born, once-married, white women living in the seven largest metropolitan areas of the United States. The third and final interview was successfully completed for 814 of the original 1,165; various tests indicated that the final sample was quite representative of the original panel.

One reason for beginning the study with women who had already had two children was that having at least two children was the almost universal experience during the baby-boom years for married women with no infecundity problems. One objective of the study was to determine how well completed fertility (fertility of women by the time of the last interview was estimated to be at least 90 percent complete) could be predicted from preferences expressed six months after the birth of the second child. The repeated interviews also allowed an estimate of the stability of family-size preferences. Instability of preferences would, of course, reduce the micropredictive value of original preferences for completed fertility. And there was indeed substantial change over the eight-year span: Only two-fifths of the women gave the same response in the first and third interviews, although most (85 percent) of the women were within one child of the desired family size reported at the first interview. There is some evidence that much of this change stems from unreliability rather than from genuine instability. Nevertheless, the consequences for lowering the potential individual correlation are the same.

As in the Kelly Study, the macropredictive validity was impressive. The average number wanted after the birth of the second child predicts very well the average size of completed families; in fact, the mean of 3.3 children was identical for both variables. From the demographic (aggregate) point of view, this is an ideal outcome. Moreover, there is little variation in aggregate predictability for religious and educational subgroups. The close correspondence at the aggregate level, however, is the result of nonrandom compensating errors. The proportion who achieved exactly the number they had wanted at the first interview was highest for Jewish women and lowest for Catholic women; was directly related to education; and, as in the Kelly Study, was consistently higher for women who planned all or most of their pregnancies than for women who planned half or fewer of their pregnancies. There is also a regression toward the mean in the relationship between desired family size and completed fertility. Women who wanted a total of 2 children, that is, who desired no more births after having their second child, had a total of 2.5 childen on the average, whereas women who wanted 6 or more children had 5.6 on the average.

At the individual level, the correlation between the wife's family-size desires after the birth of the second child and completed fertility was 0.56, accounting for 31 percent of the variance; with the husband's desires combined, the value increases to 34 percent. These values are considerably higher than the 9 percent obtained in the Kelly Study, but the time interval was considerably greater in the latter—twenty-five years from marriage compared with an average of eight years from the second birth in the Princeton Fertility Study.

The Detroit Study

In 1962 a panel study of 1,304 white, married women at zero, first, second, and fourth parities was interviewed in Detroit in the first round of a longitudinal study that culminated in 1977 after four additional contacts. In 1977, fifteen years later, with fertility essentially completed, 1,040 or 89 percent of the sample was successfully reinterviewed, providing another opportunity to evaluate the predictive validity of fertility preferences. These data have been analyzed and reported by Lolagene Coombs in a paper (Coombs 1979) that focuses on the predictive value of a measure that aims at capturing the range of preference underlying a single-valued preference statement. Essentially, women are asked to select their second and third choices in a series of paired comparisons that yields a scale labelled the I-scale. Coombs evaluates the predictive utility of the scale with a subset of 853 women who were continuously married to the same man during the entire fifteen-year period. One of her main conclusions is that underlying preference affects fertility over and above the influence of the woman's first choice. In general, the additional information on preferences obtained in the I-scale is reflected in fairly substantial differences in fertility within initial first-preference categories. For example, women whose first preference in 1962 was for three children had a mean of 2.67 births by 1977 if their I-scale value was low and a mean of 3.35 births if their I-scale value was medium. The analysis provides strong support for the usefulness of such supplementary data in fertility surveys.

The aggregate correspondence between simple first preferences and ultimate fertility in this study is fairly high: The women preferred an average of 3.86 children and experienced an average of 3.68 births, a 95 percent correspondence. The correlation across these fifteen years was 0.40. However, since the original sample contained women of different parities, the evaluation of the predictive validity of fertility preferences is influenced by the fact that women of initial higher parity are closer than others to completed parity. Particular interest therefore attaches to those women who had been married just before the study began and who had not yet had children. There were 121 zero-parity women in 1962 who expressed an initial preference for an average of 3.96 births, but by 1977 had experienced only 2.77 births. This low aggregate correspondence (72 percent) probably occurred because although in 1962 the baby-boom atmosphere still prevailed, several years later the fertility rate began the decline that accelerated sharply in the early 1970s. This is an important clue to the sensitivity of such measures to current conditions and the deviation of experience from initial preferences when conditions change.

At the individual level, the predictive value of preferences once again seems rather low. The correlation between single preferences in 1962 for zero-parity women and their eventual fertility is 0.33; the correlation is somewhat higher, 0.45, with the I-scale variable. When the I-scale value is combined with wife's education, income, and religion (Catholic–non-Catholic), the proportion of the variance of fertility explained is 0.24 (the I-scale is the dominant variable in the prediction equation). This is the highest value observed; adding first preference or expected number of births does not add to the 0.24 since their contribution is already captured with the I-scale. As Coombs concludes: "Obviously, a number of other factors enter into childbearing decisions and the process of family formation" (1979, p. 533).

The 1975 National Fertility Study

The National Fertility Study (NFS) featured three rounds. In 1965 and in 1970 there were separate national sample surveys of ever-married women of reproductive age. In 1975 a longitudinal design was introduced in which 2,361 white, once-married women first interviewed in the 1970 NFS who were in intact first marriages of less than twenty years duration, married at less than 25 years of age, were successfully reinterviewed (representing an 87 percent completion rate). The 1975 NFS included interviews with an additional 1.042 respondents married for the first time since the beginning of

1971. The basic test of the predictive validity of intended fertility was to examine the association between whether women intended any more or no more children as of 1970 and whether a birth (or current pregnancy) had occurred by the time of the reinterview five years later. At the aggregate level, 40.5 percent had intended more as of 1970 and 34 percent actually had more during the ensuing five years, constituting a 16.2 percent deficit.

This is the statistic that is critical for evaluating the usefulness of intentions for demographic forecasting. As we concluded in the report analyzing these data:

> Although some of those infertile in the interim will have a birth subsequent to the second interview, it is our judgment that their numbers will be few, principally because their mean length of open interval had by second interview reached approximately seven years. In other words, acceptance of 1970 intentions at face value would have led to a substantial overshooting of the ultimate outcome (perhaps by some 15 percent). This result should be evaluated in relation to the fact that the respondents were selected in ways that would tend to optimize predictability. This is a sample of stable marriages, avoiding the exigencies of dissolution and remarriage. The non-white population, which is probably less effective at prediction, has been omitted. There are no data for never-married women, most of whom will marry and will soon constitute the majority of the childbearing population (Westoff and Ryder 1977).

The average total fertility rate (the conventional period TFR calculated from vital statistics) for the entire population in the 1971–1975 period was one-sixth lower than the TFR at the end of 1970 (the time of the first interview). Accordingly, one interpretation of our finding would be that the respondents failed to anticipate the extent to which the times would be unpropitious for childbearing, that they made the understandable but frequently invalid assumption that the future would resemble the present—the same kind of forecasting error that demographers have often made. Perhaps answers to questions about intentions are implicitly conditional: "This is how I think I will behave if things stay the way they are now, but if they don't, I may change my mind."

The aggregate correspondence between intentions and behavior was much lower when the focus was on the timing of reproduction. Women who in 1970 reported intending more children were asked whether they intended to have a child within the next two years. Although 64 percent answered the question affirmatively, only 37 percent actually had a child or were pregnant at the end of the two years.

At the individual level the greatest "error" occurred for women who intended more in 1970, among whom 33.9 percent failed to conform to their intentions in a five-year period. The reverse error, births occurring to women who had intended not to have any more, was 12.0 percent. The net inconsistency or error of both kinds amounted to 20.9 percent. It is clear that postponement of childbearing outweighed contraceptive failure and changes of intention in the opposite direction, at least for the first half of the 1970s.

The correlation between simple intentions and fertility in the subsequent five-year period was 0.56. When information collected on how certain the respondent was about her intention was utilized, the correlation rose to 0.60. Compared with other correlations on individual data in the social sciences, these magnitudes are not bad. When duration of marriage and parity (in 1970) were added to intentions for those women who were certain about their intentions, the multiple correlation with fertility rose to 0.70. However, the duration of marriage by itself correlates (-0.55) with fertility, almost as well as do intentions.

Conclusions

What can be said about the usefulness of fertility preferences, intentions, or expectations for population forecasting? The verdict is mixed, but a few conclusions have been suggested by the studies reviewed in this chapter. A statistical summary is presented in the accompanying table (table 4–1). The first is that these attitudinal measures appear to reflect rather than anticipate changes in conditions that lead to changes in fertility rates. In this sense, they are no better than conventional period indexes of fertility. It would have been encouraging if the 1970 NFS had provided clues that fertility was going to decline in the next five years. The fact that no such clues were evident is a serious indictment of the usefulness of such information, at least for short-range population-projection purposes. If their usefulness in the short run is limited to periods of stability or little change in fertility, such information will be of little value to the demographic profession, especially when one considers that the future of fertility will increasingly be one of variations in low fertility in a population exercising a high degree of fertility control. Moreover, when one also considers that fertility rates are significantly influenced by changes in proportions married, the demographic utility of reproductive-intentions data for married women diminishes even further. On the other hand, reproductive intentions may be better measures of completed cohort fertility, as suggested by the Kelly Study and the Princeton Fertility Study. In the 1975 NFS, the 16 percent overestimate of fertility for the 1971–1975 period from 1970 reproductive-intentions data will also be lessened as some additional fertility occurs among women who intended no more births in the cohorts with some years of risk still ahead.

The question of the validity of reproductive intentions at the individual level is more difficult to evaluate neatly. On the one hand, most of the vari-

Table 4–1
Summary of the Characteristics and Main Results of Four U.S. Longitudinal Studies of Fertility

Longitudinal Study	Sample	Time of Prediction	Mean Intended or Preferred by Women	Mean Achieved	Ratio	Correlation
Kelly	145 white, once-married, fecund couples originally contacted before marriage, in the late 1930s in Connecticut	20 years	2.6	2.6	0.99	0.27 0.30 (with husbands)
Princeton	814 two-parity, once-married white women, originally resident in the seven largest metropolitan areas in 1957	5–10 years	3.3	3.3	0.99	0.56
Detroit	853 white, once-married, continuously married women first interviewed in 1962 when at zero, first, second, and fourth parity	15 years	3.9	3.7	0.95	0.40
	121 zero-parity subset of the 853		4.0	2.8	0.72	0.33
1975 NFS	2,361 white, once and continuously married women, married less than twenty years, first interviewed in 1970.	5 years	40.5% intended to have more	34.0% had more	0.84	0.56 0.60 (including certainty)

ance of fertility is unexplained by intentions. In contrast with aggregate prediction, the amount of unexplained variance increases with time. In the aggregate case, time seems to act toward balancing individual under- and overestimates of fertility, although some of this compensating mechanism may be fortuitous, as suggested in the Kelly Study. Considering the many circumstances that can change in individuals' lifetimes in ways that would influence their fertility, the fact that these correlations are not higher is certainly understandable. In any event, their validity at the individual level is at least as good as that of other social and demographic indicators.

For population forecasting, however, it is the aggregate level that is important. Here, as we have seen, the case for the usefulness of such attitudinal data is at best mixed.

References

Bumpass, Larry, and Westoff, Charles F. "The Prediction of Fertility." In *The Later Years of Childbearing,* chapter 4, pp. 41–54. Princeton, N.J.: Princeton University Press, 1970.

Coombs, Lolagene C. "Reproductive Goals and Achieved Fertility: A Fifteen-Year Perspective." *Demography* 16 (1979): 523–534.

Ryder, Norman B., and Westoff, Charles F. "The Trend of Expected Parity in the United States: 1955, 1960, 1965." *Population Index* 33 (1967): 153–168.

Westoff, Charles F. "The Predictability of Fertility in Developed Countries." *Population Bulletin of the United Nations* 11 (1978): 1–5.

Westoff, Charles F.; Mishler, Elliot G.; and Kelly, E. Lowell. "Preferences in Size of Family and Eventual Fertility Twenty Years After." *American Journal of Sociology* 62 (1957): 491–497.

Westoff, Charles F., and Ryder, Norman B. "The Predictive Validity of Reproductive Intentions." *Demography* 14 (1977): 431–453.

Westoff, Charles F.; Sagi, Philip C.; and Kelly, E. Lowell. "Fertility Through Twenty Years of Marriage: A Study in Predictive Possibilities." *American Sociological Review* 23 (1958): 549–556.

5

The Validity and Reliability of Birth Expectations: Evidence from the National Survey of Family Growth and the National Natality Survey

Gerry E. Hendershot and
Paul J. Placek

While the authors of the two preceding chapters disagreed about the usefulness of expectations for predicting lifetime births, they agreed that expectations of short-term fertility, over a period of five years or less, were not very useful. In contrast, Hendershot and Placek assert in this chapter that expectations are probably quite accurate for a five-year period in the future, even though they are not very accurate over a two-year period. Furthermore, the authors suggest that the error in two-year expectations may be consistent, and therefore itself predictable. If so, then the short-term expectations could be adjusted to provide a more accurate prediction of fertility. Of course, as Long and Wetrogan also mentioned in chapter 3, even if short-term projections are accurate, they will not be useful unless they can be produced much more quickly than they have been in the past. The notion of adjusting expectations data to improve their predictive capacity will be explored further in subsequent chapters.—*Eds*.

In many fertility surveys women are asked the number of births they expect in the future, in the belief that their responses are realistic estimates of their future fertility, estimates that allow for their own fecundity impairments, contraceptive practices, and socioeconomic prospects. The empirical basis for that belief has been investigated by many demographers, among the earliest of whom were Whelpton, Campbell, and Patterson (1966) and among the most recent of whom were O'Connell and Moore (1977), Westoff and Ryder (1977), and Monnier (1978). This study continues that research tradition by investigating the aggregate reliability, stability, and validity of women's birth expectations as reported in two surveys conducted by the National Center for Health Statistics: the National Survey of Family Growth (NSFG), and the National Natality Survey (NNS).

The NSFG elicited birth expectations by personal interview from nationally representative samples of ever-married women of reproductive age in 1973 (NSFG-I) and 1976 (NSFG-II). The NNS elicited birth expectations by mail questionnaire from the mothers of a nationally representative sample of legitimate live births occurring in 1972. Discussions of the sample design, estimating procedures, and variance estimation for the surveys are found in various publications of the National Center for Health Statistics; for instance, see Hendershot (1979) on NSFG-I and II, and Placek (1977) on the NNS.

In this study intersurvey reliability is investigated by comparing birth expectations of women with legitimate births in 1972 as measured by the NNS and the NSFG-I. Temporal stability is investigated by comparing birth expectations of women in the same populations as measured by NSFG-I and NSFG-II. Finally, predictive validity is investigated by comparing birth expectations in NSFG-I with the actual fertility of women from the same populations as reported in NSFG-II.

Intersurvey Reliability

The self-administered questionnaire mailed to mothers in the NNS sample asked if another birth were expected, and if so, the number expected. The questionnaire administered by interviewers to women in the NSFG-I sample asked for the same information but also included several structured probes for following up ambiguous responses. As in most comparisons of mail and interview surveys, the case nonresponse rate was higher for the NNS than for the NSFG-I, 29 percent compared to 19 percent; in both surveys missing data were imputed, but by somewhat different methods. There was also an eight-month difference in the midpoints of survey inquiry, January 1973 for the NNS and September 1973 for the NSFG-I. For these reasons, and possibly others, the NNS and the NSFG-I might have been expected to produce different estimates of birth expectations.

As can be seen in table 5–1, however, estimates of total births expected, the sum of children ever born, and additional births expected, are quite similar in the two surveys. For the subsample of NSFG-I women who had a legitimate live birth in 1972, whose expectations are shown in table 5–1, the estimates differ by less than 4 percent from the NNS. That difference is statistically significant, using the liberal criterion of nonoverlapping, 68 percent confidence intervals; also significant is the difference among women 15 to 24 years of age, for whom additional births expected are a large part of total births expected, although neither difference is large.[1] None of the remaining intersurvey differences in age, race, and age-race-specific total birth expectations in table 5–1 are statistically significant, although it should be noted that NSFG-I estimates of annual fertility rates for black women have large sampling variability.

In an effort to determine the reason for the small differences in total births expected between the NNS and the NSFG-I, their procedures for data

Table 5-1
Number of Women and Total Births Expected per 1,000 Women, by Race and Age [a]

Race and Age at Birth	Number of Women (in Thousands)		Total Births Expected per 1,000 Women ± 1 Standard Error		Difference: NSFG-I Less NNS	Ratio: NSFG-I Over NNS
	NNS	NSFG-I	NNS	NSFG-I		
All races,[b] 15–44 years [c]	2,833	2,643	3,067 ± 14	2,950 ± 72	−117*	0.96
15–24	1,456	1,397	2,628 ± 27	2,501 ± 82	−127*	0.95
25–29	854	813	3,085 ± 47	3,014 ± 131	−71	0.98
30–44	523	432	4,257 ± 92	4,285 ± 260	28	1.01
White, 15–44 years [c]	2,499	2,406	2,995 ± 14	2,909 ± 78	−86	0.97
15–24	1,276	1,260	2,592 ± 38	2,483 ± 90	−109	0.96
25–29	771	762	3,025 ± 50	2,996 ± 141	−29	0.99
30–44	452	384	4,082 ± 114	4,192 ± 283	110	1.03
Black, 15–44 years [c]	284	199	3,642 ± 119	3,496 ± 371	−146	0.96
15–24	160	115	2,903 ± 131	2,677 ± 366	−226	0.92
25–29	66	45	3,713 ± 255	3,957 ± 887	244	1.07
30–44	58	39	5,609 ± 398	5,395 ± 1317	−214	0.96

Source: National Center for Health Statistics.

Note: Differences marked with an asterisk (*) are greater than the sum of the standard errors of the estimates, and are statistically significant.

[a] Women 15 to 44 years of age who had a legitimate live birth in 1972; data from National Natality Survey and National Survey of Family Growth, Cycle I.

[b] Includes white, black, and other races.

[c] NNS mothers aged 14 to 43 for comparability with NSFG-I.

coding, inputing, and weighting were compared. It was discovered that range responses to the questions on additional births expected (for instance, "three or four") were coded differently in the two surveys: in the NNS, the upper end of the range was coded, but in the NSFG-I the upper and lower ends were averaged. That difference would tend to produce higher estimates in the NNS than in the NSFG-I, as was observed in table 5–1. To test the effect of this coding difference on the estimates, the NSFG-I data were recoded in the manner presumed to be most comparable to the NNS coding procedure: If a woman gave an unambiguous response when asked the number of additional births she intended, the largest number she gave, either a single number of the upper end of a range, was coded; if her response to that question was ambiguous, her response to the subsequent probe asking the largest number she expected was coded. As expected, revising the coding procedure increased the NSFG-I estimates, which are shown in table 5–2. The intersurvey difference between estimates of total births expected for all 1972 mothers is reduced to 2 percent and is not statistically significant. Neither do any of the more specific age, race, or age-race estimates in table 5–2 differ significantly between the two surveys.

Temporal Stability

The procedures for measuring birth expectations were nearly identical in NSFG-I and NSFG-II; therefore, comparing estimates for the same populations in the two surveys should reveal the extent to which women's expectations change in the thirty-two months between surveys. In comparisons of this type made by O'Connell and Moore (1977), it was found that total births expected declined by 2–3 percent between surveys conducted in 1971 and 1976, and by about 4 percent between surveys in 1967 and 1976. As shown in table 5–3, over the shorter period between NSFG-I and NSFG-II there was a smaller, nonsignificant decline of only 1 percent.

One shortcoming of the analyses reported by O'Connell and Moore and in table 5–3 is an inconsistency in the definition of the population at the two survey dates. Women who were currently married at the time of the earlier survey are compared with women in the later survey who were *first* married before the earlier survey, but who may not have been *currently* married at the time of the first survey; that is, they may have been divorced, separated, or widowed at that time. With the detailed marital history obtained in the NSFG, it is possible to eliminate those previously married women from the NSFG-II estimates, refining the comparison between the two surveys. Despite the relatively large numbers of such women (about 3.1 million), excluding them has little effect on estimates of total birth expectations: In the refined comparisons presented in table 5–4, differences between NSFG-I

Table 5–2
Number of Women and Births, Expected or Largest Intended, per 1,000 Women, by Race and Age[a]

Race and Age at Birth	Number of Women (in Thousands)		Births per 1,000 Women ± 1 Standard Error		Difference: NSFG-I Less NNS	Ratio: NSFG-I Over NNS
	NNS	NSFG-I	Expected: NNS	Intended: NSFG-I		
All races,[b] 15–44 years[c]	2,833	2,643	3,067 ± 14	2,994 ± 73	−73	0.98
15–24	1,456	1,397	2,628 ± 27	2,537 ± 83	−91	0.97
25–29	854	813	3,085 ± 47	3,073 ± 134	−12	1.00
30–44	523	432	4,257 ± 92	4,324 ± 263	67	1.02
White, 15–44 years[c]	2,499	2,406	2,995 ± 14	2,962 ± 80	−33	0.99
15–24	1,276	1,260	2,592 ± 38	2,529 ± 92	−63	0.98
25–29	771	762	3,025 ± 50	3,029 ± 143	4	1.00
30–44	452	384	4,082 ± 114	4,249 ± 287	167	1.04
Black, 15–44 years[c]	284	199	3,642 ± 119	3,462 ± 367	−180	0.95
15–24	160	115	2,903 ± 131	2,618 ± 357	−285	0.90
25–29	66	45	3,713 ± 255	3,957 ± 887	244	1.07
30–44	58	39	5,609 ± 398	5,395 ± 1,317	−214	0.96

Source: National Center for Health Statistics.

Note: Differences marked with an asterisk (*) are greater than the sum of the standard errors of the estimates, and are statistically significant.

[a] Women 15–44 years of age who had a legitimate live birth in 1972; data from National Natality Survey and National Survey of Family Growth, Cycle I.

[b] Includes white, black, and other races.

[c] NNS mothers aged 14 to 43 for comparability with NSFG-I.

Table 5-3
Number of Women and Total Births Expected per 1,000 Women, by Race and Age [a]

Race and Age in 1973	Number of Women (in thousands)		Total Births Expected per 1,000 Women ± 1 Standard Error		Difference: NSFG-II Less NSFG-I	Ratio: NSFG-II Over NSFG-I
	NSFG-I	NSFG-II	NSFG-I	NSFG-II		
All races,[b] 15–44 years	26,646	27,200	2,783 ± 25	2,758 ± 27	−25	0.99
15–19	1,028	1,422	2,376 ± 90	2,311 ± 82	−65	0.97
20–24	4,949	5,202	2,313 ± 41	2,281 ± 44	−32	0.99
25–29	6,063	6,795	2,445 ± 40	2,480 ± 42	35	1.01
30–34	5,248	6,081	2,879 ± 51	2,868 ± 52	−11	1.00
35–39	4,632	5,519	3,183 ± 60	3,268 ± 63	85	1.03
40–44	4,726	2,181	3,297 ± 62	3,454 ± 103	157	1.05
White, 15–44 years	24,429	23,918	2,737 ± 27	2,697 ± 26	−40	0.99
15–19	915	1,257	2,358 ± 100	2,277 ± 82	−81	0.97
20–24	4,469	4,583	2,283 ± 45	2,249 ± 44	−34	0.99
25–29	5,579	6,022	2,406 ± 43	2,444 ± 42	38	1.02
30–34	4,768	5,344	2,821 ± 55	2,825 ± 52	4	1.00
35–39	4,199	4,777	3,157 ± 26	3,142 ± 61	−15	1.00
40–44	4,320	1,934	3,215 ± 66	3,373 ± 102	158	1.05
Black, 15–44 years	2,081	2,802	3,326 ± 110	3,266 ± 94	−60	0.98
15–19	96	154	2,498 ± 372	2,483 ± 292	−15	0.99
20–24	451	525	2,575 ± 178	2,539 ± 162	−36	0.99
25–29	417	623	2,922 ± 212	2,818 ± 167	−104	0.96
30–34	402	605	3,534 ± 264	3,242 ± 197	−292	0.92
35–39	347	660	3,714 ± 300	4,167 ± 246	453	1.12
40–44	367	235	4,326 ± 342	4,123 ± 406	−203	0.95

Source: National Center for Health Statistics.

Note: Differences marked with an asterisk (*) are greater than the sum of the standard errors of the estimates, and are statistically significant.

[a] Women who were, in September 1973, currently or previously married and 15 to 44 years of age; data from National Survey of Family Growth, Cycles I and II.

[b] Includes white, black, and other races.

Table 5-4
Number of Women and Total Births Expected per 1,000 Women, by Race and Age[a]

Race and Age in in 1973	Number of Women (in Thousands)		Total Births Expected per 1,000 Women ± 1 Standard Error		Difference: NSFG-II Less NSFG-I	Ratio: NSFG-II Over NSFG-I
	NSFG-I	NSFG-II	NSFG-I	NSFG-II		
All races,[b] 15–44 years	26,646	24,099	2,783 ± 25	2,748 ± 28	−35	0.99
15–19	1,028	1,328	2,376 ± 90	2,301 ± 85	−75	0.97
20–24	4,949	4,693	2,313 ± 41	2,266 ± 46	−47	0.98
25–29	6,063	6,004	2,445 ± 40	2,481 ± 45	36	1.01
30–34	5,248	5,333	2,879 ± 51	2,914 ± 56	35	1.01
35–39	4,632	4,894	3,183 ± 60	3,200 ± 65	17	1.01
40–44	4,726	1,848	3,297 ± 62	3,482 ± 112	185*	1.06
White, 15–44 years	24,429	21,633	2,737 ± 27	2,707 ± 28	−30	0.99
15–19	915	1,186	2,358 ± 100	2,268 ± 84	−90	0.96
20–24	4,469	4,198	2,283 ± 45	2,236 ± 45	−47	0.98
25–29	5,579	5,413	2,406 ± 43	2,458 ± 44	52	1.02
30–34	4,768	4,792	2,821 ± 55	2,882 ± 56	61	1.02
35–39	4,199	4,359	3,157 ± 25	3,121 ± 63	−36	0.99
40–44	4,320	1,684	3,215 ± 66	3,419 ± 110	204*	1.06
Black, 15–44 years	2,081	2,016	3,326 ± 110	3,193 ± 107	−133	0.96
15–19	96	132	2,498 ± 372	2,474 ± 314	−24	0.99
20–24	451	412	2,575 ± 178	2,535 ± 183	−40	0.98
25–29	417	451	2,922 ± 212	2,753 ± 191	−169	0.94
30–34	402	411	3,534 ± 264	3,301 ± 243	−233	0.93
35–39	347	459	3,714 ± 300	4,003 ± 282	289	1.08
40–44	367	152	4,326 ± 342	4,172 ± 511	−154	0.96

Source: National Center for Health Statistics.

Note: Differences marked with an asterisk (*) are greater than the sum of the standard errors of the estimates, and are statistically significant.

[a] Women who were, in September 1973, currently married and 15 to 44 years of age; data from National Survey of Family Growth, Cycles I and II.

[b] Includes white, black, and other races.

and NSFG-II are nearly identical to those in the less-refined comparisons of table 5–3, averaging less than 1 percent for all women.

Predictive Validity

In addition to the number of additional births expected, NSFG-I obtained information about the expected timing of those births, from which the number of births expected in the two years following the interview were estimated. From the birth history obtained in NSFG-II, it was possible to estimate the number of births that actually occurred in those two years to women eligible for the NSFG-I questions on expectations—women who were currently married at the time. By comparing two-year birth expectations to actual births in the same period, the predictive validity of short-term birth expectations can be evaluated.[2] That comparison is made in table 5–5, and it indicates large and statistically significant differences between expectations and actual births: Women of all races combined bore 30 percent more children than they expected in the two years after NSFG-I; for white women the excess of births over expectations was 29 percent, and for black women it was 45 percent.

This finding contrasts sharply with that reported by O'Connell and Moore (1977), who found that women bore about 10 percent *fewer* children between 1971 and 1976 than they expected in 1971. In part the discrepancy between studies is caused by O'Connell and Moore's including in their estimates of actual births, but not of expectations, the experience of women who were divorced, separated, or widowed at the time of the first survey, whereas they were excluded in table 5–5. As might be expected, those women had low fertility in the years shortly following the earlier survey, so when they are included in the NSFG analysis, as they are in table 5–6, the estimate of actual births is lower, and the discrepancy between expectations and births is reduced; even so, the NSFG analysis in table 5–6 shows births exceeding expectations by 22 percent over the two-year period, whereas O'Connell and Moore found a 10 percent deficit over five years.

The excess may be explained in either of two ways: First, women's expectations of births in the two-year period may have risen after NSFG-I, so that they came to expect, and actually bear, about 30 percent more babies in that period than they had expected at its beginning; second, their expectations may have remained unchanged, but they had unexpected births. (Of course, for most women expectations would increase following the discovery of an unexpected pregnancy.) The second interpretation is supported by the data in table 5–7, which estimates births during the two-year period excluding births that were unwanted or wanted at a later time.[3] When the "unexpected" births are excluded in that way, actual births are within 3

Table 5-5
Number of Women and Births Within Two Years, Expected and Actual, per 1,000 Women, by Race and Age[a]

Race and Age in 1973	Number of Women (in Thousands)		Births per 1,000 Women, September 1973 to August 1975, ±1 Standard Error		Difference: Actual Less Expected	Ratio: Actual Over Expected
	NSFG-I	NSFG-II	Expected: NSFG-I	Actual: NSFG-II		
All races,[b] 15–44 years	26,646	24,415	153 ± 7	199 ± 9	46*	1.30
15–19	1,028	1,331	458 ± 61	473 ± 60	15*	1.03
20–24	4,949	4,788	283 ± 22	361 ± 28	78*	1.28
25–29	6,063	6,134	226 ± 18	280 ± 22	54*	1.24
30–34	5,248	5,403	104 ± 13	103 ± 14	−1	0.99
35–39	4,632	4,911	46 ± 10	38 ± 9	−8	0.83
40–44	4,726	1,848	15 ± 5	19 ± 11	4	1.27
White, 15–44 years	24,249	21,897	151 ± 8	195 ± 9	44*	1.29
15–19	915	1,189	467 ± 68	451 ± 59	−16	0.97
20–24	4,469	4,284	286 ± 25	353 ± 28	67*	1.23
25–29	5,579	5,520	224 ± 20	279 ± 22	55*	1.25
30–34	4,768	4,847	100 ± 14	98 ± 14	−2	0.98
35–39	4,199	4,373	43 ± 3	39 ± 9	−4	0.91
40–44	4,320	1,684	14 ± 6	18 ± 10	4	1.29
Black, 15–44 years	2,081	2,049	157 ± 31	227 ± 37	70*	1.45
15–19	96	132	411 ± 227	640 ± 234	229	1.56
20–24	451	422	255 ± 84	416 ± 109	161	1.63
25–29	417	455	238 ± 85	265 ± 85	27	1.11
30–34	402	426	119 ± 62	143 ± 66	24	1.20
35–39	347	463	52 ± 44	40 ± 34	−12	0.77
40–44	367	152	21 ± 28	42 ± 60	21	2.00

Source: National Center for Health Statistics.
Note: Differences marked with an asterisk (*) are greater than the sum of the standard errors of the estimates, and are statistically significant.
[a] Women who were, in September 1973, currently married and 15 to 44 years of age; data from National Survey of Family Growth, Cycles I and II.
[b] Includes white, black, and other races.

Table 5–6
Number of Women and Births Within Two Years, Expected and Actual, per 1,000 Women, by Race and Age [a]

Race and Age in 1973	Number of Women (in Thousands)		Births per 1,000 Women, September 1973 to August 1975, ±1 Standard Error		Difference: Actual Less Expected	Ratio: Actual Over Expected
	NSFG-I	NSFG-II	Expected: NSFG-I	Actual: NSFG-II		
All races,[b] 15–44 years	26,646	27,546	153 ± 7	187 ± 8	34*	1.22
15–19	1,028	1,425	458 ± 61	478 ± 58	20	1.04
20–24	4,949	5,308	283 ± 22	346 ± 26	63*	1.22
25–29	6,063	6,942	226 ± 18	260 ± 20	34	1.15
30–34	5,248	6,153	104 ± 13	96 ± 13	−8	0.92
35–39	4,632	5,537	46 ± 10	35 ± 8	−11	0.76
40–44	4,726	2,181	15 ± 5	17 ± 9	2	1.13
White, 15–44 years	24,249	24,207	151 ± 8	185 ± 9	34*	1.23
15–19	915	1,261	467 ± 68	450 ± 57	−17	0.96
20–24	4,469	4,679	286 ± 25	344 ± 26	58*	1.20
25–29	5,579	6,144	224 ± 20	261 ± 20	37	1.17
30–34	4,768	5,399	100 ± 14	91 ± 13	−9	0.91
35–39	4,199	4,791	43 ± 3	35 ± 9	−8	0.81
40–44	4,320	1,934	14 ± 6	16 ± 9	2	1.14
Black, 15–44 years	2,081	2,839	157 ± 31	191 ± 29	34	1.22
15–19	96	154	411 ± 227	679 ± 222	268	1.65
20–24	451	535	255 ± 84	352 ± 90	97	1.38
25–29	417	628	238 ± 85	229 ± 68	−9	0.96
30–34	402	623	119 ± 62	121 ± 50	2	1.02
35–39	347	664	52 ± 44	35 ± 26	−17	0.67
40–44	367	235	21 ± 28	27 ± 39	6	1.29

Source: National Center for Health Statistics.

Note: Differences marked with an asterisk (*) are greater than the sum of the standard errors of the estimates, and are statistically significant.

[a] Women who were, in September 1973, currently or previously married and 15 to 44 years of age; data from National Survey of Family Growth, Cycles I and II.

[b] Includes white, black, and other races.

Table 5-7
Number of Women and Births Within Two Years, Expected and Actual, Excluding Unwanted Last Births, per 1,000 Women, by Race and Age[a]

Race and Age in 1973	Number of Women (in Thousands)		Births per 1,000 Women, September 1973 to August 1975, ±1 Standard Error		Difference: Actual Less Expected	Ratio: Actual Over Expected
	NSFG-I	NSFG-II	Expected: NSFG-I	Actual: NSFG-II		
All races,[b] 15–44 years	26,646	24,415	153 ± 7	148 ± 8	–5	0.97
15–19	1,028	1,331	458 ± 61	310 ± 49	–148*	0.68
20–24	4,949	4,788	283 ± 22	274 ± 24	–9	0.97
25–29	6,063	6,134	226 ± 18	215 ± 19	–11	0.95
30–34	5,248	5,403	104 ± 13	78 ± 13	–26	0.75
35–39	4,632	4,911	46 ± 10	26 ± 8	–20*	0.57
40–44	4,726	1,848	15 ± 15	9 ± 7	–6	0.60
White, 15–44 years	24,249	21,897	151 ± 8	147 ± 8	–4	0.97
15–19	915	1,189	467 ± 68	284 ± 48	–183*	0.61
20–24	4,469	4,284	286 ± 25	278 ± 25	–8	0.97
25–29	5,579	5,520	224 ± 20	214 ± 19	–10	0.96
30–34	4,768	4,847	100 ± 14	76 ± 13	–24	0.76
35–39	4,199	4,373	43 ± 3	27 ± 8	–16*	0.63
40–44	4,320	1,684	14 ± 6	9 ± 7	–5	0.64
Black, 15–44 years	2,081	2,049	157 ± 31	153 ± 31	–4	0.97
15–19	96	132	411 ± 227	499 ± 211	88	1.21
20–24	451	422	255 ± 84	244 ± 85	–11	0.96
25–29	417	455	238 ± 85	220 ± 78	–18	0.92
30–34	402	426	119 ± 62	80 ± 50	–39	0.67
35–39	347	463	52 ± 44	18 ± 23	–34	0.35
40–44	367	152	21 ± 28	12 ± 32	–9	0.57

Source: National Center for Health Statistics.
Note: Differences marked with an asterisk (*) are greater than the sum of the standard errors of the estimates, and are statistically significant.
[a] Women who were, in September 1973, currently married and 15 to 44 years of age; data from National Survey of Family Growth, Cycles I and II.
[b] Includes white, black, and other races.

percent of expectations, a statistically nonsignificant difference. Further support for the second interpretation is found in a report by Weller and Heuser (1978) based on the NNS; they report that 35 percent of the legitimate live births in 1972 were not wanted at that time, a proportion of the same magnitude as that implied by tables 5–6 and 5–7 for the two years after NSFG-II.

Summary

Comparisons of birth-expectations data from three surveys conducted by the National Center for Health Statistics have shown:

1. The National Survey of Family Growth, Cycle I (NSFG-I), conducted by personal interview, produced slightly lower estimates of total births expected than did the National Natality Survey, conducted by mail questionnaire, but the difference was largely the result of differences in coding procedures, not in data collection techniques.
2. Estimates of total births expected from Cycle II of the National Survey of Family Growth (NSFG-II) were nearly identical to those estimated for women in the same populations in NSFG-I, about thirty-two months earlier.
3. Births actually occurring to women in the two years after NSFG-I (as reported in NSFG-II) exceeded the number expected in that period (as reported in NSFG-I) by 30 percent, but if unexpected births are not counted, expectations and actual births were not significantly different.

These findings provide evidence supporting the following conclusions:

1. Aggregate birth expectations are reliable—independent, simultaneous measurements of the same expectations using different techniques are not significantly different, provided data-coding procedures are standardized.
2. Aggregate birth expectations are stable—independent measurements at different times using the same technique are not significantly different.
3. Aggregate birth expectations are not valid—the measured number of births expected in a short period is greatly exceeded by the number of babies actually born, probably because women do not include their mistimed and unwanted births in expectations.

Of course, evidence from other studies must also be considered in evaluating these conclusions.

The predictive invalidity of birth expectations deserves further comment. Interview questions on birth expectations are intended to elicit from women realistic estimates of their future fertility, estimates that allow for their own fecundity impairments, contraceptive practices, and socioeconomic prospects. The findings of this study suggest that women do not provide realistic short-term estimates, but rather report as expected the number of children they *want* to bear in the next two years, resulting in an underestimate of their births in that period. On the other hand, O'Connell and Moore (1977) found that after five years, women's births and expectations for the period agreed quite well, within about 10 percent; if their comparison were refined by excluding women who were not currently married (that is, previously married women) at the beginning of the period, the agreement would be even better. These findings suggest that women's expectations for a five-year period are valid, but they do not correctly predict the timing of the births within that period. Women expect most of the births to occur three to five years after the interview, but they actually occur earlier. Prompted, perhaps, by these unexpectedly early births, women may improve their contraceptive practice the third to the fifth year, achieving by the end of the period about the number of births they expected at its beginning. This is a speculative interpretation of the findings, but one that needs further investigation.

The inability of women in the aggregate to predict their fertility correctly over a two-year period does not necessarily mean that their expectations are not useful in population forecasting. If, for instance, it is found that their error is consistent, their expectations may be adjusted to reflect it. In effect, demographers can expect for women those untimely births they do not expect themselves.

Notes

1. Because the purpose of the statistical comparisons was to discover differences that would then be closely examined, it was desirable to avoid disregarding small differences at the outset; therefore, narrow confidence intervals were chosen, so that even small differences would be "significant." Standard errors were estimated using equations derived from balanced half-sample pseudo-replication estimates of selected standard errors; a discussion of the technique as applied to NSFG-I is in French (1978).

2. The comparison is not precise because the two-year periods do not coincide exactly. The expectations are for the two years following the interview; since the interviews occurred over an eight-month period, July 1973 through February 1974, the calendar period in which the births were expected was July 1973 through February 1976. The two-year period for

which actual births are counted begins with the midpoint of interviewing for NSFG-I, September 1973, and ends with August 1975. The effect of this small discrepancy is assumed in this study to be negligible.

3. Although the wantedness of all pregnancies was measured in NSFG-II, only the wantedness of the latest birth was available for analysis in preparing this report. Therefore, only births that were unwanted or wanted later, and were also the woman's latest birth, are excluded from the estimates of actual births in table 5-7. Since some women had an earlier, unwanted birth in the same period, the actual number of unwanted births is somewhat larger than the number excluded.

References

French, Dwight K. "National Survey of Family Growth, Cycle I: Sample Design, Estimation Procedures, and Variance Estimation." *Vital and Health Statistics,* series 2, no. 76 (1978).

Hendershot, Gerry E. "Use of Family Planning Services by Currently Married Women 15-44 Years of Age: United States, 1973 and 1976." *Advance Data,* no. 45 (1979).

Monnier, Alain. "Projets de Maternité et Comportements Reéls: Une Enquête Longitudinale (1974-1976)." *Population* 33 (1978): 813-853.

O'Connell, Martin, and Moore, Maurice J. "New Evidence on the Value of Birth Expectations." *Demography* 14 (1977): 255-264.

Placek, Paul J. "The Incidence of Sterilization Following Delivery of Legitimate Live Births in Hospitals: United States." *Monthly Vital Statistics Report* 26 (1977): supplement.

Weller, Robert H., and Heuser, Robert L. "Wanted and Unwanted Childbearing in the United States: 1968, 1969, and 1972 National Natality Surveys." *Vital and Health Statistics,* series 21, no. 32 (1978).

Westoff, Charles F., and Ryder, Norman B. "The Predictive Validity of Reproductive Intentions." *Demography* 14 (1977): 431-453.

Whelpton, Pascal K.; Campbell, Arthur A.; and Patterson, John E. *Fertility and Family Planning in the United States.* Princeton, N.J.: Princeton University Press, 1966.

6

A Model for Forecasting Fertility from Birth-Expectations Data

Ronald Demos Lee

In earlier chapters we have seen that the record of fertility expectations as predictors of completed cohort fertility has been very good, while the record has been something less than perfect in predicting short-term period fertility. In this chapter Lee suggests that the latter failure has resulted from positing a simple relationship between expectations and fertility, when the relationship is really more complex. Most importantly, he says, it must be recognized that women's expectations may change in response to changing social and economic conditions. Furthermore, he points out that when expectations of total births change, expectations of short-term additional fertility must change even more and faster to compensate for already completed fertility that was geared to earlier, different expectations. For instance, if a cohort of women began childbearing aiming at having an average of two children, the pace of their fertility may have been rather slow; if, however, their expectations jumped to three children, then the pace of fertility would have to be very rapid to reach that target in the remaining years of childbearing. To an observer in the latter period, it might seem that current fertility is much higher than expectations implied, but that would overlook past fertility and the trend in expectations.

Using actual trends in fertility and expectations, Lee develops a model that relates changing expectations to current (period) fertility. The model fits the actual trends to date quite well and seems to resolve some apparently anomalous observations. For instance, it had been observed that changes in actual fertility had preceded changes in fertility expectations, suggesting that expectations are the effect and fertility the cause. But Lee's model shows that as a turning point is approached, the rate of change in expectations slows. While expectations are changing slowly, women have an opportunity to compensate for their earlier fertility excess or deficit; when the compensation is complete (that is, cumulative fertility is in line with current expectations), current fertility will change (up or down) to the "normal" level implied by that expectation.

Lee proposes that fertility forecasting be undertaken in two steps. First, the future trend in expectations themselves must be forecast. This might be done by simply extrapolating recent past trends, or by taking into account known relationships between social and economic conditions and expectations. Once the trend in expectations is forecast, Lee's model of expectations and fertility can be used to forecast fertility itself. Lee acknowledges that his model is too simple to be realistic—for instance, it assumes that all women marry, and at the same age. However, the model has already given good results, and the author is confident that through successive elaborations it can be made even better.—*Eds.*

This research was supported by Grant HD12331 from NICHD.

Introduction

Basic Questions

Are survey data on fertility expectations useful for understanding and fore-casting temporal changes in fertility rates? This is a broad question that can be better answered by posing three related, but more sharply focused, questions:

1. Is it useful to conceptualize childbearing as a process by which cohorts of women move toward a target level of completed fertility?
2. Do survey data provide a useful estimate of a cohort's contemporary target?
3. Is the target of a cohort relatively invariant over its reproductive years?

It is important to note that these questions are quite distinct, and in particular that one does *not* have to accept the notion of a fixed fertility target in order to believe that the notion of a target is useful, and that survey data can measure it well. Often the debate over the usefulness of expectations data is transformed into a debate about their stability over time. But such data are still useful if the third question is answered in the negative, as I believe it must be; their exploitation is more complicated in this case, but it also leads to new insights.

The purpose of this chapter is to develop a conceptual and mathematical framework for analyzing and forecasting fertility when the cohort targets are changing. A number of intriguing and unforeseen generalizations about the relation of rates to goals emerge from this study. A fairly detailed method for forecasting fertility is also presented. It must be stressed, how-ever, that the model is preliminary and simple, and that it does violence to demographic reality in several respects, to be noted later in this chapter. While the generalizations will almost certainly survive the refinement of the model, the forecasting procedures are not yet of practical use. As elabo-rated here, they should be viewed as describing an approach that will ulti-mately prove useful, but only after some additional details have been dealt with.

Background

The pioneering work on fertility expectations was done in the United States in 1955 with the express intention of improving forecasts of fertility (Freed-man, Whelpton, and Campbell 1959). Since then there have been sixteen additional fertility surveys of national scope in the United States and many in other countries. In the words of a recent United Nations publication that presented comparative data from twelve nations: "The usefulness of such surveys for . . . improving the reliability of population forecasts, has gradually become their main objective" (United Nations 1976, p. 97). Clearly, considerable resources are being devoted to fertility surveys with the expectation that they can, in fact, be used for forecasting. How, then, are they to be used for this purpose?

The basic notion is that each woman has a relatively fixed target for completed fertility and that this target can be elicited through direct questioning. The responses, aggregated for birth cohorts, then provide a basis for forecasting the completed fertility of each cohort. After taking into account the children already born at the time of the survey, and making some assumptions about timing, it is possible to forecast period fertility rates that are consistent with the stated targets. Women not yet old enough to be surveyed are generally assigned the targets of the youngest women interviewed.[1]

Inherent Limitations

Expectations data, if they are useful predictors, should be very closely related to current fertility behavior, after taking cumulated fertility (children already born) into account. Indeed, later in this chapter (see equation 6.20) a procedure for estimating fertility goals indirectly from observable vital statistics is suggested. But if this is so, then expectations data cannot contain much information that is not already implicit in the observable current and past fertility of women; that is, surveyed expectations cannot provide much information beyond what is already the basis for all nonexpectational approaches to forecasting. For this reason it should be no surprise that expectations data have not so far yielded any dramatic advantage for forecasting in comparison to other methods—they should not be expected to do so. Furthermore, if the use of expectations methods is inappropriately wed to the assumption of constant cohort expectations over the reproductive cycle, then resulting forecasts might well be a good deal worse than those based on more flexible methods that permit examination of trends.

Inherent Advantages

Nevertheless, there are several ways in which expectations data are useful for forecasting purposes. First, variations in timing and spacing may confound the relation of expectations to current behavior, so that the cohort expectations data may in fact contain important information that cannot be derived easily from observable demographic behavior. Second, cohort goals are the most relevant fertility measure from a theoretical point of view, and they lend themselves most naturally to explanation and forecasting through socioeconomic behavioral models or simple trend analysis. Third, the use of cohort goals makes it possible to take advantage of extraneous information, such as trends in contraceptive techniques and failure rates or sex preselection technologies, information that otherwise would be difficult to exploit systematically. Fourth, asymmetries and nonlinearities, such as those that arise from the irreversibility of fertility, may be taken explicitly into account. These reasons are sufficient to justify continued exploration of the utility of expectations data for forecasting purposes.

The Controversy

Although the use of expectations data for forecasting purposes appears on the surface to be a reasonable and straightforward approach, it is the subject of considerable controversy. It will be worthwhile to provide a brief overview of this literature before proceeding.

Numerous studies have assessed the extent to which individual women, when reinterviewed, were found to have experienced fertility in accordance with their earlier stated expectations. The usual finding has been that fertility expectations of women, as measured in the base period, are fairly good predictors of subsequent fertility, and typically dominate socioeconomic characteristics as predictors. In the aggregate, there is often a close relation between average expectations and average fertility. However, such aggregate cancellation of discrepancies appears to be typical only of periods when expectations are themselves fairly stable. In a recent study, Westoff and Ryder (1977b) found substantial aggregate inconsistency between intentions and performance for U.S. women interviewed in 1970 and again in 1975. They concluded that the expectations data would have been no better guide than the total fertility rate (TFR) itself in 1970. This is in accord with their earlier view: "Our conclusion is that . . . [expected parity] is a small and untrustworthy addition to our stock of projection procedures" (Ryder and Westoff 1971, p. 48).

A recent study by Moore and O'Connell (1978, p. 24), on the other hand, compared fertility projected in 1960 using expectations data to actual parity in 1976. The maximum error for an age group, which occurred for the cohort aged 20 to 24 in 1960, was only 4 percent. This seems to offer impressive evidence for the utility of these data for forecasting purposes. One wonders, however, whether this similarity of expected and subsequent behavior might have occurred only because of the special period—one of declining fertility goals—over which it was examined. The cohorts analyzed bore, on the average, something like 0.5 unwanted birth per woman, an excess fertility that must have been offset in large part by a decline in desired completed fertility.[2] Had contraceptive failure been anticipated and incorporated into the original forecast, the projected fertility would presumably have overstated substantially the later reproductive performance.

This point can be seen more clearly in a longitudinal study of Detroit women having a first, second, or fourth birth in 1961.[3] Their actual fertility by 1977 almost exactly matched their expected fertility in 1962, as in the Moore and O'Connell study; however, the number of births wanted "if life could be lived over" declined sharply—by 0.75 child between 1962 and 1977. If we confine our attention to women who had no births reported as unwanted over this period, the completed parity in 1977 is 0.54 child less than the expected in 1962, for women with one or two births when first surveyed. For women with *no* births in 1961, the shortfall is 0.93 birth.

There have been several attempts to relate the survey data on expectations to levels and changes in aggregate period fertility. In a well-known paper, Easterlin observed that the period fertility rates declined well before either ideal of expected fertility, and concluded that ". . . changes in behavior precede those in attitudes, rather than vice versa" (Easterlin 1973, p. 209). Easterlin's conclusion was cited with approval by Westoff (1978, p. 3).

Blake and Das Gupta (1975, pp. 239–240) found that the difference in marital fertility between 1960 and 1970 was largely attributable to changed attitudes, a view with which Ryder (1978a, p. 453) has implicitly concurred. However, Ryder imputes only a minor role to changing reproductive goals in the baby boom, as opposed to the "bust."

Finally, Lee (1977; in press a, b), found a close consistency of aggregate rates and birth expectations for ages 25 to 39 over the period 1955–1975, and provided a formal model linking rates and expectations. He showed that it was not inconsistent for period rates to show turning points before measures of reproductive goals, since period rates should be related to *additional* expected fertility, not to *total* expected fertility. This work will be discussed in more detail later in this chapter.

This literature is consistent with the following summary: The expectations of individuals are moderately good predictors of their subsequent behavior, although many revise their expectations upward or downward in subsequent years. Average expectations are quite good predictors of subsequent average fertility during periods when expectations are stable, although unwanted fertility confuses the comparison. However, since 1965 expectations have dropped rapidly and therefore have been a poor guide. In short, current expectations are congruent with current behavior when properly interpreted, but may not be a good indication of future expectations or desires.

It is clear from the studies just reviewed, and from other evidence, that there have been substantial changes over time in the United States in the fertility goals of a given cohort, as well as between cohorts. This is true even for average fertility-*expectations* data, which have enormous inertia at the older ages; it would presumably be much more true if we restricted our attention to the expectations of women who still wanted additional children at each age (nonterminators);[4] and it is demonstrably more true for the number of children wanted if life could be lived over, a measure that is at least *conceptually* independent of children already born. Attitudinal data apparently mirror couples' *current* plans and explain their *current* behavior, but that is all. It would be premature, however, to conclude that expectations data are not useful for forecasting purposes. Rather, the way in which they are used must be reexamined.

Plan for This Chapter

This chapter suggests that a two-step procedure should be employed: First, future trends in cohort goals and contraceptive failure rates should be forecast; second, these forecasts should be combined with base-period data on children ever born to develop forecasts of duration-specific marital fertility rates for future years.

The next section of this chapter develops the basic mathematical model relating period fertility rates to changing cohort goals; some nonobvious and often counterintuitive aspects of the relationship will be derived or illustrated. All the analysis in this section abstracts from the complications of contraceptive failure and the irreversibility of fertility. In the following section, on forecasting procedures, actual computational procedures for forecasting marital fertility flows when forecasts of goals have already been made are developed. In this section, contraceptive failure and irreversibility are explicitly taken into account.

Moving-Target Model

The Basic Model

In two previous papers (Lee 1977, and in press a) I have developed an analytic framework relating period fertility behavior to fertility goals. The first of these papers dealt with fertility when the reproductive goals of a cohort were unchanging, taking account of contraceptive failure both in number and in timing. The second paper dealt with the effects of changing reproductive goals on both aggregate period fertility and cohort fertility. It ignored the problem of contraceptive failure but discussed problems arising from the irreversibility of fertility. Here I will not attempt to recapitulate the findings in any detail but will instead present the principal results for the simplest models, for perfectly contracepting populations with reversible fertility. These restrictions will be removed in the next section.

The starting point of the analysis is the observation that current fertility should be related not to the desired completed fertility (D), but rather to the additional desired fertility (A). The difference, of course, lies in variations in the numbers of children already born, or cumulated fertility, (C):

$$A = D - C \qquad (6.1)$$

If we consider two groups of women with identical targets (D), we would expect the group with lower cumulated fertility (C), and hence greater additional desired births (A), to have a higher current birth rate. This will be equally true whether the groups of women have different cumulated fertility because they differ by age or because they differ in the pace of their earlier childbearing. Of course, the current timing of fertility will also play a role, but, other things being equal, we would expect A, not D, to matter.

The relationship of period fertility to A can be illustrated with U.S. data for the past twenty or so years, a period for which we have abundant survey measures of fertility goals. Figure 6-1 shows a scatter plot of current *wanted* marital fertility against additional expected fertility, for white women aged 18 to 39 in selected years, 1955-1975. There is a strong and nearly proportional relationship. The slope of the line suggests that for each additional expected birth, there are about 0.2 births each year. The line is drawn to pass through the origin; had the birth rates not been adjusted for unwanted births, we would expect a positive vertical intercept, indicating that children would be born even when none were wanted.

Figure 6-1 was based on fertility and expectations for women of all ages grouped together. However, it is convenient to begin by modeling the behavior of separate age groups, and then to derive the all-age measures by summing these (or integrating over age). In fact, the relation between wanted period fertility flows and additional expected births holds quite well for all individual age groups over 25, with only small variations in the factor of proportionality. For present purposes let us assume that the relation holds for *all* age groups with an identical factor of proportionality, which we will take to be 0.2 (see Lee 1977). Future work should be based on more realistic assumptions.

This specification might seem to imply the implausible: that birth intervals are inversely proportional to additional desired fertility, and are thus, for example, only half as long when women want twice as many additional births. But this is not so. The marital fertility rate can be factored into two multiplicative components: the proportion, p, of all women who

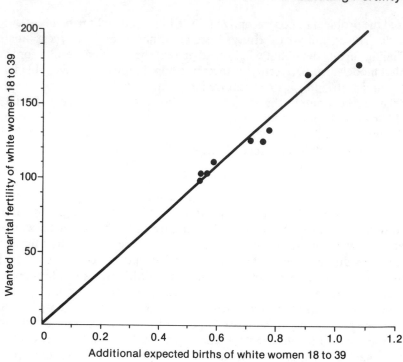

Note: Legitimate live births to married women aged 15 to 44 were taken from U.S. Public Health Service, *Natality,* Vital Statistics of the United States, 1975, vol. 1 (Washington, D.C.: U.S. Government Printing Office, 1979). These were multiplied by 1.36 = (45 − 15)/(40 − 18) to get a rate more nearly representative of married women aged 18 to 39. For each preceding year, the average proportion of nonterminators among white married women 18 to 39 was calculated from Maurice Moore and Martin O'Connell, "Perspectives on American Fertility," *Current Population Reports,* Special Studies, Series P-23, no. 70 (1978), with interpolation for 1972–1974. This was multiplied by the post-termination birth rate given in Norman Ryder, "A Model of Fertility by Planning Status," *Demography* 15 (1978a):449, with some interpolation, and the assumption of a constant rate of 0.04 after 1970 (versus 0.05 for 1966–1970 and 0.09 for 1961–1965). This was subtracted from marital fertility to get *wanted* marital fertility. Additional expected fertility of white women was calculated from Moore and O'Connell, "Perspectives on American Fertility," p. 24, for 1955–1965, excluding 1962–1964. For 1967–1974 it was calculated from U.S. Bureau of the Census, "Fertility of American Women: June 1977," *Current Population Studies,* series P-20, no. 325 (1978), p. 2. For 1962–1964 it was calculated from Ronald Freedman and Larry Bumpass, "Fertility Expectations in the U.S.: 1962–64," *Population Index* 32(1966):181–197. The years represented for expectations data are 1955, 1960, 1962–1964, 1965, 1967, 1971, 1972, 1973, and 1974; the wanted-marital fertility data refer to the following year in each case: 1956, 1961, and so on. The line is drawn by eye and is constrained to go through the origin.

Figure 6-1. Wanted Marital Fertility and Additional Expected Fertility of U.S. Married White Women, Aged 18 to 39, for Selected Years, 1955–1975

want additional births, called *nonterminators,* and the birth rate to these women, *m* (which is roughly equal to the inverse of the desired birth interval). Empirically, it is the proportion of nonterminators (*p*) that varies over time in association with additional desired fertility; the birth rate to nonterminators (*m*) has been relatively constant.

The Model Applied to a Cohort

Now consider a birth cohort of women, all of whom are assumed to marry, and to marry at the same age. Let x be their duration of marriage, and let $g(x)$ be their fertility rate at duration x. Then it follows from the preceding discussion and definitions that

$$g(x) = 0.2A(x) = 0.2[D(x) - C(x)] \tag{6.2}$$

which says that current annual births are 20 percent of all additional wanted births.

Cumulated births up to duration x, $C(x)$, are just the sum (integral) of the earlier annual birth rate of this cohort:

$$C(x) = \int_0^x g(x)\,dx \tag{6.3}$$

From this it is clear that the change over time (or duration) in $C(x)$, denoted $C'(x)$, is just given by the current fertility rate:

$$C'(x) = g(x) \tag{6.4}$$

We are seeking an expression for the way that fertility, $g(x)$, changes over time (and age). Since $g(x)$ is roughly proportionate to $A(x)$, it is useful to begin by considering how $A(x)$ evolves over time. From equation 6.1 we have, by differentiating:

$$A'(x) = D'(x) - C'(x) \tag{6.5}$$

This just says that the change in additional wanted fertility is equal to the change in desired completed fertility minus the change in cumulated fertility. But note that the change in cumulated fertility is just the birth rate, $g(x)$ (see equation 6.4), and that $g(x)$ is just $0.2A(x)$ (see equation 6.2), so that

$$A'(x) = D'(x) - 0.2A(x) \tag{6.6}$$

This last is a differential equation that can be solved for $A(x)$, giving the following:

$$A(x) = e^{-0.2x}\left[\int_0^x e^{0.2u} D'(u)\,du + k\right] \tag{6.7}$$

For any specified time path of $D(x)$, this can be solved explicitly for $A(x)$. The constant k is found by using the initial condition that at time of marriage ($x = 0$), the additional desired fertility, $A(0)$, and total desired fertility, $D(0)$, are equal:

$$A(0) = D(0) \tag{6.8}$$

For example, if we assume that the reproductive goal of this cohort is constant over its reproductive years, so that $D(x) = D$ for all x and $D'(x) = 0$, then we get for $A(x)$:

$$A(x) = e^{-0.2x}D \tag{6.9}$$

In this case additional desired fertility declines exponentially toward 0 at the rate of 20 percent per year. Marital fertility, which is proportional to $A(x)$, will likewise decline exponentially. In fact, this is a fairly good description of the shape of cohort marital-fertility schedules when fertility goals are steady (see Lee 1977).

When the reproductive target is constant for a cohort, there is a typical relationship, by age, between marital fertility rates and the desired completed family size:

$$g(x) = 0.2e^{-0.2x}D \tag{6.10}$$

However, if the target has changed for the cohort, then the cohort will, in a sense, find itself unexpectedly ahead of or behind schedule, and it will reduce or increase its birth rate accordingly. In this case, the relation of $g(x)$ to $D(x)$ is no longer simple; instead, it depends on the whole history of the changes in $D(x)$. The women bearing children in the late 1950s had been revising their family-size targets upward; consequently, their cumulative fertility was low relative to these targets, and they had unusually high birth rates compared to their targets. On the other hand, in the late 1960s women had been revising their fertility goals downward, and therefore their cumulative fertility, which had been geared to higher goals, was unusually high; this led to low additional desired fertility, and low birth rates (see Lee in press a). This can be shown analytically using the preceding model, as follows.

Suppose that the fertility target of a cohort, D, has been changing linearly since the time of marriage. Then at duration x, $D(x)$ is given by

$$D(x) = D(0) + dx \qquad (6.11)$$

where d is the change per year in $D(x)$, so that $D'(x) = d$. What will be the time path of the birth rate in this case?

Substituting $D'(u) = d$ into equation 6.7 and solving, we have

$$A(x) = e^{-0.2x}[5d(e^{0.2x} - 1) + k] \qquad (6.12)$$

Using $A(0) = D(0)$ to find k and to eliminate it from equation 6.12 gives

$$A(x) = e^{-0.2x}D(0) + 5d(1 - e^{-0.2x}) \qquad (6.13)$$

Using $g(x) = 0.2A(x)$, this finally gives

$$g(x) = 0.2e^{-0.2x}D(0) + d(1 - e^{-0.2x}) \qquad (6.14)$$

Equation 6.14 may be used to compare the fertility of cohorts with currently equal desired completed family size, but with different histories of changes in it. Suppose, for example, that one cohort wanted 3.5 children at marriage, but that it gradually reduced its desired number by 0.1 child per year for the next five years, and therefore currently wanted 3.0. Thus $D(0) = 3.5, d = -0.1, x = 5$. Then their current fertility, calculated from equation 6.14, would be $g(5) = 0.8e^{-1} - 0.1$. Similar calculations show that for a cohort initially wanting 2.5 children, but revising their goal upward to 3.0 over their first five years, the birth rate would be $0.4e^{-1} + 0.1$. Evaluating these, and including the birth rate to a cohort constantly wanting 3.0 children, gives:

Past History of Target	Current Target	Current Fertility
Rising	3.0	0.247
Constant	3.0	0.221
Falling	3.0	0.194

In other words, three groups of women with identical fertility targets, but with different past histories of changes in targets, would typically have quite different current fertility rates. This is a formal explanation of the example given earlier of the mid-1950s versus the mid-1960s, with similar fertility targets but quite different current rates. Such variation in the relation between fertility targets (D) and current fertility (g) is typically included in the catch-all phrase "changes in timing" (see, for example, Ryder 1978b; Ward and Butz 1978). However, this is a potentially misleading term because one usually looks for the sources of timing variations in current conditions, whereas in this instance the explanation derives from past demographic changes and is largely unrelated to the pace at which those women who currently want additional children are having them.

Total Fertility and Targets

So far only the fertility of a single cohort has been discussed; now it will be useful to aggregate over cohorts cross-sectionally to derive a summary measure of period fertility. Since we have been assuming that all women marry at the same age, a good summary of marital fertility is provided by summing (integrating) over all marriage durations in a given year. (Of course, this ignores the potentially important source of variation in period rates arising from changes in nuptiality.) In fact, if all women marry, and marry at the same age, then the "total marital fertility rate" so defined will be exactly equal to the total fertility rate. Formally, let $g(x, t)$ be the marital fertility of women with marriage duration x at time t. Then the total fertility rate in year t, denoted $TF(t)$, is given by

$$TF(t) = \int_0^\beta g(x, t)dx \qquad (6.15)$$

where β is the greatest duration of marriage at which births still occur (say $\beta = 20$ for convenience). If $A(x, t)$ is the additional desired fertility of women age x at time t, then

$$TF(t) = 0.2\int_0^\beta A(x, t)dx = 0.2\Gamma(t) \qquad (6.16)$$

Equation 6.16 defines $\Gamma(t)$ which is not a conventional measure; $\Gamma(t)/\beta$, however, is readily interpretable as the average additional desired fertility per married woman, the variable used in the scatter plot of figure 6-1.

In order to derive actual values of $TF(t)$ it is necessary to assume specific values for $D(x, t)$, the numbers of children desired by each age or duration group at each instant. The usual assumption in most demographic work has been that D varies across cohorts but is constant over time for a given cohort. It is helpful, however, to work with the opposite assumption: that D varies over time but is the same across all ages at a given time. Whatever assumptions are made, however, the framework outlined previously will permit the calculation of the implied time path of cohort fertility and of the total fertility rate.

In Lee (in press a), the behavior of TF for different time paths of D, assumed the same for all age/duration groups, is derived. That analysis will not be repeated here, but the model for the case of a linear change in family-size desires is provided for illustration. D should now be regarded as a function of time rather than of marriage duration, so let s or t index time, and:

$$D(s) = a + ds \qquad (6.17)$$

For a cohort at duration x in year t the target is then $D(t) = a + dt$, and at the time of marriage, x years previously, the target would have been $D(t - x) = a + dt - dx = D(t) - dx$. Using equation 6.13 with the substitution of $D(t - x)$ for $D(0)$, we get

$$A(x, t) = e^{-0.2x}(D(t) - dx) + 5d(1 - e^{-0.2x}) \qquad (6.18)$$

This describes the additional desired fertility of the different cohorts in year t. Note, for example, that for the just-married cohort we have $x = 0$ and equation 6.18 implies that $A(0, t) = D(t)$, as it should since they as yet have no children.

Now it is necessary to find $\Gamma(t)$ by summing over all durations:

$$\Gamma(t) = \int_0^\beta A(x, t)dx$$

$$= \int_0^\beta [e^{-0.2x}(D(t) - dx) + 5d(1 - e^{-0.2x})]dx \qquad (6.19)$$

The solution to this, after multiplying by 0.2 to get the TF, is

$$TF(t) = D(t)(1 - e^{-0.2\beta}) + d\beta(1 + e^{-0.2\beta}) - (2d/0.2)(1 - e^{-0.2\beta})(6.20)$$

The terms $e^{-0.2\beta}$ represent the proportion of unattained fertility when a cohort ages out of the reproductive years: with $\beta = 20$, this is only about 0.02, and can be ignored. Then, again taking $\beta = 20$, equation 6.20 simlifies to:

$$TF(t) = D(t) + 10d \qquad (6.21)$$

This result establishes that when the fertility target is unchanging ($d = 0$), total fertility equals the target. If the target is rising at a rate of, say, 0.1 child per year ($d = 0.1$) then total fertility will be 1 child greater than the target (for example, 4 children per woman instead of 3), and when the target is declining at 0.1 child per year, total fertility will be 1 child below the target.

Two other kinds of time paths of D are interesting to examine, although the analytic derivation will not be given here. The first is a movement from a high plateau to a low plateau, such as might occur during a demographic transition. Figure 6-2 shows this kind of change for D and the implied change for TF. Note that TF starts roughly equal to D, and then falls more rapidly than D (reaching a trough part way through the transition, when the rate of decline in D begins to slacken), and then rises again to approximate equality with D after the transition ends. Of course this pattern would be altered if the roles of contraceptive failure and the irreversibility of fertility were taken into account, but figure 6-2 displays what might nonetheless be an important component of fertility change during a transition.

It is also interesting to examine the case of a long swing in the fertility goal, such as apparently occurred over the course of the baby boom/bust in the United States. Such a change can be analytically represented by a sinusoidal time path for D, and the surprising results are shown in figure 6-3. The two outstanding features are that turning points in TF precede those in D rather than following them, and that the amplitude of the swings in TF far exceeds that of the swings in D: Small changes in fertility targets produce large changes in period fertility flows (for the analytic derivation see Lee in press a).

A number of generalizations emerge from this type of analysis, of which the most important are:

1. When D is rising, then the TF is greater than D; when D is falling, the TF is less than D; and when D is constant, the TF equals D.
2. When D fluctuates, turning points in the TF may actually *precede* turning points in D by several years, rather than following them as one might have expected.
3. A mere slowing down or speeding up in the rate of change in D may be enough to cause a turning point in the TF.
4. Fluctuations in D are amplified in their effects on the TF.

These results suggest that the relation of aggregate period fertility to the aggregate desired completed family size is very complicated and often counterintuitive. Therefore, assessing the consistency of these two kinds of information about fertility is also difficult, and basing fertility forecasts on expectational data is complicated as well. In the next section some procedures are developed, based on the kind of analysis just presented, that could be used to forecast fertility using expectational data drawn from surveys.

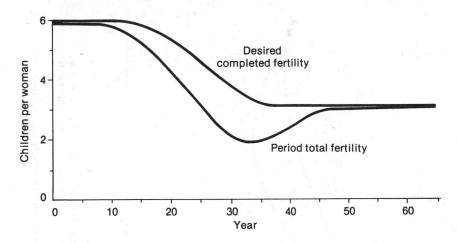

Note: Desired completed fertility is assumed to follow a segment of a sinusoidal path as it falls from 6.0 to 3.0 children per woman over the course of thirty years (from year 10 to year 40 on the scale).

Figure 6–2. Changes in Period Total Fertility When Desired Completed Fertility Moves from a High to a Low Level

Forecasting Procedures

Basic Strategy

When women state a number of additional expected births, it is presumably based on some kind of implicit forecast of what the future economic, social, and psychological environment will be like. Since these aspects of the environment and indeed of one's own psyche are notoriously difficult to forecast, it is not surprising that women revise their plans and expectations as time passes and more information becomes available. Such revision demonstrably affects not only women as individuals but also the central tendency of whole cohorts of women. For this reason it is inadequate to take the latest average stated expectation of a cohort as the basis for forecasting their future fertility. Instead, the expectations or targets should themselves be forecast first. If expectations of an age group or of a cohort have been declining, this provides some evidence that they will continue to decline in the future. A forecast of expectations should be made as are forecasts of other variables; by a careful inspection and analysis of past patterns, with or without the help of formal statistical procedures and behavioral models.

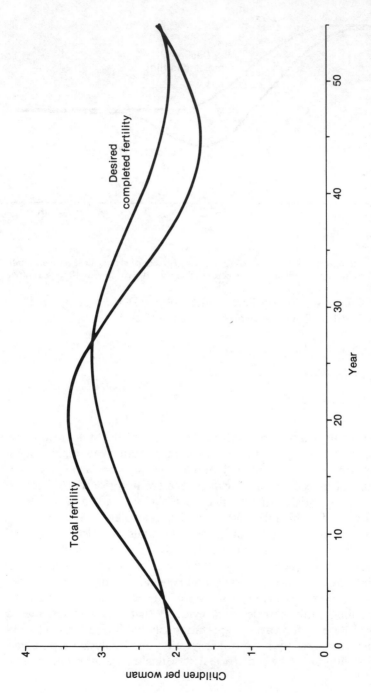

Note: The length of the cycle (trough to trough) is fifty years, and desired completed fertility varies from 2.1 to 3.1 children per woman. The time path of *TF* was calculated from equation 25 of Ronald Lee, "Aiming at a Moving Target: Period Fertility and Changing Reproductive Goals," *Population Studies* (in press).

Figure 6–3. The Time Path of Period Total Fertility When Desired Completed Fertility Fluctuates Sinusoidally

Forecasting Expectations

For most populations, of course, long time series of measures of expectations do not exist; the United States is very unusual in having a twenty-five-year series on expectations data (not without gaps, to be sure), plus an even longer series on ideal family size. This problem may not be insurmountable, however. Lee (1977) shows that, at least for the United States, it is possible to construct quite reliable estimates of expected completed fertility using only data on current marital fertility and on children ever born. We recall that according to equation 6.2:

$$g(x,t) = 0.2[D(x-1,t-1) - C(x-1,t-1)] \qquad (6.22)$$

where a one-year lag between changes in plans and changes in flows is added. This equation can be rewritten to express $D(x,t)$ as a function of $g(x+1,t+1)$ and $C(x,t)$:

$$D(x,t) = C(x,t) + 5g(x+1,t+1) \qquad (6.23)$$

This measure is affected by current unwanted births in g, but it is not distorted by past unwanted births since here, as in direct survey measures, these will show up as a component both of expected completed fertility (D) and of births to date (C), and they therefore do not affect additional expected births, $A = D - C$.

The estimator will, unfortunately, be vulnerable to variations in the desired birth interval, which is one component of timing. However, experience with U.S. data suggests that this may not be a serious problem.

While an estimator like equation 6.23 may provide a useful and simple way to reconstruct trends in birth expectations for countries with inadequate survey data, it should not be used without testing and calibration on such data as are available. In particular, the coefficient 0.2 was chosen to fit U.S. data, for ages 25 and over, on desired birth intervals and on additional births expected per nonterminator; different coefficient values would probably be more appropriate in other settings.

Let us now suppose that a past series of values of $D(x,t)$ is available. This could then be used to develop forecasts of $D(x,t)$ for future years, using any of a number of methods. The techniques of Box and Jenkins (1970) might be applied to model the internal structure of the time series as a basis for forecasting, or behavioral models like those of Easterlin (for an application using the moving target framework see Lee in press b) or Butz and Ward (1979) might be employed. Alternatively, an intelligent inspection of the plotted data might serve; in the case of the United States, this procedure would probably suggest that expectations will continue at their current levels of close to 2.1 for the younger cohorts.

The Mechanics of Forecasting

Suppose now that we have developed forecasts of $D(x,t)$ so that this can be taken as given. We will also have information on base-period values of $C(x,t)$, births to date. If s denotes the base year of the forecast, then $C(x,s)$ and $D(x,s+i)$ for $i = 0, \ldots$ are given. The first step is to calculate additional expected fertility:

$$A(x,s) = D(x,s) - C(x,s) \tag{6.24}$$

for each duration group x. Then the next year's marital fertility is given as

$$g(x+1,s+1) = 0.2A(x,s) \tag{6.25}$$

This is the desired forecast for year $s+1$. The next step is to calculate $C(x + 1, s + 1)$ as the basis for the next year of the forecast:

$$C(x+1,s+1) = C(x,s) + g(x+1,s+1)$$
$$C(0,s+1) = 0 \tag{6.26}$$

Then the procedure is repeated:

$$A(x,s+1) = D(x,s+1) - C(x,s+1) \tag{6.27}$$

and so on. This permits calculation of duration-specific marital fertility as far into the future as the forecasts of $D(x,t)$ permit.

Forecasting With Contraceptive Failure

If information on contraceptive failure rates is available, this may be incorporated in the forecast. Let $Q_1(x,t)$ be the unwanted-birth rate to terminators (that is, women wanting no more births). Let $Q_2(x,t)$ be the timing failure rate to nonterminators (that is, women wanting at least one additional birth). The time series of past values of Q_1 and Q_2 must be used to forecast future values of $Q_1(x,s+1)$; in what follows, these future values of Q_1 and Q_2 will be taken as given. Data on these for the U.S. population have been generated by Ryder and Westoff in various publications (see, for example, Ryder and Westoff 1972; Westoff 1976; Ryder 1978a).

It is also necessary to introduce two new parameters of central importance. The desired birth rate of nonterminators (roughly equal to the reciprocal of the desired birth interval) is denoted m. While it could be allowed to vary by duration and time, for simplicity we will take it to be constant. U.S. data suggest a value of about 0.3 for m (see Lee 1977). The other parameter is α, the average number of additional children expected per nonterminator, given by $A(x,t)/p(x,t)$, where $p(x,t)$ is the proportion of women at duration x in year t who want additional children. Although α could also vary by duration and time, for the United States, except at young ages, it is close to 1.5; and this value will be assumed for present purposes. On reflection it should be clear that A, g, α, and m are related by

$$g/A = m/\alpha \text{ or } 0.2 = 0.3/1.5 \qquad (6.28)$$

It also follows from the definition of α and p that:

$$p(x,t) = A(x,t)/\alpha \qquad (6.29)$$

Thus knowledge of the parameter α makes it possible to calculate the proportions of terminators and nonterminators, and therefore to know the proportions of each cohort at risk to timing failures or to unwanted births.

Some additional notation will be necessary. Let $C^*(x,t)$ be the number of *wanted* births ever born (including timing failures but not number failures). Let $A^*(x,t)$ be additional wanted births. Let $g^*(x,t)$ be the *fully planned* birth rate (excluding number and timing failures). Further, let $g(x,t)$ retain its previous meaning—it includes all births and is the observed marital fertility rate. $D(x,t)$ is defined as desired completed fertility and therefore excludes unwanted births. It is assumed to be the same for terminators and nonterminators at each duration. All these matters are discussed in detail in Lee (1977).

The forecast proceeds as follows:

$$A^*(x,s) = D(x,s) - C^*(x,s) \qquad (6.30)$$

$$g^*(x+1,s+1) = (m/\alpha)A^*(x,s) = 0.2A^*(x,s) \qquad (6.31)$$

This gives the *planned* birth rate. But to this must be added unwanted births, occurring at the rate $Q_1(x+1,s+1)$ to a proportion $1 - p(x,s) = 1 - A^*(x,s)/\alpha$ of these women, and timing failures, occurring at the rate $Q_2(x+1,s+1)$ to a proportion $p(x,s) = A^*(x,s)/\alpha$ of these women:

$$g(x+1,s+1) = g^*(x+1,s+1) + Q_1(x+1,s+1)(1 - A^*(x,s)/\alpha)$$
$$+ Q_2(x+1,s+1)A^*(x,s)/\alpha \qquad (6.32)$$

This can be slightly simplified to:

$$g(x+1,s+1) = A^*(x,s)[0.2 + (Q_1(x+1,s+1) \qquad (6.33)$$
$$- Q_2(x+1,s+1))/\alpha] + Q_1(x+1,s+1)$$

If the number and timing failure rates were equal, which might not be too far wrong given that nonterminators are only at risk about half the time, then equation 6.33 would simplify to:

$$g(x+1,s+1) = 0.2A^*(x,s) + Q_1(x+1,s+1) \qquad (6.34)$$

Either equation 6.33 or 6.34 yields the desired forecast of fertility. The final step is to update the values of wanted births to date, $C^*(x,t)$, and then forecast for period $s+2$:

$$C^*(x+1,s+1) = C^*(x,s) + g^*(x+1,s+1) \qquad (6.35)$$

$$A^*(x+1,s+1) = D(x+1,s+1) - C^*(x+1,s+1) \qquad (6.36)$$

and so on.

Forecasting with Irreversibility of Fertility

The final refinement is to take into account the irreversibility of fertility. This is important for two reasons: first, because there has so far been an implicit assumption that when C was greater than D, and therefore A was negative, the flow of births would also be negative. Skeptics may view this as unrealistic. In fact, it is necessary to distinguish between positive and negative A not only in the aggregate, but also at the individual level. Second, given the growing use of sterilization for contraceptive purposes, it may be unrealistic to assume that women can switch from terminator to nonterminator status if they revise their fertility desires upwards. The first kind of problem becomes important in an era of declining fertility targets, when a cohort may accumulate a number of "no-longer-wanted" children, denoted $U(x,t)$, who were wanted when conceived but would not be wanted if the decision could be rescinded in the light of subsequent information. The second kind of problem becomes important when fertility goals are being revised upward, as during the 1950s. Here we will deal only with the first kind of problem.

It is necessary to elaborate on the earlier notation: Let $C^{**}(x,t)$ be the number of still-wanted births, and let $A^{**}(x,t)$ be the additional wanted births, given by $D(x,t) - C^{**}(x,t)$. Note that births to date are now made up of three components: C^{**}, U, and cumulated unwanted births. I assume that $C^{**}(x,s)$ is known (procedures for calculating it may be found in Lee in press b). Then we proceed as follows:

$$A^{**}(x,s) = D(x,s) - C^{**}(x,s) \tag{6.37}$$

$$g^*(x+1,s+1) = 0.2A^{**}(x,s) \tag{6.38}$$

$$g^*(x+1,s+1) = g^*(x+1,s+1) + Q_1(x+1,s+1)$$
$$+ A^{**}(x,s)[0.2 + (Q_1(x+1,s+1)$$
$$- Q_2(x+1,s+1))/\alpha] \tag{6.39}$$

So far this closely parallels the previous method. Now, however, it is necessary to calculate the increment to no-longer-wanted births, $U(x+1,s+1)$, if $D(x+1,s+1)$ is less than $D(x,s)$. If D is declining, then terminators (in proportion A^{**}/α) will each acquire a number of no-longer-wanted children equal to the decline in D. Furthermore, there will be some women who will become terminators between time s and time $s+1$ (say halfway between, on average). These considerations lead to the following equation for $C^{**}(x+1,s+1)$, to be used only when D is declining:

$$C^{**}(x+1,s+1) = C^{**}(x,s) + g^*(x+1,s+1)$$
$$- [D(x,s) - D(x+1,s+1)]\{[1 - p(x,s)]$$
$$+ 0.5[p(x,s) - p(x+1,s+1)]\} \tag{6.40}$$

where $p(x,s) = A^{**}(x,s)/\alpha$ and $p(x+1,s+1) = A^{**}(x+1,s+1)/\alpha$. The difficulty here is that $A^{**}(x+1,s+1)$ is not known until $C^{**}(x+1,s+1)$ has been found, so further manipulation of equation 6.39 is necessary. After a good deal of algebra, the following expression for C^{**} can be derived:

$$C^{**}(x+1,s+1) = D(x+1,s+1) + \left(g^*(x+1,s+1) \right.$$
$$\left. + A(x,s)\{[D(x,s) - D(x+1,s+1)]/3 - 1\} \right)/$$
$$\{[D(x,s) - D(x+1,s+1)]/3 + 1\} \tag{6.41}$$

This can be evaluated using known values, and permits the iteration of the procedure for period $s+2$ and so on.

If D is not declining, then the problem of irreversibility does not arise, and

$$C^{**}(x+1,s+1) = C^{**}(x,s) + g^*(x+1,s+1) \qquad (6.42)$$

Some Problems with This Approach

The moving-target model was developed with an eye toward analytic tractability and therefore simplicity. For forecasting purposes, the resulting distortions of reality are a serious problem, and some of the simplifying assumptions must be modified or dropped altogether. It cannot be assumed that all women marry, and do so at exactly the same age, and remain married throughout their reproductive life. Separate accounting systems must be incorporated for women marrying at different ages, not marrying at all, getting divorced, and so on. Such problems are, however, incidental to the main thrust of the ideas presented here. More central is the problem that the coefficient used, 0.2, is not really invariant by marriage duration; in fact, at durations below five or six years, the true coefficient is much less than 0.2. For these durations, at least, a different specification is necessary. One possibility would be to make g, the fertility flow, a linear (rather than proportional) function of A, additional expected births, with the coefficient depending on marriage duration. This procedure gives a good fit to U.S. data, but is rather unappealing from a theoretical point of view. A more appealing approach is to develop the analysis in terms of the *distribution* of women by desired completed family size, rather than in terms of the mean of this distribution. Using the distributions is, of course, a much more data-demanding approach, but it is the most natural approach from a theoretical point of view.

Conclusions

Target fertility provides a powerful analytic framework for the study of fertility, and surveys provide useful measures of targets. But because the target of a cohort may vary substantially over time, the use of survey data is not at all straightforward. For example, it would be a mistake to derive fertility flows from the cohort targets by imposing on them some standard age- or duration-specific distribution of fertility. Current fertility depends, via additional desired fertility, on a cohort's entire history of changing reproductive goals, not solely on its current target.

Furthermore, if a cohort's goal has changed in the past, it is likely to continue to change in the future. For forecasting purposes one should not take the most recently expressed birth expectations of a cohort as definitive; to do so would be conceptually similar to the old procedure of forecasting future age-specific rates at whatever their base-year level happened to be. A more appropriate approach is to forecast the future expectations of a cohort based on an analysis of its past expectations.

Once this has been done, there remains the difficult task of translating a series of changing cohort goals into a series of age- or duration-specific fertility rates. This chapter has provided a simple model for this purpose, and has shown how it could be used to forecast fertility while making allowance for contraceptive failure and irreversibility of fertility. However, for practical purposes, a more flexible and more detailed model is required; and such a model has not yet been developed.

Notes

1. For more detailed discussion of procedures see Freedman, Whelpton, and Campbell (1959); Whelpton, Campbell, and Patterson (1966); Shryock and Siegel (1973); or U.S. Bureau of the Census (1975).

2. For estimates of the unwanted births cumulated by these cohorts through 1970, see Westoff and Ryder (1977a, p. 262).

3. The data on these women at several dates in the 1960s were gathered by Ronald Freedman and Lolagene Coombs; the reinterview study in 1977 was undertaken by Deborah Freedman. They have generously made their as-yet-unpublished data available to me; see Freedman (1977, 1978).

4. Unfortunately, the necessary data are almost never tabulated separately for terminators and nonterminators in published sources. For the assertion about "wanted if life could be lived over," see Freedman (1978).

References

Blake, Judith, and Das Gupta, Prithwis. "Reproductive Motivation Versus Contraceptive Technology: Is Recent American Experience an Exception?" *Population and Development Review* 2(1975):229–249.

Box, George, and Jenkins, Gwilym. *Time Series Analysis: Forecasting and Control.* San Francisco: Holden-Day, 1970.

Butz, W.P., and Ward, M.P. "The Emergence of Countercyclical U.S. Fertility," *American Economic Review* 69(1979):318–328.

Easterlin, Richard. "Relative Economic Status and the American Fertility Swing," in *Family Economic Behavior,* edited by Eleanor Sheldon, pp. 170–223. Philadelphia: J.B. Lippincott, 1973.

Freedman, Ronald. "Notes on Trends in Expectations, Parities and Prefer-

ences for Detroit Women." Research Memorandum, University of
Michigan Population Studies Center, 1977.
———. "Consistency of 'Wantedness' Statements over Time." Working
Paper, University of Michigan Population Studies Center, 1978.
Freedman, Ronald, and Bumpass, Larry. "Fertility Expectations in the
U.S.: 1962–64." *Population Index* 32(1966):181–197.
Freedman, Ronald; Whelpton, Pascal, K., and Campbell, Arthur A. *Family
Planning, Sterility and Population Growth.* New York: McGraw-Hill,
1959.
Lee, Ronald. "Target Fertility, Contraception and Aggregate Rates:
Toward a Formal Synthesis." *Demography* 14(1977):455–479.
———. "Aiming at a Moving Target: Period Fertility and Changing
Reproductive Goals." *Population Studies* (in press a).
———. "A Stock Adjustment Model of U.S. Marital Fertility, 1947–74."
In *Research in Population Economics, III,* edited by Julian Simon and Peter
Lindert, Greenwich, Conn.: JAI, in press b.
Moore, Maurice, and O'Connell, Martin. "Perspectives on American
Fertility." *Current Population Reports,* Special Studies, series P-23,
no. 70 (1978).
Ryder, Norman. "A Model of Fertility by Planning Status." *Demography*
15(1978a):433–458.
———. "Components of Temporal Variations in American Fertility."
Paper presented at Symposium on Recent Changes in Demographic
Patterns in Developed Countries, London, 1978b.
Ryder, Norman B., and Westoff, Charles F. *Reproduction in the United
States, 1965.* Princeton, N.J.: Princeton University Press, 1971.
———. "Wanted and Unwanted Fertility in the U.S.: 1965 and 1970." In
Demographic and Social Aspects of Population Growth, edited by
Charles Westoff and Robert Parke, pp. 467–488. Washington, D.C.:
Commission on Population Growth and the American Future, 1972.
Shryock, Henry, and Siegel, Jacob. *The Methods and Materials of
Demography.* Washington, D.C.: U.S. Government Printing Office,
1973.
United Nations. *Fertility and Family Planning in Europe Around 1970.*
Population Studies, no. 58 (1976).
United States Bureau of the Census. "Projections of the Population of the
United States: 1975 to 2050." *Current Population Reports,* series P-25,
no. 601 (1975).
———. "Fertility of American Women: June 1977." *Current Population
Reports,* series P-20, no. 325 (1978).
United States Public Health Service. *Natality.* Vital Statistics of the United
States, 1975, vol. 1. Washington, D.C.: U.S. Government Printing
Office, 1979.

Ward, Michael, and Butz, William. *Completed Fertility and Its Timing.* Santa Monica, Calif.: Rand Corporation, 1978.

Westoff, Charles F. "The Decline of Unplanned Births in the United States." *Science,* 9:January 1976, pp. 38–41.

Westoff, Charles, "The Predictability of Fertility in Developed Countries." *Population Bulletin of the United Nations* 11(1978):1–5.

Westoff, Charles F., and Ryder, Norman B. *The Contraceptive Revolution.* Princeton, N.J.: Princeton University Press, 1977a.

Westoff, Charles F., and Ryder Norman B. "The Predictive Validity of Reproductive Intentions." *Demography* 14(1977b):431–453.

Whelpton, Pascal K.; Campbell, Arthur A.; and Patterson, John E. *Fertility and Family Planning in the United States.* Princeton, N.J.: Princeton University Press, 1966.

7

Changes in Parity Orientation from 1970 to 1975

Norman B. Ryder

In chapter 6 Lee argued that forecasting fertility requires some knowledge of how and why fertility expectations are changing. Those questions are addressed in this chapter by Norman Ryder, using data from the 1970 and 1975 National Fertility Studies. Since many of the women interviewed in 1975 had also been interviewed in 1970, Ryder is able to perform longitudinal as well as cross-sectional analyses. That is, he can compare changes between 1970 and 1975 for individual women and for the aggregates of all women.

A principal finding in the study is that orientations toward family size, whether measured by ideal family size, desired family size, or intended family size, declined between 1970 and 1975, both in the aggregate and for most individuals. While this trend was mentioned by others as well, Ryder's evidence is stronger by virtue of the variety of measures and subgroups he considers.

Having established the downward direction of change in fertility orientations, Ryder considers its causes. Specifically, he disaggregates the decline in family-size ideals, desires, and intentions into three factors: marriage duration, cohort, and period. Although these separate effects are difficult to distinguish empirically, their conceptual distinction is easily understood: A marriage-duration effect implies that women married for different lengths of time have different fertility orientations, even though they were born at the same time and lived through the same historical period. A cohort effect implies that women born at different times differ in orientation, even though they have been married for equal durations and were exposed to the same historical influences. Finally, a period effect implies that women living in different historical periods have different fertility orientations, even though born at the same time and married for the same duration.

The very interesting results of Ryder's analysis are that marriage duration had negligible effects on fertility orientations, while cohort and period effects are significant and about equal. That is, the number of children intended (desired, idealized) by women in 1975 was lower than the number in 1970 because (1) the 1975 women included some born later than any in the 1970 sample, among whom lower numbers of children were intended; and (2) 1975 was somehow different from 1970 or at least was perceived to be.

This chapter is a report of the 1975 National Fertility Study, codirected by Charles F. Westoff and the present author, under contract to the National Institute of Child Health and Human Development, Center for Population Research. It was presented at the annual meetings of the Population Association of America, Philadelphia, April 1979.

In another approach to the problem of explaining changes in fertility orientations, Ryder investigates the causal relationships between the three different measures of orientations-intentions, desires, and ideals. He concludes from that analysis that, if anything, intentions are the cause of ideals and desires, not vice versa. Thus measures of attitudes, such as ideals and desires, do not offer much promise as tools for forecasting fertility expectations.—*Eds.*

National-sample surveys in the United States since 1955 have documented the contributions to fertility variations arising from two sources—changes in reproductive intentions and changes in the capacity to fulfill those intentions. Although there have been dramatic developments in both areas, most of our research to date has emphasized the latter—increase in the use of methods of fertility regulation, the shift from less to more effective methods, the improvement in contraceptive efficacy, and the consequent reduction of ill-timed and unwanted births. So substantial has been the progress in the effective employment of means to achieve reproductive ends that we are now approaching a situation in which actual fertility will be the same as intended fertility. If so, our research responsibilities should shift in the direction of improvement of our understanding of reproductive intentions.

Expectations and intentions, although similar, are not identical. The discrepancy between them is limited to past unwanted births (the incidence of which is much smaller than it used to be) and anticipated future unwanted births (few respondents anticipate any). Since our judgment is that the appropriate strategies for investigating intended and unintended fertility are likely to be quite different, and the correlates dissimilar, we focus here on intentions.

In this chapter we consider the relationships among three kinds of information—intended parity, ideal parity, and desired parity—in terms of the face value of the questions producing them and in terms of their empirical interconnections. The purpose of the chapter is to determine the kind of information provided by the responses to questions about ideal parity and desired parity, marginal to the statements of reproductive intentions themselves, which we may be able to use to improve our understanding and prediction of changes in those intentions.

The Data

The evidence presented in this chapter comes from the 1970 and 1975 National Fertility Studies (NFS). The respondents are a national sample of white women, in an intact first marriage of duration less than twenty-five years at time of survey, and with wife's age at marriage less than 25 years.

Those with marital duration between five and twenty-four years in 1975 were reinterviews of women first interviewed in 1970. The characteristics of the sample are examined elsewhere (Westoff and Ryder 1977, appendix).

Before looking at the evidence, we consider the questions in terms of the research purposes that led to their inclusion in the surveys. Intended parity is the key variable, relative to which the meaning of the others is to be examined, because it is regarded as the immediate attitudinal precursor to reproductive behavior. The code for intended parity is the sum of the outcomes of two questioning procedures. Each past birth is classified as "intended" or "unintended." An unintended birth is determined by a negative response to the following question: "Think back to just before you found out you were pregnant again. At that time did you and your husband intend to have any more children eventually, or did you intend to have no more children?" The same procedure was used for any current pregnancy. The wording here is that of the 1975 questionnaire. The procedure was somewhat different in 1970; the implications are examined in Ryder (1979). Although the information is necessarily ascertained after the fact, the design of the question is an attempt to elicit from the respondent a prospective state of mind.

If the respondent thinks she is able to have any more children, she is also asked about possible future births. The questions are as follows: "Do you and your husband intend to have any more children eventually, or do you intend to have no more children?" If the answer is affirmative, the next question is: "How many more children do you intend to have?" If the answer is equivocal, the next question is: "Well, which do you think is the more likely: that you will decide to have another child, or that you will decide not to have another child?" The sum of past intended births and additional intended births is what we here call intended parity.

The question on ideal parity is the first one in the questionnaire, identically worded in 1970 and 1975. "What do you think is the *ideal* size of a family—a husband, a wife, and how many children?" The purpose of the question is to provide the respondent with the opportunity to indicate the relative place of parental and nonparental pursuits in her value system, in abstraction from consideration of actual circumstances. The conceptual advantage of this question, if it works well, is that intended parity presumably reflects some compromise between a couple's reproductive orientation, on the one hand, and the actual and projected contextual constraints, on the other. If ideal parity serves as an index of the former, uncontaminated by considerations of the latter, then it can serve analytically as one of the determinants of intended parity and predictively as a clue to the direction of change in reproductive intentions if the context were to improve. The formulation conveys the further implication that one's reproductive orientation is relatively stable over time, and that short-run variations in intentions are primarily attributable to changes in the context within which decisions must be made.

The question on desired parity is located late in the questionnaire, subsequent to the classifications of births and the ascertainment of future intentions. The wording, identical in 1970 and 1975, is: "Given the circumstances of your life, how many children *in all* would you really consider the most desirable for you and your husband?" The potential utility of the response presumably differs between those respondents who may intend to have an additional birth and those who do not. For the former, one would expect intended and desired parity to be the same. If there is a difference, it may represent an opportunity for the respondent to register doubt concerning the reproductive intention she has expressed (and thus provide the analyst with information that may improve prediction).

For those who unequivocally intend no future childbearing, the distinction between intended and desired parity would seem to be clear. The decisions implicit in past intended births were predicated on the current and projected circumstances (and the reproductive orientation) prevailing at that time; the question on desired parity provides a retrospective view—as things have turned out, do those past decisions look sensible?

We have not mentioned one obvious way in which there would be a departure of intended parity from what would be considered ideal or desirable—the case of the respondent balked by infecundity in her ambition for another child. For the most part we have avoided this problem in the subsequent analysis by confining our tabulations to those women who report they are fecund, that is, those from whom we have ascertained future reproductive intentions.

The research strategy described here may or may not have been translated into a successful outcome with the questions we employed. One objective of this chapter is to try to answer this question.

Cross-Sectional Analysis

The first presentation treats the 1970 and 1975 data as independent cross sections; subsequently we exploit the longitudinal aspect of the design. For purposes of comparability, the universe is defined in terms of the lowest common denominator of the two studies. Beyond the specifications already listed, we excluded from the 1975 data set, for present purposes, sixty respondents who would have been too old to be eligible for the 1970 study.

Some responses to the questions on ideal and desired parity were non-numerical. The proportions were small: 0.5 percent in 1970 and 1.0 percent in 1975 for ideal parity; 0.2 percent in 1970 and 1.1 percent in 1975 for desired parity. There was no relationship between the disposition to give such responses and the two independent variables—religion and marital duration—used in the analysis. These responses were deleted.

Some responses to these two questions took the form of a range (such as—and particularly—"two or three"). The proportions were small: 1.3 percent in 1970 and 1.8 percent in 1975 for ideal parity; 1.2 percent in 1970 and 1.5 percent in 1975 for desired parity. In the cross-sectional analysis, these responses were used at their midvalue.

As previously noted we have no value for intended parity for respondents who said they were unable to have another child. Moreover, a substantial proportion of respondents in 1970 (but only a small proportion in 1975) gave a noncommittal response to the question of whether a past birth was intended or unintended. (In 1970 but not in 1975, the interviewer used a permissive approach in reaction to hesitant or ambivalent responses.) For present purposes, we have treated intended parity for these respondents as indeterminate and have excluded them from the tabulations. Table 7–1 shows the proportion of respondents, by marital duration, excluded from the calculations of intended parity because they were nonfecund or gave noncommittal responses.

The magnitude of exclusion is substantial, particularly in 1970 and particularly in the higher durations. The increase in noncommittal exclusions with duration presumably occurs because ambivalence about intention is more likely with a birth of higher order. The comparable tabulation by religion (not shown) indicated that Catholics were more likely to be noncommittal than non-Catholics, presumably because of their higher fertility. The increase in nonfecund exclusions by duration has an obvious explanation, but the lower level in 1975 than in 1970 deserves a comment. Since only those not currently using contraception were asked whether they were

Table 7–1
Percentage Nonfecund and Percentage Noncommittal about Whether a Birth Was Intended, by Marital Duration

Duration	Nonfecund		Noncommittal		Number of Respondents	
	1970	1975	1970	1975	1970	1975
0–4	1	1	7	1	1,017	1,042
5–9	5	2	14	2	857	705
10–14	7	5	23	4	741	638
15–19	16	10	25	6	634	554
20–24	23	15	25	6	564	404
Total	9	5	18	3	3,813	3,343

Source: U.S. National Fertility Studies, 1970 and 1975.

able to have a child, a rise in the proportion currently using, such as occurred between 1970 and 1975, would lead to a decline in registered non-fecundity, all other things being equal. The comparable tabulation of non-fecundity, by religion (not shown) indicated that Catholics were more likely to be classified as nonfecund than non-Catholics, presumably because they were less likely to be reported as current contraceptive users.

Because we were concerned that the considerable proportions excluded from intended-parity calculations might affect comparisons with the other parameters, we prepared table 7-2. This gives the mean values of ideal and desired parity for those with a determinable intention, and, parenthetically, for all respondents. It is reassuring that there is so little consequence. We produced the subsequent tabulations for this section on both bases, that is, for respondents with determinable intentions, and for all respondents reporting ideal or desired parity. Since there were no significant discrepancies, we have chosen to display only the latter.

Several findings may be noted from table 7-2. Although the similarity of the three parity measures is perhaps more interesting than their differences, desired parity tends to be somewhat higher than either ideal or intended parity; this holds in both time periods and for both religion subgroups. All three parity measures decline substantially from 1970 to 1975: The decline is larger for desired parity than for the other two and is larger for Catholics than for non-Catholics. Finally all three measures show substantially higher values for Catholics than for non-Catholics. (Parenthetically, one detail of the calculations in table 7-2 and subsequent tables should be mentioned. Rather than produce means for all respondents, regardless of marital duration, which would give greater weight to the lower durations in which there are more respondents, we have followed the practice of calculating means for each quinquennial duration, and showing the mean of these means. This weights the duration groups equally.)

Table 7-2
Mean Ideal, Desired, and Intended Parity, for Those with a Determinable Intention, by Religion

	Total		Non-Catholic		Catholic	
	1970	1975	1970	1975	1970	1975
Ideal	2.79	2.57	2.68	2.47	3.09	2.86
	(2.82)[a]	(2.58)	(2.71)	(2.47)	(3.15)	(2.88)
Desired	3.00	2.66	2.85	2.54	3.49	3.00
	(3.06)	(2.68)	(2.87)	(2.56)	(3.59)	(3.04)
Intended	2.77	2.48	2.61	2.36	3.27	2.85

Source: U.S. National Fertility Studies, 1970 and 1975.

[a]Numbers in parenthesis are mean ideal and desired parity for all respondents.

In tables 7-3 and 7-4 we show the means for each of the three kinds of parity, by religion and marital duration, 1970 and 1975. Table 7-3 is presented conventionally in columns for periods and rows for durations; an implicit third variable is concealed. In each row (for each marital duration), the change from one period to the next is also a change from one marriage cohort to the next, so that the observed difference is attributable to a combination of what one may call a period effect and a cohort effect. Similarly, in each column (for each period) the change from one marital duration to the next is also a change from one marriage cohort to another. (In this case increase in duration is associated with a decrease in cohort.) The challenge in such a tabulation is to separate the effects of change from

Table 7-3
Mean Ideal, Desired, and Intended Parity, by Religion and Marital Duration

	Total		Non-Catholic		Catholic	
	1970	1975	1970	1975	1970	1975
Ideal						
0–4	2.69	2.40	2.60	2.31	2.94	2.64
5–9	2.61	2.39	2.50	2.34	2.90	2.53
10–14	2.84	2.54	2.69	2.42	3.20	2.90
15–19	3.00	2.72	2.82	2.58	3.51	3.07
20–24	2.98	2.83	2.93	2.69	3.19	3.27
Mean	2.82	2.58	2.71	2.47	3.15	2.88
Desired						
0–4	2.83	2.43	2.71	2.34	3.15	2.67
5–9	2.80	2.43	2.61	2.33	3.33	2.68
10–14	3.09	2.60	2.89	2.45	3.57	3.04
15–19	3.33	2.94	3.06	2.80	4.05	3.30
20–24	3.25	3.02	3.08	2.87	3.87	3.49
Mean	3.06	2.68	2.87	2.56	3.59	3.04
Intended						
0–4	2.57	2.28	2.47	2.18	2.85	2.54
5–9	2.62	2.28	2.46	2.21	3.13	2.45
10–14	2.85	2.33	2.65	2.17	3.35	2.81
15–19	2.83	2.73	2.67	2.60	3.33	3.10
20–24	2.95	2.81	2.79	2.64	3.68	3.35
Mean	2.77	2.48	2.61	2.36	3.27	2.85

Source: U.S. National Fertility Studies, 1970 and 1975.

Table 7–4
Numbers of Respondents for Table 7–3

	Total		Non-Catholic		Catholic	
	1970	1975	1970	1975	1970	1975
Ideal						
0–4	1,014	1,034	737	755	277	279
5–9	852	700	627	502	225	198
10–14	738	632	525	473	213	159
15–19	631	544	464	393	167	151
20–24	560	399	440	302	120	97
Total	3,795	3,309	2,793	2,425	1,002	884
Desired						
0–4	1,017	1,033	739	752	278	281
5–9	854	693	627	497	227	196
10–14	741	631	528	471	213	160
15–19	630	554	463	399	167	155
20–24	563	396	440	301	123	95
Total	3,805	3,307	2,797	2,420	1,008	887
Intended						
0–4	941	1,025	694	747	247	278
5–9	696	677	524	484	172	193
10–14	521	579	371	441	150	138
15–19	384	471	291	343	93	128
20–24	308	327	251	250	57	77
Total	2,850	3,079	2,131	2,265	719	814

period to period, from cohort to cohort, and from duration to duration. It is not difficult to defend these three sources of influence as independently significant. Marriage cohorts may have distinctive socialization experiences that affect their responses throughout their subsequent lives. There may also be a tendency for responses to increase or decrease systematically with advancing age (with increasing marital duration). Finally, the circumstances of a particular period may make their impact on the responses of all constituent marriage cohorts (at their respective marital durations).

Nevertheless, without an assumption that goes beyond the bounds of the data themselves, it is not possible to produce a unique set of measures of separate period, cohort, and duration effects. The essence of the problem is that the three variables are linked in an identity: cohort + duration = period. We have devised a procedure for cutting the Gordian knot, based on

Table 7-5
Period (P), Cohort (C) and Duration (D) Effects in Table 7-3

	Column Effect ($P + C$)	Row Effect ($C - D$)	Period Effect (P)	Cohort Effect (C)	Duration Effect (D)
Ideal					
Total	−0.25	−0.11	−0.13	−0.12	−0.01
Non-Catholic	−0.24	−0.10	−0.13	−0.11	−0.01
Catholic	−0.27	−0.15	−0.13	−0.14	+0.01
Desired					
Total	−0.38	−0.15	−0.20	−0.18	−0.02
Non-Catholic	−0.31	−0.14	−0.16	−0.15	−0.01
Catholic	−0.56	−0.22	−0.30	−0.26	−0.04
Intended					
Total	−0.28	−0.12	−0.14	−0.13	−0.01
Non-Catholic	−0.25	−0.11	−0.13	−0.12	−0.01
Catholic	−0.42	−0.21	−0.21	−0.21	−0.00

Source: U.S. National Fertility Studies, 1970 and 1975.

what we regard as a defensible assumption from various standpoints. The resultant procedure can be described briefly. We assume linearity for the column and row variables, and fit a plane $Y = a + b_1 X_1 + b_2 X_2$ by the customary least-squares technique, where X_1 is the row variable and X_2 is the column variable. Then b_1 is the difference of the duration effect and the cohort effect and b_2 is the sum of the period effect and the cohort effect. To obviate the circumstance that we have only two equations in three unknowns, the assumption is that the period effect is the sum of the cohort effect and the duration effect. The justification for this assumption is presented in the appendix.

The results of this exercise are presented in table 7-5. For all three variables, and for both religion subgroups, there is approximate equality of the period and cohort effects, together with negligible duration effects. The effects are equal in magnitude for ideal and intended parity, and appreciably larger for desired parity. We make the following inferences from these data, recognizing that they are contingent on the propriety of the estimating technique. First, the small size of the duration effect suggests that the three parity measures are robust, in the aggregate, over the course of the life cycle. Second, approximately one-half of the decline in these variables between 1970 and 1975 is attributable to a period effect, which we would interpret as inherently a short-run phenomenon (whereas a cohort effect manifests an inherently long-run phenomenon). If so, this had important predictive implications. Third, the greater sensitivity to change manifested by desired parity is what one would expect from a question that (unlike that of ideal parity) makes explicit the consideration of current circumstances and (unlike that of intended parity) has no cumulative character to it.

The triviality of the duration effect is a null finding of more than routine interest. There are biases in the data we are examining. Since these are intact marriages, each marriage cohort experiences a process of attrition (marital dissolution) with advancing duration; those selected in this way may be distinctive with respect to their parity orientations. Since intended parity can only be determined for those who are neither nonfecund nor noncommittal, this is another selective process with advancing duration. In the third place, the deletion of respondents on the basis of age, as noted above, implies an upper limit on age at marriage, for those in the highest duration group, of 23 rather than 25. Finally, the respondents in durations of five to twenty-four years in 1975 differ from the rest in that they submitted to reinterview. In light of all these possible ways in which the results may have been affected by selectivity with advancing duration, it is gratifying to observe a miniscule duration effect.

The final set of cross-sectional data to be considered are the correlations shown in tables 7–6, 7–7, 7–8, and 7–9. In order to determine the strength of relationship among the three parity variables, we have calculated the zero-order correlations for each pair of variables in turn, and then the partial correlations for each pair with the third variable held constant. The sets of zero-order correlations (the two columns on the left of tables 7–6, 7–7, and 7–8) show for each pair moderately strong correlations of approximately equal magnitude, and only a weak tendency to decline with advancing duration.

Table 7–6
Correlation of Ideal and Desired Parity, Zero Order, and with Intended Parity Controlled, by Marital Duration

	Zero Order		Intended Parity Controlled	
	1970	1975	1970	1975
0–4	0.75	0.62	0.51	0.30
5–9	0.67	0.69	0.44	0.49
10–14	0.68	0.69	0.49	0.48
15–19	0.60	0.65	0.40	0.52
20–24	0.62	0.63	0.48	0.46
Total	0.69	0.67	0.47	0.46

Table 7–7
Correlation of Desired and Intended Parity, Zero Order, and with Ideal Parity Controlled, by Marital Duration

	Zero Order		Ideal Parity Controlled	
	1970	1975	1970	1975
0–4	0.70	0.69	0.35	0.47
5–9	0.68	0.65	0.46	0.41
10–14	0.68	0.68	0.47	0.45
15–19	0.65	0.54	0.50	0.32
20–24	0.65	0.64	0.51	0.48
Total	0.68	0.65	0.46	0.43

Table 7–8
Correlation of Intended and Ideal Parity, Zero Order, and with Desired Parity Controlled, by Marital Duration

	Zero Order		Desired Parity Controlled	
	1970	1975	1970	1975
0–4	0.71	0.66	0.39	0.41
5–9	0.61	0.60	0.29	0.28
10–14	0.58	0.61	0.22	0.26
15–19	0.53	0.50	0.22	0.24
20–24	0.47	0.49	0.11	0.16
Total	0.60	0.59	0.25	0.28

Table 7–9
Numbers of Respondents, Table 7–6, 7–7, and 7–8

	1970	1975
0–4	938	1,009
5–9	692	661
10–14	518	569
15–19	379	464
20–24	307	319
Total	2,834	3,022

The partial correlations in the right-hand columns of these three tables tell a quite different story. Ideal and desired parity remain reasonably well correlated despite control of intended parity; desired and intended parity remain reasonably well correlated despite control of ideal parity; there are no noteworthy differentials on a duration-specific basis in either of these. But the control of desired parity sharply attenuates the correlation of ideal and intended parity, and that relationship becomes progressively weaker with advancing duration. (All these correlations were also calculated for Catholics and non-Catholics separately; these results are not shown because no significant differences emerged.)

Where we simply let the data speak for themselves without consideration of presumed conceptual content, the evidence in table 7-10 would suggest that desired parity is intermediate between ideal parity, on the one hand, and intended parity on the other, and that the link between ideal and intended parity is primarily indirect. A cross-sectional analysis of similar variables, but with a somewhat different methodology, arrived at the same result, using data from the 1965 National Fertility Study (Ryder and Westoff 1971).

Reconsideration of the Content of the Variables

On the basis of the evidence presented so far, several difficult questions arise—questions that provoke a more detailed examination of conceptual distinctions among the variables. Consider first the relationship between ideal and intended parity. These were represented above as being differentiated primarily on the ground that the ideal-parity question abstracted from realistic considerations, permitting a relatively open expression of strength of reproductive orientation, whereas intended parity derived from a compromise between reproductive orientation and the contextual constraints perceived and projected at the time of decision. In light of this distinction, it is disconcerting to see how little difference there is between mean ideal parity and mean intended parity. Admittedly, an ideal life without constraints (the perfect husband, the best of health, unlimited income, and so forth) would produce a fantasy response; the low level of ideal parity indicates that respondents do assume some compromise with reality.

Yet despite the similarity of the means for ideal and intended parity, the partial correlation between these, with desired parity controlled, is weak. Three considerations may be mentioned as possible explanations. First, the referent for the ideal-parity question is not the respondent but "a family." The answer may be in terms of a person like the respondent, or the average member of her community, or the population at large. Second, the question on ideal parity does not specify for whom it would be ideal. Surely one

Table 7–10
Mean Ideal, Desired, and Intended Parity, by Religion and Marriage Cohort

	Total		Non-Catholic		Catholic	
	1970	*1975*	*1970*	*1975*	*1970*	*1975*
Ideal						
1951–1955	2.90	2.83	2 79	2.68	3.21	3.14
1956–1960	2.76	2.66	2.63	2.53	3.12	3.00
1961–1965	2.57	2.51	2.48	2.41	2.89	2.85
1966–1970	2.66	2.38	2.54	2.33	2.94	2.57
Mean	2.72	2.60	2.61	2.49	3.04	2.89
Desired						
1951–1955	3.21	3.01	3.03	2.85	3.74	3.48
1956–1960	3.00	2.83	2.82	2.70	3.47	3.17
1961–1965	2.77	2.55	2.61	2.41	3.33	3.05
1966–1970	2.77	2.37	2.62	2.28	3.16	2.61
Mean	2.94	2.69	2.77	2.56	3.42	3.08
Intended						
1951–1955	2.79	2.80	2.58	2.59	3.44	3.43
1956–1960	2.77	2.70	2.62	2.55	3.18	3.10
1961–1965	2.51	2.31	2.36	2.18	3.02	2.77
1966–1970	2.53	2.25	2.41	2.17	2.84	2.45
Mean	2.65	2.52	2.49	2.37	3.12	2.94
Number of respondents						
1951–1955		321		241		80
1956–1960		422		306		116
1961–1965		532		411		121
1966–1970		626		446		180
Total		1,901		1,404		497

Source: U.S. National Fertility Studies, 1970 and 1975.

would expect somewhat different responses depending on whether the perspective was that of the mother, the father, the children, the nation, or perhaps even the world. Perhaps the extensive publicity given to problems of population growth may have led some respondents to think less of what fertility signifies for the family itself and more of what it signifies for the population as a whole. Third, reproductive orientations may not be stable over time, at least not as captured by the ideal-parity question. (To anticipate a result from the next section, the correlation between ideal parity in 1970 and in 1975 for the same respondents is only +0.53.) The respondent may have a different view at the time of the interview than prevailed at the time she was making reproductive decisions.

The next difficult question to consider is why desired parity is substantially greater than intended parity (regardless of religion, marital duration, or time period). If the principal distinction between desired and intended parity were that the former was retrospective and the latter prospective ("If I knew then what I know now"), one would expect that a worsening of the context within which reproduction takes place (a reasonable inference from the decline of all measures between 1970 and 1975) would lead to statements of desired parity distinctly below those of intended parity. Several possible explanations may be suggested for this anomaly. If the respondent's record contains one or more unintended births, she may use her answer to the desired-parity question to indicate that she does not now regret the coming of those children—that in retrospect they are wanted. Conversely, many respondents may have wanted another child but deferred the decision until it was too late, that is, until the respondent felt too old for another round of motherhood. Since there is no reference in the desired-parity question to when the desired children would occur, it is not an unreasonable finding that more would be desired but no more intended.

Those suggestions apply to respondents who intend no more children. For those in earlier stages of the life cycle, the desired-parity question may offer an opportunity for the respondent to express some reservation about the reproductive intention previously specified—perhaps indicating that her own desires differ from the decision that she and her husband have jointly reached. Alternatively, despite the specification of "the circumstances of your life," the respondent may answer more in terms of her wishes than of reality.

That possibility is raised by the closeness of the relationship between desired parity and ideal parity. Taking the questions at face value, one's inclination would be to anticipate a reasonably strong relationship between ideal and intended parity, on the one hand, and between intended and desired parity, on the other hand, but only a weak relationship between ideal and desired parity. The contrary finding suggests two possibilities. Either reproductive orientations (in abstraction from reality) are unstable over time, so that desired and ideal parity are linked by the circumstance that they both express attitudes as of the time of the interview (unlike intended parity, which refers back to the time of decision); or ideal as well as desired parity is sensitive to the current contextual constraints. It would be important to replace such speculations as these with evidence—provided one could be assured that either ideal or desired parity played either an explanatory or a predictive role with respect to reproductive intentions. That question is addressed in the final section of this chapter.

Longitudinal Analysis

In the remainder of this chapter, the focus is on reinterviewed respondents, and on the study of changes in the orientation variables through time for the same individuals. In particular, we want to try to answer the question of the causal direction of the relationships between ideal and intended parity, and between desired and intended parity—to establish the extent to which responses to the questions about ideal and desired parity provide information that can help us understand or predict changes in intended parity.

In all, 2,361 respondents were reinterviewed. They belonged to the marriage cohorts of 1951–1970, interviewed at durations 0–20 in 1970 and 5–25 in 1975. Not all these women are represented in the subsequent analysis. First we deleted all those who reported, either in 1970 or in 1975, that they were unable to have any more children. The practical reason for this is that we did not ask these women their reproductive intentions; the theoretical reason is that, even if we had, the suspicion would remain that under the circumstances their answers concerning ideal and desired parity might be tinged with irresponsibility. Second, we omitted from the calculations the small number of respondents who failed to give a single-valued numerical response to either the desired- or ideal-parity question.

Third, a substantial proportion of respondents in 1970 (as indicated in table 7–1) gave an equivocal response to the question of whether a particular birth was intended or unintended. For the reinterviewed women, we have two reports of that information, as collected at first interview and at reinterview. Accordingly, we avoided the problem of noncommittal responses in 1970 by using the 1975 reports, for which the comparable proportion was small. This had a further important advantage. For a substantial proportion of respondents, a birth reported in the first interview as intended, was reported in the reinterview as unintended; for another substantial (albeit smaller) proportion, the reverse occurred. This was one reason for the decline in intended parity between 1970 and 1975 (as reported in table 7–3, but it was a reason we wanted to exclude from the present analysis in order to focus on changes between 1970 and 1975.

The tabulations that follow are based on the 1,901 respondents remaining after the deletion of these three categories. The information presented in tables 7–10 and 7–11 is parallel to that contained in tables 7–3 and 7–5. Here, however, it is appropriate to use the marriage-cohort rather than marital-duration designation for the row variable, and to begin with the earliest cohort. The data in table 7–10 confirm the findings reported on a cross-sectional basis. All three variables have registered declines from 1970 to 1975. The decline is somewhat greater for desired than for intended parity, and somewhat greater for intended than for ideal parity. The decline is greater for Catholics than for non-Catholics in all three cases.

Table 7–11
Period (P), Cohort (C) and Duration (D) Effects in Table 7–10

	Column Effect (P + D)	Row Effect (C – D)	Period Effect (P)	Cohort Effect (C)	Duration Effect (D)
Ideal					
Total	– 0.13	– 0.12	– 0.12	– 0.12	– 0.00
Non-Catholic	– 0.12	– 0.10	– 0.12	– 0.11	– 0.01
Catholic	– 0.15	– 0.14	– 0.15	– 0.15	– 0.00
Desired					
Total	– 0.25	– 0.19	– 0.23	– 0.21	– 0.02
Non-Catholic	– 0.21	– 0.17	– 0.20	– 0.19	– 0.01
Catholic	– 0.35	– 0.23	– 0.31	– 0.27	– 0.04
Intended					
Total	– 0.14	– 0.15	– 0.14	– 0.15	+ 0.01
Non-Catholic	– 0.12	– 0.12	– 0.12	– 0.12	– 0.00
Catholic	– 0.18	– 0.26	– 0.21	– 0.24	+ 0.03

Source: U.S. National Fertility Studies, 1970 and 1975.

Since the Catholic values were substantially greater than those for non-Catholics, the implication is that there has been some convergence.

Table 7–11 has been prepared with the same methodological orientation as was used in constructing table 7–5. In the present situation the column variable manifests the combined result of increase in period and increase in duration (for each marriage cohort) whereas the row variable manifests the combined result of increase in marriage cohort and decrease in duration (for each period). Although the algebra of the equations producing separate period, cohort, and duration effects is a little different, the implicit assumptions are the same.

As was the case with the cross-sectional tabulations, there are strong and approximately equal period and cohort effects for all three variables, and the duration effect is negligible. If we are correct in interpreting the period effect as short-run, transitory, and reversible, then something like one-half the change in each kind of parity between 1970 and 1975 can be so described. That the period effect is much smaller for ideal than for desired parity is evidence that the former is less responsive to changes in context than the latter (as one would expect from the form of the questions) but the temporal variability in ideal parity (quite apart from the succession of cohorts) is sufficient to raise some doubts about its meaning. Although the

Table 7–12
Correlation of Ideal Parity, 1970 and 1975; Correlation of Desired Parity, 1970 and 1975; Correlation of Intended Parity, 1970 and 1975, by Religion and Marriage Cohort

	Total	Non-Catholic	Catholic
Ideal			
1951–1955	0.58	0.54	0.61
1956–1960	0.53	0.50	0.52
1961–1965	0.53	0.44	0.63
1966–1970	0.47	0.49	0.41
Total	0.53	0.50	0.54
Desired			
1951–1955	0.62	0.63	0.57
1956–1960	0.57	0.56	0.53
1961–1965	0.60	0.52	0.67
1966–1970	0.44	0.47	0.32
Total	0.57	0.55	0.53
Intended			
1951–1955	0.99	0.98	0.98
1956–1960	0.94	0.93	0.95
1961–1965	0.82	0.78	0.84
1966–1970	0.55	0.57	0.46
Total	0.83	0.81	0.84

period effect for intended parity is smaller than that for desired parity, it is nevertheless remarkably large, considering that the substantial part of intended parity that had occurred prior to first interview is excluded from the possibility of contributing to the variations reported here.

The results shown in table 7–12 speak directly to the question of the temporal stability of each measure at the individual level. These are the correlations between the response to the ideal-parity question given at first interview and the response to the same question by the same woman five years later at second interview—and likewise for desired parity and intended parity. Regardless of marriage cohort or religion subgroup, the correlations for ideal parity and for desired parity are low, although a little lower for the more recent than for the more distant cohorts. We repeated the kinds of correlation reported in tables 7–6, 7–7, and 7–8 for the present data set and found that the correlation between ideal and desired parity was 0.67 in 1970 and 0.66 in 1975. In other words, there is a stronger relationship between ideal and desired parity at the same observation time than there is between ideal parity in 1970 and that in 1975, or between desired parity in 1970 and that in 1975.

The correlations of intended parity for 1970 and 1975 are substantially higher, but for an obvious reason. Whereas ideal and desired parity are unrestricted in principle with respect to the possibilities of variation from one time to another, intended parity may be thought of as having two components in 1970—intended births that had occurred by then, and additional intended births—and two components in 1975—intended births that had occurred by 1970, and the sum of intended births since then and additional intended births as of 1975. In other words, the variables being correlated have a common component, and one that is a progressively larger proportion of the total with advancing duration (the earlier the marriage cohort). The correlation of intended parity, 1970 and 1975, for marriage cohort 1966–1970 does not depart substantially from its counterparts for desired and ideal parity.[1]

Which Is Cause and Which Effect?

The final task is to attempt to use our panel data to resolve what may be the thorniest issue in any field of knowledge in which one is forced to rely on nonexperimental data. We observe a relationship between two variables. In the data examined in this chapter, the correlation between ideal and intended parity is 0.59 in 1970 and 0.55 in 1975. As is well known, that observation does not permit us to choose among three alternative explanations: (1) ideal parity is a cause of intended parity; (2) intended parity is a cause of ideal parity; (3) both ideal and intended parity are effects of some third variable. We approach this question from the viewpoint of improvement in prediction. Our aim is to predict a change in intended parity, say from 1970 to 1975, by using information about the individual that is available to use in 1970. Suppose intended parity at 1970 is y, and the change from 1970 to 1975 is dy. We also know the respondent's ideal parity in 1970, say x. Now we would not want to calculate the correlation between dy and x, to determine whether knowledge of ideal parity helped to predict change in intended parity, because it is not unlikely that the change in intended parity, dy, is a function of its initial value, y, and we know there is a correlation between y and x. Accordingly, we first calculate the relationship between dy and y, as measured (in a prediction sense) by the coefficient of determination, $r^2_{dy \cdot y}$ —the proportion of variance in dy that is explained by y. Then we measure the improvement in prediction achieved by regressing dy on y and on x, say $R^2_{dy \cdot y, x}$, incorporating ideal parity in 1970 in the prediction equation. Then the value $R^2_{dy \cdot y, x} - r^2_{dy \cdot y}$ gives the improvement in prediction of change of intended parity, by considering ideal parity, over and above what can be achieved with the information y (intended parity at first interview).

This exercise has been performed for successive marriage cohorts, and separately by religion. The results are shown in the left-hand panels of table 7-13. Of the fifteen cases considered, only one, the marriage cohort of 1966–1970 (all women) shows a statistically significant improvement (as measured by the appropriate F test) at the 5 percent level. Even in that case, the improvement in prediction is very small. We conclude that ideal parity cannot be considered a cause of intended parity, because the change in intended parity is insensitive to ideal parity, beyond whatever derivative effect there may be, by way of its correlation with intended parity.

Table 7–13
Contribution of Ideal Parity 1970 (x) to Prediction of Change in Intended Parity (dy), Given Intended Parity 1970 (y); and Contribution of Intended Parity 1970 to Prediction of Change in Ideal Parity (dx), Given Ideal Parity 1970

	$r^2_{dy \cdot y}$	$R^2_{dy \cdot y, x} - r^2_{dy \cdot y}$	$r^2_{dx \cdot x}$	$R^2_{dy \cdot x, y} - r^2_{dx \cdot x}$
Total				
1951–1955	0.01	0.00	0.18	0.05**
1956–1960	0.04	0.00	0.21	0.06**
1961–1965	0.19	0.01	0.23	0.08**
1966–1970	0.25	0.01*	0.34	0.03**
Total	0.09	0.00	0.24	0.05**
Non-Catholic				
1951–1955	0.00	0.01	0.24	0.02**
1956–1960	0.05	0.00	0.29	0.03**
1961–1965	0.23	0.00	0.31	0.03**
1966–1970	0.22	0.01	0.36	0.02**
Total	0.11	0.00	0.30	0.02**
Catholic				
1951–1955	0.03	0.02	0.14	0.06*
1956–1960	0.03	0.02	0.12	0.12**
1961–1965	0.12	0.00	0.12	0.19**
1966–1970	0.31	0.00	0.29	0.07**
Total	0.06	0.00	0.15	0.11**

* = significant at the 1 percent level.
** = significant at the 5 percent level.

Now we turn the question around and ask what relationship there is between ideal and intended parity, where the question concerns improvement of prediction of change in ideal parity, say dx. First we calculate the coefficient of determination of dx as a function of x, and then recalculate it, including y in the regression as well. The results are shown in the righthand panels of table 7-13. In this case, again using the appropriate F test, we find that all of the fifteen improvements in prediction are statistically significant, and all but one of them at the 1 percent level. The cautious conclusion from this finding would be either that ideal parity is the effect and intended parity the cause, or that both are influenced by some third variable. The latter alternative, however, would seem to be ruled out by the previous finding of a null result when one considered the determinants of change in intended parity.

Accordingly, we conclude that the reason for the correlation between ideal and intended parity is that intended parity is the cause and ideal parity the effect. The significance of this can be expressed as follows. If, in 1970, a respondent gives discrepant answers to the two questions of ideal and intended parity, the future consequence of that discrepancy is for ideal parity to be pulled toward intended parity, but not for intended parity to be pulled toward ideal parity. We are not, of course, entitled to generalize beyond the particular slice of history examined here—the experience of the 1970-1975 period. Nevertheless, on the basis of these data, we see no advantage, in the analysis of reproductive intentions, to an inquiry into ideal parity, since the latter is an effect rather than a cause of the former.

Now we examine the same problem with respect to the relationship between desired and intended parity. In this data set, there is a correlation of 0.68 in 1970 and of 0.64 in 1975 between desired and intended parity. In the lefthand panels of table 7-14, we show the improvement in the prediction of change in intended parity when we employ desired parity as of 1970 as well as intended parity as of 1970. In this case, five of the fifteen calculations are statistically significant. While this is a more impressive demonstration than that obtained for ideal parity, it proves on closer examination to be of minor analytic importance. Two of the five statistically significant changes in coefficient of determination apply to the earliest marriage cohort, for which the mean change in intended parity from 1970 to 1975 was +0.01. The other three statistically significant changes are also small in magnitude. We have noted in the preceding text that questions of desired and intended parity are very close to being the same question for those who intend more children (those in the earlier marital durations). The small improvements in prediction registered for the marriage cohort of 1966-1970 suggest the extent to which the desired-parity question, for this subset of women, conveys usable information marginal to that provided by the intended-parity question itself.

Table 7-14
Contribution of Desired Parity 1970 (z) to Prediction of Change in Intended Parity (dy), Given Intended Parity 1970 (y); and Contribution of Intended Parity 1970 to Prediction of Change in Desired Parity (dz), Given Desired Parity 1970

	$r^2_{d \cdot y}$	$R^2_{dy \cdot y,z} - r^2_{dy \cdot y}$	$r^2_{dz \cdot z}$	$R^2_{dz \cdot z,y} - r^2_{dz \cdot z}$
Total				
1951–1955	0.01	0.00	0.14	0.10**
1956–1960	0.04	0.00	0.24	0.05**
1961–1965	0.19	0.01	0.19	0.06**
1966–1970	0.25	0.01**	0.30	0.05**
Total	0.09	0.00	0.21	0.06**
Non-Catholic				
1951–1955	0.00	0.03**	0.12	0.15**
1956–1960	0.05	0.00	0.24	0.04**
1961–1965	0.23	0.00	0.24	0.03**
1966–1970	0.22	0.02**	0.24	0.05**
Total	0.11	0.01	0.20	0.06**
Catholic				
1951–1955	0.03	0.05*	0.18	0.04*
1956–1960	0.03	0.02	0.24	0.07**
1961–1965	0.12	0.00	0.13	0.11**
1966–1970	0.31	0.00	0.42	0.04**
Total	0.06	0.00	0.23	0.07**

* = significant at the 5 percent level.
** = significant at the 1 percent level.

The right-hand set of panels in table 7-14 shows the results when the calculations proceed in the opposite direction. That is to say, we consider the prediction of change in desired parity first using the information about desired parity in 1970 and then adding into the regression the information about intended parity in 1970. All fifteen of the cases are statistically significant and all but one of them at the 1 percent level. On the basis of the evidence in table 7-14, we conclude that intended parity is causally prior to desired parity. We see no advantage, in the analysis of reproductive intentions, to an inquiry into desired parity, since the latter has been shown to be an effect rather than a cause of the former. Again we are obliged to make the qualification that this result has been obtained solely for the 1970–1975 time interval.

Conclusion

In this chapter we have examined the relationships between intended parity, on the one hand, and desired and ideal parity on the other. Using data from the 1970 and 1975 National Fertility Studies, for white women in intact first marriages, we examined the variations in the three parity-orientation variables over time, separately by marriage duration, and for non-Catholics and Catholics. Although the means for all three variables are similar in each survey, desired parity is systematically higher than the other two. The means for all three variables are much higher for Catholics than for non-Catholics, although the difference is smaller in 1975 than in 1970.

Using a newly developed procedure, we have distinguished among period, (marriage) cohort, and (marital) duration effects in our tabulations. For all three variables, the duration effect is negligible, and the period and cohort effects are strong and approximately equal. We interpret this as signifying that about one-half of the registered decline in each variable should be considered as short-run in character.

The variables, at the zero-order level, are moderately strongly correlated with one another. When partial correlations are calculated for each pair, with the third controlled, the link remains reasonably strong between ideal and desired parity, and between intended and desired parity, but is substantially attenuated between ideal and intended parity. These findings cast doubts on the interpretation of the variables, and on their relationship to one another, that one would otherwise infer from the wording of the questions, taken at face value.

We used the longitudinal feature of the data to explore the relationships between ideal parity in 1970 and in 1975 ($r = +0.53$), and between desired parity in 1970 and in 1975 ($r = +0.57$); these are weaker relationships than those that prevailed between desired and ideal parity in either 1970 or 1975. Although there was a substantially higher correlation ($r = +0.83$) between intended parity in 1970 and in 1975, this reflected primarily the substantial common component of the two values for each individual.

The final presentation evaluated the extent to which one could better predict change of intended parity between 1970 and 1975, knowing ideal parity, and the extent to which one could better predict change of ideal parity between 1970 and 1975, knowing intended parity. Since the answer was clearly negative in the former case and clearly affirmative in the latter case, we concluded that intended parity is causally prior to ideal parity. The same procedure, applied to desired and intended parity, produced the conclusion that intended parity is also causally prior to desired parity.

The evidence presented in this paper leads to the conclusion that questions concerning ideal and desired family size are pointless for the purpose of understanding or predicting reproductive intentions.

Note

1. Note that the effect of a common component on correlation can readily be indicated in a simplified situation. Suppose the two variables are $x = a + b$, and $y = a + c$. Assume that there are zero correlations among a, b, and c. Then if x and y have the same coefficient of variation as a (a plausible and innocuous assumption), the correlation of x and y is the product $p'p''$, where p' and p'' are the proportions a constitutes of x and y respectively, despite zero correlation between b and c.

References

Ryder, Norman B. "Consistency of Reporting Fertility Planning Status." *Studies in Family Planning* 10(1979):115–128.

Ryder, Norman B., and Westoff, Charles F. "Orientations toward Numbers of Children." In *Reproduction in the United States,* pp. 19–35. Princeton, N.J.: Princeton University Press, 1971.

Westoff, Charles F., and Ryder, Norman B. "The Predictive Validity of Reproductive Intentions." *Demography* 14(1977):431–453.

Appendix 7A

The data in the various panels of table 7-3 are values of a variable for particular row and column values. We fitted surface $Y = a + b_1 X_1 + b_2 X_2$ to these data, where X_1 is the row variable and X_2 the column variable. The model is linear; the variables are treated as independent; the solution is by ordinary-least-squares procedures. The row regression coefficient (b_1) shows the difference between the duration effect (say d) and the cohort effect (say c). The column regression coefficient (b_2) shows the sum of the period effect (say p) and the cohort effect. This gives two equations in three unknowns: $p + c = b_2$ and $d - c = b_1$. This is the familiar situation of underidentification. It arises from the circumstance that marital duration is defined as the difference between the marriage cohort and the period, what one may call an identity crisis. The root of the problem is that we are operating at a primitive level of analysis, with three black boxes, each containing unspecified influences. Were we able to specify the relevant content of any one of the black boxes, in its own terms, the statistical problem would vanish.

As a step in summarizing such tables, it is worthwhile to determine whether the variations in the table can be explained by only one variable. If the row effect is zero, then a sufficient description is $p = b_2$ (with the other two effects zero); if the column effect is zero, a sufficient description is $d = b_1$; if the sum of the row effect and the column effect is zero, a sufficient description is $c = (b_2 - b_1)/2$. This merely codifies the procedure one might follow in examining the tabulations by eye. Should one of the three indicated conditions approximately apply, the specified solution is recommended on the principle of parsimony.

A general resolution of the problem requires commitment to a model. My own preference with variables referring to lifetime reproductive performance is to make a first approximation to the representation of the surface by acting as if the period effect were zero, and to examine the residuals for period-specific patterning. This is equivalent to a classification of the cohort effect as long-run and the period effect as short-run. The more difficult question of a duration patterning to the period effect is unanswered.

This approach fails when one is working, as in the present situation, with only two periods of observation, since there is no way to discriminate between the short run and the long run in such case. Rather than resolve the predicament by fiat, it seems preferable to employ some assumption that treats the three effects evenhandedly. I chose an assumption on the basis of the following line of argument. In most regressions, the dependent variable is a function of various independent variables (such as income, education, occupation, and the like), which are in fact highly intercorrelated. The independent effect of each is established by calculating partial regression coefficients. In effect, these eliminate the overlap that is manifest at the zero-order level. Now the three variables—period, cohort, and duration— inherently overlap, by courtesy of the identity relating them. The proposal is to resolve the underidentification problem by introducing the equation that would minimize the magnitude of the three effects and thus eliminate their redundancy. Since an effect may have positive or negative sign, I chose to minimize the sum of squares of the three effects. To minimize $c^2 + p^2 + d^2$, substitute $b_2 - c$ for p, and $c + b_1$ for d (from the two available equations given previously). Then the derivative of $c^2 + (b^2 - c)^2 + (c + b_1)^2$ with respect to c is $6c + 2(b_1 - b_2)$. This is zero when $c = (b_2 - b_1)/3$, and the other two effects become $p = (2b_2 + b_1)/3$ and $d = (b_2 + 2b_1)/3$.

One can simply achieve this result by using, as the third equation, $p = c + d$. Exactly the same outcome can also be achieved by two other different routes: (1) set each of the three effects (p, c, d) in turn equal to 0, calculate the values for the other two from the available equations, and then strike an average of the three sets of results; (2) set each pair of effects equal in turn ($p = c, p = d, c = d$) and strike an average of the three sets of results. What all three approaches have in common is evenhandedness with respect to treatment of the separate effects.

In considering the results displayed in table 7–5 (derived by the procedure just outlined) I was disconcerted by the similarity from panel to panel: period and cohort effects approximately equal, and duration effect negligible, with all effects negative. The concern that this might be an artifact of the particular solution was dispelled by the following results. An additional set of data is available from the cross-sectional analysis: expected parity, defined as the sum of past births (whether intended or unintended) and additional intended births. With this variable, those who are nonfecund are coded as 0 for additional intended births. The mean values of expected parity by period and duration are as follows:

	1970	1975	
0–4	2.58	2.59	$b_1 = +0.2195$
5–9	2.65	2.35	$b_2 = -0.2800$
10–14	3.11	2.60	$p = -0.1135$
15–19	3.26	3.13	$c = -0.1665$
20–24	3.27	3.10	$d = +0.0530$

This outcome differs from those shown in table 7-5, and the difference is intelligible in terms of the special features of expected parity. The variable has two components, one of which (past births) is necessarily nondecreasing with advancing duration. Although the other component, additional intended births, may decrease with advancing duration, that result tends to be counterbalanced by the occurrence of additional unintended births. Thus there is good reason for anticipating a positive duration effect for expected parity, despite a negative duration effect for intended parity. Moreover, the cumulative character of expected parity is such that one would expect a less-pronounced period effect (since it can operate only at the margin) but a more-pronounced cohort effect (since the incidence of unintended as well as intended births can decline from cohort to cohort). The data show a period effect that is less for expected than for intended parity, and a cohort effect that is greater for expected than for intended parity. While this proves nothing about the validity of the proposed procedure, it is reassuringly plausible.

The problem of underidentification is ubiquitous in demographic analysis. Many of our variables are created by observing the times of occurrence of two events, and then subtracting to get the length of interval between those times. More common than the triad of period, marriage cohort, and marital duration, is its temporal counterpart—period, birth cohort, and age. A nontemporal example is the triad of age, age at marriage, and marital duration. In every such situation, three variables are potentially influential. It is not uncommon to find the analyst ignoring one of the three, perhaps because of the form in which the data are presented (highlighting the row and column, but forgetting the implicit diagonal) or perhaps because it is assumed that the third variable is trivial in its effect. One virtue of the expository device proposed here is that it brings to the fore the possible effects of all three rather than of a particular two variables.

8

Adjusting Stated Fertility Preferences for the Effect of Actual Family Size, with Application to World Fertility Survey Data

Thomas W. Pullum

In chapter 7 Ryder showed that the fertility desires and ideals of American women were higher than their intended fertility. He also suggested that ideals and desires were influenced significantly by intentions; that is, the decline in ideals and desires between 1970 and 1975 was a response to the decline in intentions. The change in intentions, in turn, was a response to changes in social and economic conditions (and to changes in birth-cohort composition of the reproductive population). While Ryder is not so confident as is, for example, Lee, that intentions (or expectations) provide useful information about actual future fertility, he does not regard them as mere rationalizations, but as orientations at least loosely rooted in social and economic conditions and having an effect on fertility-related behavior.

In this chapter by Thomas Pullum, the social and demographic setting is much different. Sri Lanka, like many developing nations, has high fertility, and yet women's fertility orientations are moderate to low. In consequence, fertility often exceeds the desires of individual women; and when that happens, the tendency, according to Pullum, is for women to elevate their desires. That is, the response to unwanted fertility is rationalization rather than the implentation of more effective contraception.

Pullum's problem, given this rationalization, is to estimate what would happen to fertility in Sri Lanka if the situation were changed so that women would implement their true fertility desires. In other words, what is the true value of their present fertility desires, after removing the effects of their rationalization of unwanted previous fertility?

Three approaches to answering the question are presented, of which the last is most appealing. In that approach, Pullum argues that rationalization is unlikely to affect women's preferences for the *next* birth, even when it might seriously affect their preferences for total births. If so, Pullum demonstrates a simple way to use that information to estimate the average family size that would result if unrationalized preference were successfully implemented.

Pullum emphasizes that he is talking about stated *preferences* about fertility, not about future fertility itself. The objective is different from that of

The research described in this chapter was supported by a contract from the International Statistical Institute to the University of Washington.

estimates of their actual future fertility. The difference is partly conceptual—preferences are normative, while expectations include both normative and objective elements. In other words, preferences are what women really want in the absence of obstacles, while expectations are what they want in view of obstacles they are likely to encounter.

The difference is empirical as well as conceptual. In a society like that of Sri Lanka, women have so little knowledge and control of the determinants of their own fertility that they have little basis for *expecting* fertility of any particular level. Their fertility is determined by forces beyond their knowledge or out of their control. In the United States, on the other hand, women have sufficient, albeit variable and imperfect knowledge and control, so they can assess the obstacles to attaining their fertility preferences and their ability to overcome these obstacles.

In the context of this book, therefore, the significance of this chapter is its suggestion that there are different fertility regimes in which the relationship between women's fertility orientations—ideals, preferences, desires, intentions, and expectations—and that their future fertility may differ significantly.

Pullum uses data from the 1974 Fertility Survey of Sri Lanka, one of the many fertility surveys conducted in developing countries with the sponsorship of the World Fertility Survey. Those surveys, and many surveys being undertaken in developed countries concurrently, used similar designs and procedures. This standardization has made it possible to compare fertility processes in different countries to a greater extent than ever before. Thus the analysis presented here by Pullum can be replicated for twenty or more other countries at about the same time.—*Eds.*

The purpose of the research to be described briefly in this chapter is to improve our measurement of group differences in fertility preferences. The source of data assumed to be available is a cross-sectional survey, with personal fertility preferences measured by questions such as:

1. Do you want to have another child sometime?
2. Thinking back to the time before you became pregnant with your last child, had you wanted to have more children?
3. If you could choose exactly the number of children to have in your whole life, how many would that be?

In addition, of course, some fertility and socioeconomic characteristics are assumed to be available. The various country surveys of the World Fertility Survey (WFS) furnish these kinds of data, and in fact serve as both the stimulus and the illustration for the suggestions to be offered here. Some analysis of these questions as applied in Asia has already been published by Cho (1978). Many other surveys include essentially the same information. If more is known so that, for example, the consistency and predictive power of the responses and how this varies from one group to another can be measured, then the strategies to be suggested may require modification. See, for example, Coombs (1974) regarding more extensive forms of these questions.

Many authors have commented on the reliability and validity of these questions. See, for example, Knodel and Prachuabmoh (1973) and Pullum (1980). These issues will not be raised here, except for the one that is the central theme of this chapter.

Some of the uses that others have made of these questions will be listed in order to make it clear that preferences are here regarded as dependent variables. First, applying a rational model of fertility behavior, some researchers have used stated preferences as indicators of need for family-planning services. Women who believe themselves capable of having more children, but who want no more (or whose actual family size is at least as large as their stated ideal), are assumed to be in need of contraception. They make up a target group for information about or easier access to modern contraception. WFS (and others) usually find large numbers of women in developing countries who want no more children but show resistance to modern contraception. It is unclear whether the source of this discrepancy is in the nature of the preference data (for example, a lack of validity), in the formulation of the rational behavior model, or in the objective characteristics of the family-planning program. At any rate, this use of stated preferences as indicators of contraceptive need is probably the primary use.

Second, and related, the relationship between stated preferences and actual fertility leads to estimates of unwanted fertility. For example, Westoff et al. (1979) used the WFS survey of Panama to estimate the numbers of unwanted births.

By contrast, this chapter considers the fertility preference as a dependent variable. The basic question is this: Can we use the stated preferences to infer what would be the mean completed fertility of a group of women if they could implement their preferences throughout the family-building career? We shall propose and compare three different strategies for making such inferences.

Obviously, this would be a trivial problem if stated preferences could be taken at face value. If this were possible, we would simply calculate the average stated desired family size within each subgroup (possibly within cohorts as well to allow for time trends). We note, however, that data from developing countries generally show a strong positive correlation between desired and actual family sizes. If this correlation is entirely the result of implementation of earlier preferences—that is, if the women who have large families are precisely the women who wanted large families, and similarly for small families—then this correlation is to be expected and would not bear on the procedure of averaging the response within subgroups.

Our premise here is that at least some of the correlation between actual and desired family size results from rationalization of actual family size, originating either in the psychological need to reduce the inconsistency between attitudes and behavior, or in the social situation of the interview. Such rationalization can raise the response relative to what it would have been with an alternative actual family size. The highly fertile woman may decline to say that she has had any unwanted births, or may understate their number. The very concept of unwanted fertility implies that there are failures in implementation and is consistent with the notion of rationalization.

Rationalization could also lower the stated preference of women who had fewer children than originally desired. It will be assumed that in a developing country this type of bias is infrequent, but it might be substantial in a country such as the United States.

When comparing original preferences in a U.S. sample with their recalled values twenty years later, Westoff, Mishler, and Kelly (1957) stated:

> . . . there is a definite tendency among individuals whose recalled preference differs from their original preference, for the error [to be] in the direction of their actual number of children. . . . This error is considerable. . . . Thus the correlation between actual number of children and recalled family-size preferences are much inflated.

As a corollary there will also, of course, be an inflation in the correlation between actual family size and the currently stated preference.

In a cross-sectional survey it is patently impossible to say which effect, implementation of preferences or rationalization of actual fertility, is responsible for the correlation between actual and desired family sizes. Our approaches will bypass a statement about the balance of the two effects, but will only be useful if there is, in fact, some degree of rationalization.

The three approaches will be applied to the 1975 Fertility Survey of Sri Lanka conducted by the World Fertility Survey and the Department of Census and Statistics of Sri Lanka. That survey included 6,812 ever-married women. A description of Sri Lanka and of the survey will not be given here; reference may be made to the country report on the survey (Sri Lanka, 1978). In that sample, the mean desired family size was 3.75, with a relationship to actual family size that is illustrated in figure 8-1. The product-moment correlation between the two variables was 0.74. The three procedures will first be described for the sample as a whole, and then differentials between subgroups will be examined.

First Procedure

Whatever the balance between implementation and rationalization, it will be assumed that recently married women will not rationalize their

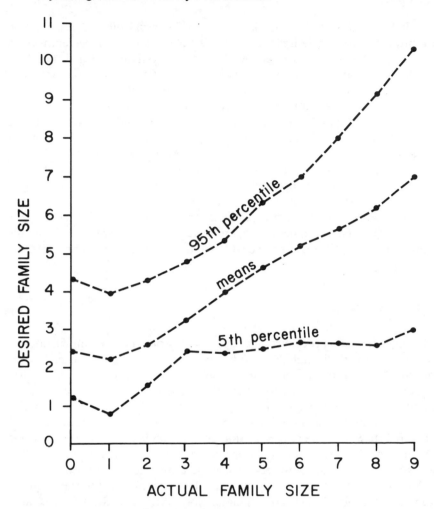

Figure 8-1. Mean and Range of Stated Desired Family Size According to Actual Family Size, Sri Lanka, 1975

responses. Except for the usual problem of validity, these responses may be taken at face value as the desired completed family size of the respondents. At the very short marital durations, in which women have few children and have had little opportunity to have children, the desire and behavior should agree only for those women who wish to remain childless or to have very small families; such women are (by any measure) a small minority in most developing countries. Thus a recently married woman is not likely to have raised her stated preference in order to justify originally unwanted children.

In Sri Lanka, women married less than five years showed a correlation of only 0.17 between desired and actual fertility. Less than 1 percent wanted fewer than they had, and 83 percent wanted more than they had. For each of the later marital duration intervals above ten years, by contrast, only about one-quarter of the women wanted more children than they had. Because rationalization is more likely when there is more face evidence of unwanted fertility, it appears indeed that the women married less than five years have the least biased responses. (Our conclusions would not be much affected by using less than the first five years of marriage or venturing a couple of years into the next marriage cohort; an interval of exactly five years is used simply for convenience.) For the 1,295 women in this youngest marriage cohort, the mean desired family size was 2.54.

An incidental reason for focusing on this cohort is that if there are any trends in fertility preferences, it will represent the most recent levels; by the same token, it will not then recover the former preferences of the older women.

Second Procedure

The remaining two procedures make use of all women in the sample, not just those with short marital durations. The first of these will be called the *rationalization model*. For each woman i, her stated desired family size willl be labeled s_i and her current family size will be c_i. We shall assume a number t_i which is the desired family size "adjusted" for actual family size or the response that would have been given if no rationalization had occurred. It will not be suggested that such a number can be estimated for the individual woman, but a relationship among these three quantities—two measured and one unmeasured—will be hypothesized. Specifically, it will be assumed that if the actual family size is less than or equal to the hypothesized adjusted ideal, then no rationalization occurs and the stated ideal is equal to the adjusted ideal (plus an error term). But if the actual family size *exceeds* the underlying personal ideal, then the response will have been adjusted upward in proportion to the amount of excess or unwanted fertility. Formally, the rationalization model states that:

$$s_i = t_i + e_i \qquad\qquad \text{if } c_i \leq t_i$$

and

$$s_i = t_i + b(c_i - t_i) + e_i \qquad \text{if } c_i > t_i$$

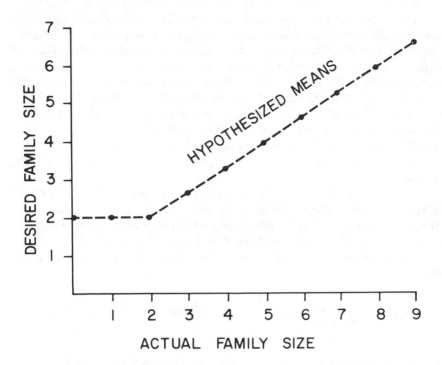

Note: The slope in the figure is merely illustrative.

Figure 8-2. Hypothesized Pattern of Mean Desired Family Size (Unadjusted) as a Function of Actual Family Size, When the Adjusted Preference in the Rationalization Model is for Two Children.

Here b is the constant of proportionality, assumed to be positive, and e_i represents random error and unmeasured sources of variation.

Figure 8-2 shows, for example, the relationship between s_i and c_i that would be expected for women whose adjusted ideal is actually two children. Such women would give a response s_i of two children as long as they had only zero, one, or two children. Afterwards, each additional child would raise the response. (There would, of course, be a scatter in the actual responses, partly because of the "error" term and partly because of the confinement to integer responses.)

Not only is it impossible to estimate t_i for each individual women, it is also impossible (without adding more assumptions) to estimate the proportion of women whose adjusted ideal is variously no children, one child, two children, and so on. In order to modify this model to permit some estimation, t_i will be replaced by t, which will be interpreted as approximately the mean value of the distribution of t_i in the population. If there is little dispersion in the values of t_i, the approximation should be a good one. If there is dispersion, it will be entirely consolidated with the error term in the first equation and mostly but not entirely consolidated with the error term in the second equation. Some bias in the estimates will result from this assumption.

With this modification, the quantities t and b may be estimated by least-squares procedures. Recognizing that the responses s_i and c_i are integers, define $n(j,k)$ to be the number of women in the sample who state they want j children and who have k children. That is, there are $n(j,k)$ women for whom $s_i = j$ and $c_i = k$. The sum of the squares to be minimized is then

$$SS(b,t) = \sum_k \left[\sum_{j<t} n(j,k)(j-t)^2 + \sum_{j>t} n(j,k)[j-t-b(k-t)]^2 \right]$$

For any given value of t, this sum of squares will be minimized with

$$b = \left[\sum_k \sum_{j>t} n(j,k)(j-t)(k-t) \right] / \left[\sum_k \sum_{j>t} n(j,k)(k-t)^2 \right]$$

Thus b can be expressed as a function of t; the minimizing value of t is found iteratively. (Note that this sum of squares is discontinuous in the neighborhood of integer values of t. The value of t that will be selected is either (1) the value at which there exists a horizontal tangent to SS, or (2) if SS does not have any horizontal tangent, then the integer value of t at which SS is minimized, even though discontinuous.)

For Sri Lanka's 1975 survey, the minimizing value of t is 2.51. That is, upward adjustment seems to begin on the average at this family size, although for individual women it must of course begin at some whole number such as 2 or 3. The coefficient b is estimated to be 0.676; for every child above the desired family size, the response is biased upward by two-thirds of a child. The increase is remarkably regular.

In the sample as a whole, this model accounts for 55.1 percent of the variance in the stated response s_i, using two parameters. By comparison, a one-way analysis of variance in which the response variable is considered within family-size categories 0, 1, 2, . . . , 10+ (and which therefore makes maximum use of the actual family-size distribution) accounts for 56.3 percent of the variance using eleven parameters.

The rationalization model cannot be tested against other models to which it is not hierarchically related. However, the model is parsimonious and its parameters are interpretable.

Third Procedure

So far the only question used has been the one on the personal ideal family size. We now turn to the standard WFS questions on desire for another child and desire for the latest pregnancy. Rationalization of originally unintended births is unlikely to affect the entirely prospective question about desire for another child. It may indeed bias the response to the question on desire for the latest pregnancy. However, it can be shown that estimates obtained under the present procedure are relatively insensitive to any such bias.

I have described elsewhere (Pullum 1980) the present procedure, that of a synthetic family-building cohort. In brief, the proportion of women at each actual family size who state they would like to continue childbearing is treated as a parity progression ratio. These proportions are used to generate the family-size distribution that would result if an artificial cohort passed through the family-building process. The mean of this distribution, which may be described as the mean completed family size of the synthetic cohort, is of particular interest.

The procedure may be described in more detail as follows. First the parity progression ratio p_i, referring to transitions from family size i to $i + 1$, is estimated as the proportion of (1) those women who wanted their last child or pregnancy who (2) want another child. Udry, Bauman, and Chase (1973) proposed using simply the proportion of *all* women at parity i who want another child in developing estimates of unwanted fertility. That simpler proportion has the defect of including in its denominator women who would never have achieved parity i if their preferences had been implemented. See Lightbourne (1977) for a critique.

In our estimate p_i, the women who are undecided about another child are classified with those who want more. However, those undecided about their latest child are classified with those who did *not* want their latest child. This allocation of the "undecided" cases gives the maximum possible value to the estimated parity progression ratio. The upward shift is quite small for Sri Lanka because only about 4 percent gave the undecided response.

These ratios are defined for $i = 0, 1, \ldots, I$, where I is the maximum observed parity for which $p_i > 0$. Let P_i be the expected proportion of women in the synthetic cohort who will have completed family-size i. These women will start their reproductive careers with no children and will progress sequentially to their ith child, stopping there, so that

$$P_i = (1 - p_i) \prod_{j=0}^{i-1} p_j$$

The mean completed family size will then be

$$M = \sum_i iP_i = \sum_i F_i \qquad \text{where } F_i = \prod_{j=0}^{i} p_j$$

The measure is comparable to the expectation of life in a stationary population that is subjected to a specific regime of mortality. Just as that quantity is free of the observed age structure and reflects only the age-specific probabilities of dying in an interval of age, M is free of the parity composition of the sample. The variance of the distribution is given by

$$S^2 = \sum_i i^2 P_i - M^2$$

Table 8–1 gives for Sri Lanka the estimated parity progression ratios p_i, the proportion who would stop at each parity, P_i, and the mean and standard deviations. The mean is 2.55 children and the standard deviation is 1.09. The completed family-size distribution of the synthetic cohort is shown graphically in figure 8–3.

Alternative estimates of the parity progression ratios in a synthetic cohort can be developed using the data on current family size, desire for the latest birth, and desire for another child. All of these synthetic estimates, including the procedure described previously, must be used cautiously, with the recognition that these three types of data cannot possibly tell us with certainty the first parity at which each women would have stated (or will state) that she wants no more children. The present procedure, for example, may be shown under plausible assumptions to be unbiased if there is no implementation of preferences. But if preferences are being implemented, then each current parity will include an accumulation of women who intentionally stopped at that parity long before the date of the survey. These accumulations will inflate the denominator of each p_i and will bias downward each estimated parity progression ratio. In Sri Lanka there is little evidence of an accumulation of women who stopped at their desired family size many years before the survey, and the bias is not believed to be substantial, at least not for the total and not for most socioeconomic subgroups.

Table 8-1
Calculation of the Synthetic Family-Size Distribution for the Entire Sample of Women Who Are Married and Fecund or Sterilized for Contraceptive Purposes, Sri Lanka, 1975

Actual or Synthetic Family Size, i	Sample Size (Weighted)	p_i	P_i
0	356	0.983	0.017
1	933	0.862	0.136
2	754	0.581	0.355
3	600	0.358	0.316
4	323	0.225	0.137
5	214	0.195	0.032
6	115	0.111	0.007
7	72	0.123	0.001
8	35	0.329	0.000
9	32	0.108	0.000
10	11	0.000	0.000

Notes: Mean of synthetic distribution = 2.547; standard deviation = 1.089; see text for definition of symbols.

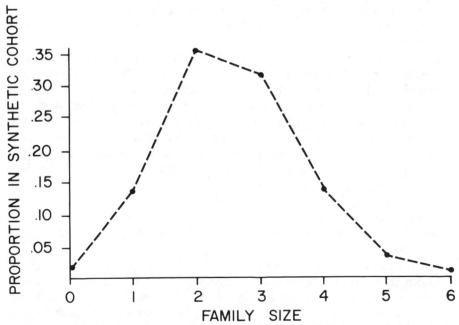

Figure 8-3. The Completed Family-Size Distribution of the Synthetic Cohort, Sri Lanka, 1975

Differentials

To summarize, the three methods used so far imply a mean desired family size for Sri Lanka of 2.54, 2.51, and 2.55. Despite their very different uses of data and the restriction of the first procedure to a subsample, the estimates are within 2 percent of one another. We now turn to differences between some of the main subgroups of Sri Lanka. The original motivation for these procedures, it will be recalled, was to be able to compare subgroups free of the possible bias of achieved fertility.

For this purpose only two illustrative background variables will be drawn from the Sri Lanka survey: *religion*, with four categories, and *region of residence*, with six categories. These two variables appear to be the most important sources of variation in most dependent variables of the Sri Lanka survey. The four religious groups are Buddhists, Hindus, Muslims, and Christians. Among all the ever-married women in the survey, these comprised 66, 19, 7, and 8 percent, respectively. The six regions are described as follows: Zone I is metropolitan Colombo, entirely urban; Zone II is the rest of the southwest lowlands, and shares many of Colombo's modern characteristics. Zone IV is the east coast, with a high proportion of Muslims; Zone V is the northern tip, closest to India, and has a high proportion of Hindus. Zone VI consists of the central mountainous area, where the tea estates are located. These estates are worked by Indian Tamils who are, of course, Hindus. The remainder of the island, Zone III, consists of dry lowlands.

The first two columns of table 8-2 give the deviation of each zone and religious group from the overall family size and from the unadjusted, stated desired family size. Actual family size is defined to be the number of living children, including any current pregnancy, as in the rationalization model. For the overall sample, ideal family size slightly exceeds actual family size (3.75 compared with 3.57). This apparent inconsistency with our earlier discussion results mainly from accumulated deaths of children to older, high-parity women. The mean number of children ever born, 3.96, does exceed the overall desired family size.

In general, the pattern of deviations is the same in both these columns, as would be expected from the high correlation at the individual level. There are some correspondences, however, to which we shall return later in this chapter.

The remaining three columns give the differentials in desired family size under the three procedures described earlier. Not only is there close agreement in the overall estimated means (2.54, 2.51, and 2.55), there is also close correspondence in the deviations. Without exception, the signs of the deviations agree in all three procedures. To interpret these patterns of

Table 8-2
Actual Family Size and Desired Family Size, Unadjusted and Adjusted, for Sri Lanka, 1975

	Mean of Actual Family Size	Unadjusted Ideal Family Size for Total Sample	Procedure 1 (Marital Duration 0-4)	Procedure 2 (Rationalization Model)	Procedure 3 (Synthetic Cohort)
Mean	3.57	3.75	2.54	2.51	2.55
Deviations					
Zone I	−0.24 (6)	−0.37 (6)	−0.15 (5)	−0.12 (5)	−0.33 (6)
Zone II	−0.23 (5)	−0.32 (5)	−0.19 (6)	−0.28 (6)	−0.20 (5)
Zone III	+0.34 (1.5)	+0.32 (2)	+0.03 (4)	+0.13 (4)	+0.20 (6)
Zone IV	+0.34 (1.5)	+0.42 (1)	+0.09 (2)	+0.20 (3)	+0.22 (2)
Zone V	−0.03 (4)	+0.25 (3)	+0.36 (1)	+0.49 (1)	+0.69 (1)
Zone VI	+0.03 (3)	+0.07 (4)	+0.08 (3)	+0.24 (2)	+0.05 (4)
Buddhist	+0.05 (2)	+0.01 (2)	−0.03 (3)	−0.01 (3)	−0.01 (3)
Hindu	−0.23 (4)	−0.05 (3)	+0.10 (2)	+0.09 (2)	+0.10 (2)
Muslim	+0.34 (1)	+0.49 (1)	+0.34 (1)	+0.49 (1)	+0.45 (1)
Christian	−0.15 (3)	−0.36 (4)	−0.22 (4)	−0.32 (4)	−0.29 (4)

Note: Numbers in parentheses represent ranks.

deviations, two strategies will be followed. The procedures will first be compared with one another and then with the unadjusted desired family size.

First, consider the degree of agreement among the three in their ranking of the regions. Under all three procedures, the largest positive deviation is found for zone V, the northern tip of the island. That is, the adjusted desired family size is greatest in zone V by all three procedures. Zone IV receives ranks 2, 3, and 2; zone III ranks 4, 4, and 3; and zones I and II share ranks 5 and 6. Zone VI receives a range of ranks (3, 2, and 4) and is less easily classified. However, at the very minimum, there is consensus that the adjusted ideal family size is greatest in zone V; intermediate in zones IV, VI, and III; and lowest in the more-developed part of Sri Lanka, zones I and II.

Turning to religion, there is perfect agreement in rank order. Under all three procedures, Muslims prefer the largest families, followed in order by Hindus, Buddhists, and Christians. There is also better agreement as to the magnitudes of the deviations within religious groups than within zones; however, within both sets of categories the correspondence is clear.

In general, the differentials for the unadjusted ideal family size (in column 2 of table 8-2) also agree with these conclusions. However, the two discrepancies will be noted. (If there were no discrepancies, there would be little point in making the adjustments.) In the case of the breakdown by region, the unadjusted responses suggest that the desired family size is largest in zone IV, rather than zone V, and that zone V is third in rank rather than first. This reversal, centering on zones IV and V, is unambiguous. Some other shifts, although noticeable, are less pronounced. We infer that the order of the zones in column 2 is affected by their order in column 1 through rationalization (women in zone IV have larger actual families than those in zone V), and our three procedures have all compensated for this bias.

In the case of religion, there is a reversal involving the Buddhists and the Hindus. The unadjusted responses for the total family size give them ranks 2 and 3 rather than ranks 3 and 2, respectively, on which the adjusted measures agreed completely. Again we infer that the differentials in actual family size are being mimicked through rationalization. For one reason or another, the Buddhists have larger families than the Hindus, by an average of 0.28 children, and they state that they want larger families, on the average; but we infer that if stated preferences could be implemented, then the Buddhists would have *smaller* families than the Hindus.

Conclusions

A few concluding remarks will be made. First, questions of sampling variation have been ignored because of an emphasis on differences between procedures rather than on inferences about the overall population of Sri Lanka. Certainly, some of the deviations described above are not significantly different from zero or from one another.

Second, it may appear that the adjustment procedures are only suitable for categorical data. On the contrary, each of them can be applied to interval-level variables. Appendix 8A develops approximate formulas for estimating sampling variation and for including interval-level predictors under the synthetic-cohort approach.

Third, it must be emphasized that the three procedures do not use all women equally in the calculations. The first procedure, being confined to women currently in their first five years of marriage, will consist disproportionately of women who are young, of low parity, of better education, and so on. It has already been suggested that such women are precursors of future preferences, but if there are trends in preferences, they will not be representative (in levels, at least) of the whole sample. The second procedure, the rationalization model, because it is estimated by least squares, will be disproportionately affected by women whose actual and desired family sizes are far apart. Some of these will be women who are just starting childbearing and others will be high-parity women who say they wanted small families. The third procedure, the synthetic cohort, can be shown to be most affected by preferences of women with small families. In Sri Lanka, in fact, women with more than six children do not even affect the results in the second decimal place.

For some purposes, such as the delivery of family-planning services, it may be sufficient to know the distribution of women who want no more children. By this measure, in Sri Lanka the sharpest difference is between zones IV and V, where respectively 65 and 45 percent of the women want no more, although in table 8-2 these two zones showed very similar ideal-size preferences. There would be no question that family-planning services are needed more in zone IV than in zone V. Here, however, another kind of question has been asked, namely, how many children would women have if their preferences could be implemented, net of the possibly biasing effect of their actual family size? The policy relevance of these results is admittedly more remote, with implications for the *consequences* of fully available and implemented family-planning services, rather than for their immediate *need*. It is also suggested that explanations of actual fertility differentials, at the aggregate level at least, may sometimes be improved if they are developed in two steps—first, an explanation of the adjusted desired family size, and second, an explanation of departures from that level.

References

Cho, Lee-Jay. "Fertility Preferences in Five Asian Countries." *International Family Planning Perspectives and Digest* 4(1978):2-8.

Coombs, Lolagene C. "The Measurement of Family Size Preferences and Subsequent Fertility." *Demography* 11(1974):587-611.

Goodman, Leo A. "On the Exact Variance of Products." *Journal of the American Statistical Association* 55(1960):708-713.

Knodel, John, and Prachuabmoh, Visid. "Desired Family Size in Thailand: Are the Responses Meaningful? *Demography* 10(1973):619-637.

Lightbourne, Robert "Family Size Desires and the Birth Rates They Imply." Unpublished Ph.D. dissertation, Department of Sociology, University of California, Berkeley, 1977.

Pullum, Thomas W. "Illustrative Analysis: Fertility Preferences in Sri Lanka." *World Fertility Survey Scientific Reports* 9(1980):1-36.

Udry, J. Richard; Bauman, Karl E.; and Chase, C.L. "Population Growth Rates in Perfect Contraceptive Populations." *Population Studies* 27(1973):365-371.

Westoff, Charles F.; McCarthy, James; Goldman, Noreen; and Mascarin, Felix. "Sterilization in Panama." *International Family Planning Perspectives* 5(1979):111–117.

Westoff, Charles, F.; Mishler, Elliot G.; and Kelly, E. Lowell. "Preferences in Size of Family and Eventual Fertility Twenty Years After." *American Journal of Sociology* 62(1957):491–497.

Appendix 8A:
Statistical Properties of
the Synthetic-Cohort
Procedure

In order to facilitate the application of the synthetic-cohort procedure to sample data, two of its statistical properties will be developed. The first will be an estimate of the sampling error in M, the mean of the synthetic family-size distribution. With this estimate it is possible to test for the statistical significance of a difference between two subgroups. Second, it will be shown how variation in M can be related to an interval-level variable.

Estimating the Standard Error of M

Let Θ_i be the population value of the ith parity progression ratio, which would be obtained if our procedure could be applied to the entire population. Let p_i be the sample estimate based on a sample of size n_i (the denominator of p_i), which is regarded as a binomial random variable with $E(p_i) = \Theta_i$ and $\text{Var}(p_i) = \Theta_i (1 - \Theta_i)/n_i$.

Under the synthetic-cohort procedure described in chapter 8, the variables $p_0, p_1, \ldots p_I$ are statistically independent. The following comments will apply to any similar procedure having this property. The mean of the synthetic-cohort distribution in the population is

$$\mu = \sum_{i=0}^{I} i(1 - \Theta_i) \prod_{j=0}^{i-1} \Theta_j$$

which is estimated from a sample with

$$M = \sum_{i=0}^{I} i(1 - p_i) \prod_{j=0}^{i-1} p_j$$

If we define

$$F_i = \prod_{j=0}^{i} p_j$$

then it is easily shown that

$$M = \sum_{i=0}^{I} F_i$$

The variance of M is then

$$\text{Var}(M) = \text{Var}(\sum_{i=0}^{I} F_i) = \sum_{i=0}^{I} \text{Var}(F_i) + 2\sum_{i=0}^{I} \sum_{j=i+1}^{I} \text{Cov}(F_i, F_j)$$

The covariance terms in this expression can be eliminated as follows because of the independence property of the p_i. For $j > i$, we have

$$F_j = F_i \prod_{k=i+1}^{j} p_k$$

and

$$E(F_j) = E(F_i)E(\prod_{k=i+1}^{j} p_k) = E(F_i)[\prod_{k=i+1}^{j} E(p_k)] = E(F_i)\prod_{k=i+1}^{j} \Theta_k$$

A similar factorization of $E(F_i F_j)$ is possible.
Therefore

$$\text{Cov}(F_i, F_j) = E(F_i F_j) - E(F_i)E(F_j) = [E(F_i^2) - E(F_i)]^2 \prod_{k=i+1}^{j} \Theta_k$$

$$= \text{Var}(F_i) \prod_{k=i+1}^{j} \Theta_k$$

Because of this simplification,

$$\text{Var}(M) = \sum_{i=0}^{I} \text{Var}(F_i) \left[1 + 2 \sum_{j=i+1}^{I} \prod_{k=i+1}^{j} \Theta_k \right]$$

The problem now is to estimate $\text{Var}(F_i)$. For this purpose we apply the general formula for the variance of a product of independent random variables (see, for example, Goodman 1960). Letting $m_i = E(p_i)$ and $\sigma_i^2 = \text{Var}(p_i)$ and writing the general formula in recursive form, we have

$$\text{Var}(F_i) = (m_i^2 + \sigma_i^2)\text{Var}(F_{i-1}) + \sigma_i^2 \prod_{j=0}^{i-1} m_j^2 \text{ for } i = 1, \dots, I$$

with $\text{Var}(F_0) = \sigma_0^2$.

Stating m_i and σ_i^2 in terms of Θ_i and n_i for binomial variables, we obtain

$$\text{Var}(F_i) = \left[\Theta_i^2 + \frac{\Theta_i(1 - \Theta_i)}{n_i} \right] \text{Var}(F_{i-1}) + \frac{\Theta_i(1 - \Theta_i)}{n_i} \left[\prod_{j=0}^{i-1} \Theta_j \right]^2$$

Finally, noting that the sample estimate of

$$\prod_{k=i+1}^{j} \Theta_k$$

will be F_j / F_i, we have

$$\text{Vâr}(M) = \text{Vâr}(F_i) \left[1 + \frac{2}{F_i} \sum_{j=i+1}^{I} F_j \right]$$

where $\text{Vâr}(F_i)$ is calculated recursively by

$$\text{Vâr}(F_i) = \left[p_i^2 + \frac{p_i(1 - p_i)}{n_i} \right] \text{Vâr}(F_{i-1}) + \frac{(1 - p_i)}{n_i p_i} F_i^2$$

$$\text{for } i = 1, \ldots I$$

with $\text{Vâr}(F_0) = p_0(1 - p_0)/n_0$.

When this formula is applied to the data for Sri Lanka in table 8-1, assuming simple random sampling, we obtain $\text{Var}(M) = 0.0025$; the estimated standard error is 0.05. (This calculation ignores the effects of the stratified cluster design of the sample and is to be considered as illustrative.)

Adapting M to a Regression Framework

In this chapter the variation in M from one subgroup to another was evaluated by calculating its value within each subgroup. This was acceptable in Sri Lanka because all the predictors were categorical variables. Other surveys, however, could include interval-level predictors. It might also be desirable to include interval-level covariates, such as age or marital duration. This appendix will describe the inclusion of such variables. For simplicity, it will be assumed that there is only one interval-level predictor; the extension to more than one or to combinations of categorical and interval-level variables is exactly parallel to the extension from simple linear regression to multiple regression and analysis of covariance, etc.

Instead of simply calculating p_i within each parity i, it is necessary to do a regression within each parity. Exclude completely those women who did not want their last birth. Define a dichotomous variable D to be 1 if a women wants an additional child and 0 if she does not. Earlier, we calculated p_i as the proportion of women of parity i who have $D = 1$. Let x be a continuous variable, evaluated for all women in the sample, and regress D on x. Let $D_i = a_i + b_i x$ represent the regression, to be repeated for all parities i, $i = 0, 1, \ldots, I$. Such an estimate is interpretable if we regard D_i as an estimate of an underlying probability of a positive response. Following this interpretation, we rewrite the regression as $p_i(x) = a_i + b_i x$, where $p_i(x)$ is the estimated parity progression ratio as a linear function of x. In the same manner, P_i, F_i, and M may be regarded as functions of x. The slope of $M(x)$ at x will be

$$b(x) = \frac{dM}{dx} = \frac{d}{dx} \sum_{i=0}^{I} F_i = \sum_{i=0}^{I} \frac{dF_i}{dx}$$

It is easily shown that:

$$\frac{dF_i}{dx} = F_i \sum_{j=0}^{i} [b_j / p_j(x)]$$

Substituting this into the equation for $b(x)$ and then evaluating at the mean value of x, we obtain

$$b^* = b(\bar{x}) = \sum_{i=0}^{I} F_i \left(\sum_{j=0}^{i} b_j / p_j \right)$$

Here p_j and F_i will simply be the same as when x is ignored, and b_j will come from the within-parity regression of D on x. This b^* may be regarded as the impact on M of a unit change in x in the vicinity of the mean.

It will be preferable, if the facilities for logit regression are available, to estimate a and b for the regression

$$\ln \frac{p_i(x)}{1 - p_i(x)} = a_i + b_i x.$$

This equation has the property that

$$\frac{dp_i(x)}{dx} = b_i p_i(x)[1 - p_i(x)]$$

It then follows that the impact of a unit change in x in the vicinity of its mean is

$$b^{**} = \left.\frac{dM}{dx}\right|_{x=\bar{x}} = \sum_{i=0}^{I} F_i \sum_{j=0}^{i} b_j (1 - p_j)$$

where p_j and F_i are as when x is ignored and b_j comes from the within-parity logit regression on x. Note that b^* and b^{**} are in different scales and need not be similar in value for the same data.

This procedure will apply for any synthetic-cohort estimates that are calculated from nonoverlapping subsets of women.

Part III
Trends and Patterns in Birth Expectations

9 Findings from Census-Bureau Surveys

Maurice J. Moore

While the articles in part II contained considerable information on trends and differences in birth expectations, their focus was largely methodological—they inquired into the validity and reliability of expectations and into techniques for adjusting expectations to improve their usefulness in fertility forecasting. In part III the emphasis shifts to substantive patterns in fertility expectations, although the authors do not lose sight of the methodological issues raised earlier.

In this chapter by Maurice Moore, the focus is on trends in birth expectations primarily as measured by the Current Population Surveys of the census bureau. During the period covered by those data (1971-1979), the expected lifetime fertility of young women has been consistently and significantly higher than the total fertility, that is, the number of births to women in a lifetime if current period fertility rates persisted. Moore interprets this as indicating that the low current fertility rates of that period would not continue, that current fertility would turn upward in the near future. This observation is consistent with Lee's analysis in chapter 5; Lee's model predicted that in a period of declining lifetime fertility expectations, women's current fertility will be very low as they try to undercompensate for the earlier fertility, the pace of which they now regard as having been too fast and too early.

In addition to describing the downward trend in average expectations, Moore examines the distribution of women by particular numbers of children expected. He shows, for instance, that most of the overall decline in expectations is accounted for by the decline in expectations of large families (four or more children). There has been little increase, according to Moore, in the popularity of childless or one-child families. Of course, the result of these trends in expectations of large and small families is a convergence on expectations of moderate-sized families, especially the two-child family. By the end of the 1970s, a majority of young women (25 to 29 years of age) expected to have borne two children at the end of their childbearing years.—*Eds.*

As part of the Johnson administration's antipoverty program, funds were made available through the Office of Economic Opportunity for a special survey to assess the extent and correlates of poverty in the United States. This Survey of Economic Opportunity, which was conducted by the Bureau of the Census in 1967, was the first government-administered interview survey to ask about the number of children expected in the future. Similar questions were not asked again in census-bureau surveys until June 1971, when the Current Population Survey (CPS) for that month included the birth-expectations questions as part of a survey of marriage and fertility histories. Since 1971 every June CPS has included questions about child-bearing to date and that expected in the future. This series of census-bureau surveys, extending over twelve years, covers both the early 1970s, in which very rapid declines occurred in annual measures of fertility, as well as the later 1970s, in which comparative stability seems to have set in.

The earliest (Freedman, Whelpton, and Campbell 1959) and most con-sistent use of birth-expectations data is to provide an estimate of completed childbearing for birth cohorts of women who are in their early or middle reproductive years. The thought behind this approach is that cohort mea-sures of anticipated fertility, such as average lifetime expected fertility, pro-vide a more reliable vehicle for predicting the future course of population growth than does the extrapolation of annual fertility measures from birth registrations. Whether or not birth expectations are the best vehicle, or even a good one, for making such a prediction, they do provide evidence of the increasingly well-established fact that the fluctuations in cohort fertility are likely to be substantially less than those suggested by annual measures of fertility (see, for example, Ryder 1974).

Figure 9–1 illustrates the relationship between the annual total fertility rate, a measure of fertility for synthetic cohorts, and the average number of births expected by real cohorts of women who were 18 to 29 years old on the survey dates shown. Although lifetime birth expectations are available for complete cohorts of women (of all marital statuses) only since 1976, the data plotted in figure 9–1 for wives shows the general relationship that would exist if all women were included. In the late 1950s, when birth rates reached levels not seen in the United States since the early 1900s, expecta-tions data for women in their late teens and twenties were indicating that the total fertility rate, with its conditional implication of lifetime averages around 3.7 births per woman, was substantially in excess of what would actually occur. Women themselves were "expecting" to complete their reproductive lives with an average around 3.2 children per woman. The pas-sage of time since then, with which women 18 to 29 in 1955 become 40 to 51 years old in 1977, has established the reasonable accuracy of the women's predictions in this instance; the June 1977 CPS showed all women 40 to 49 years old had averaged 3.1 children per woman, and ever-married women averaged 3.2 (Bureau of the Census 1978).

In the 1950s and 1960s there were no annual measures of expected childbearing comparable to the CPS in the 1970s. Quinquenniel measures were provided first by the Growth of American Families (GAF) studies in 1955 and 1960, then by the National Fertility Surveys (NFS) in 1965 and 1970. Although measures from 1955 to 1970 occurred five years apart, it appears from the data plotted in figure 9–1 that annual birth rates began to decline several years before a corresponding decrease appeared in the life-

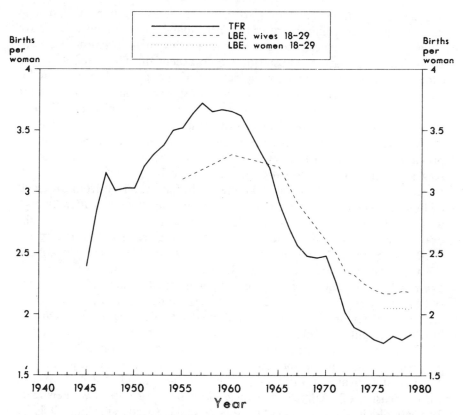

Sources: Total fertility rates for 1945-1977 are from National Center for Health Statistics, various volumes of *Natality*, Vital Statistics of the United States, vol. 1, and *Monthly Vital Statistics Report* 27, no. 11 (1979): supplement. Total fertility rates for 1978 and 1979 are unofficial estimates calculated at the Bureau of the Census. Lifetime births expected for 1955 and 1960 are from Ronald Freedman and Larry Bumpass, "Fertility Expectations in the United States: 1962-1964," *Population Index* 32(1966):table 3; for 1965, from unpublished data from the National Fertility Survey; for 1967 and 1971-1979, from Bureau of the Census, "Fertility of American Women: June 1979," *Current Population Reports*, series P-20, table 1.

Figure 9-1. Total Fertility Rate (TFR), 1940-1979, and Lifetime Births Expected (LBE), 1955-1979

time expectations of wives 18 to 29 years old. Setting aside for the moment the issue of comparability of the two fertility measures, the annual total fertility rate, which was well above the cohort-expectations measure in the late 1950s and early 1960s, fell below the cohort measure in the latter part of the 1960s and has been substantially below it in the 1970s.

Assuming this comparison tells us something, what is it? One possible interpretation is that birth expectations are no more than a lagging measure of American fertility. According to this interpretation, women's expectations about childbearing are, after the fact, adapted to the reality they have already begun to experience and to shape with their practical decisions about family formation. Those who would accept this view are looking to expectations data for near-term indications of changes in direction and/or levels of annual-fertility measures. One must admit that neither lifetime birth expectations (figure 9–1) nor expectations of future births (table 9–1) have proven to be sensitive predictors of birth rates on a year-to-year basis.

On the other hand, if one can be content to accept birth expectations as previews of completed fertility for real groups of women still in various stages of their reproductive lives, then the data of figure 9–1 may be *indicative* of the future. In 1955 and 1960 one might have inferred from the levels of lifetime expected births that annual birth measures were artificially high and would not long be sustained at levels then current; one might draw the opposite conclusion about the very low levels that have persisted through the 1970s. Since 1975 the annual total fertility rate has fluctuated around the average of 1.8 births per woman. In the same period, however, the average number of lifetime births expected per married woman 18 to 29 years old has been approximately 2.2. Even when women of *all* marital statuses are included (figure 9–1), the average has not fallen below 2.0. On this basis, one might be cautious about expecting birth rates to continue as low as they currently are, although the expectations data also indicate that no new baby boom is on the horizon, in any meaningful sense of the term.

Is it statistically appropriate to compare the annual total fertility rate with a measure of lifetime birth expectations by the group of women 18 to 29 years old in the corresponding survey year? Strictly speaking, it is an apples-and-oranges type of comparison. The total fertility rate is the summation of actual age-specific rates in a given year for women 10 to 49 years old. It may be regarded as a statement about what levels of completed fertility *would* occur, *if* a group of women experienced the rates for that year throughout their reproductive lives. It has nothing to do with births expected in the future or by a specific cohort of women. Averages of lifetime expected births, on the other hand, state the completed level of fertility expected by a given group of women; they take into account actual cumulative fertility to date and personal projections about future childbearing. Expected childbearing is hypothetical too, but in a different way than the total fertility rate; expectations depend for their predictive accuracy on the degree to which a group of women in the remainder of their reproductive years actually attain the averages they expected.

Still, the comparison of the total fertility rate with averages of lifetime birth expectations is not without some justification; 70 percent or more of the total fertility rate in any given year is attributable to the rates for women 18 to 29 years old in that year (derived from National Center for Health

Table 9–1
Future Births Expected per 1,000 Wives

Survey Year	Age of Wives at Survey Date		
	18 to 24 Years	25 to 29 Years	30 to 34 Years
1967	1,679	725	238
1971	1,423	670	187
1972	1,327	645	166
1973	1,367	631	181
1974	1,317	644	185
1975	1,354	657	182
1976	1,323	633	174
1977	1,334	706	194
1978	1,338	728	216
1979	1,312	750	224

Source: Bureau of the Census, "Fertility of American Women: June 1979," *Current Population Reports,* series P-20, table 1 (by subtraction).

Statistics 1979, table 4). Moreover, *in the longer run,* it is impossible for women to fulfill expectations at a 2.0- to 2.1-children-per-woman average while the total fertility rate remains, year after year, at the 1.8 level. The comparison illustrated in figure 9–1 is meant to highlight the cautions that current survey data provide about assuming an indefinite continuation or even lowering of current annual fertility rates.

Declines in Average Expected Parity

Over the twelve-year period in which census-bureau surveys have been taken, the level of average lifetime births expected has declined sharply (table 9–2). In 1967 wives in their early twenties expected an average of 2.9 children per woman; women then in their early thirties, who were some of the most prolific contributors to the baby boom, expected a lifetime average of 3.3 children per woman, over 90 percent of which were children already born at the time of the 1967 survey. By the time of the 1971 survey, significant decreases occurred in the average number of lifetime births for each of the three age groups shown in table 9–2.

As time passes, women in one age group gradually move into the next. Women 20 to 24 in 1967 were 25 to 29 in 1972. Thus the reproductive goals of a younger age group automatically become those of an older age group with the passage of time, to the extent that goals remain stable over time.

Table 9–2
Lifetime Births Expected per 1,000 Wives

	Age at Survey Date		
Survey and Year	18 to 24	25 to 29	30 to 34
1967 SEO	2,852	3,037	3,288
1971 CPS	2,375	2,619	2,989
1972 CPS	2,255	2,452	2,915
1973 CPS	2,262	2,387	2,804
1974 CPS	2,165	2,335	2,724
1975 CPS	2,173	2,260	2,610
1976 CPS	2,141	2,202	2,536
1977 CPS	2,137	2,197	2,468
1978 CPS	2,166	2,215	2,424
1979 CPS	2,164	2,193	2,282

Source: Bureau of the Census, "Fertility of American Women: June 1979," *Current Population Reports,* series P-20, table 1 (by subtraction).

Average lifetime expectations for wives 20 to 24 years old seem to have become relatively constant around 2.1 to 2.2 children per woman, beginning around 1974. The same level was reached around 1976 by wives 25 to 29 years old. Wives in the 30- to 34-year age group at each survey are currently approaching the 2.2 level, which is 1 child per woman less in 1979 than in 1967.

Changes in Parity Distribution

In 1967 wives expected an average of about 3 children per woman, as discussed above. By 1979 the corresponding average was slightly above 2 children per woman. Table 9–3 focuses on wives 25 to 29 years old, to indicate the parity distributions underlying the averages of table 9–2. The age group 25 to 29 was chosen for two reasons: (1) the vast majority of women in this age group have already married for the first time and are consistently included in the survey universes, and (2) a large portion (25 to 35 percent) of their expected lifetime childbearing remains to be completed.

In 1967 one woman in three expected to have three children in her lifetime; the next most commonly expected parity (29 percent) was two children. As of 1979, the norm had shifted to two children and was even more strongly established, with one woman in two expecting a two-child family. The three-child family was in a distant second place (21 percent).

Table 9-3
Distribution of Expected Lifetime Parity for Wives 25 to 29 Years Old

Survey and Year	Total	Number of Lifetime Births Expected (Percentage Distribution)						Lifetime Births Expected per 1,000 Wives
		None	1	2	3	4	5+	
1960 GAF	100.0	4.0	7.0	25.0	27.0	20.0	17.0	3,400
1967 SEO	100.0	2.2	5.1	29.3	33.5	17.7	12.3	3,037
1971 CPS	100.0	3.2	6.8	44.1	27.6	11.7	6.6	2,619
1972 CPS	100.0	4.0	7.9	48.5	26.6	9.5	4.6	2,452
1973 CPS	100.0	4.1	9.1	49.9	24.1	8.7	4.0	2,387
1974 CPS	100.0	4.7	9.5	51.7	22.3	8.0	3.9	2,335
1975 CPS	100.0	4.9	11.7	50.4	23.3	6.9	2.9	2,260
1976 CPS	100.0	6.4	11.2	51.5	21.8	6.5	2.6	2,202
1977 CPS	100.0	6.3	11.6	50.4	22.7	6.8	2.2	2,197
1978 CPS	100.0	6.0	11.6	50.8	22.2	7.0	2.5	2,215
1979 CPS	100.0	5.3	12.9	51.9	21.3	6.0	2.6	2,193

Sources: (1960) Ronald Freedman and Larry Bumpass, "Fertility Expectations in the United States: 1962–1964," *Population Index* 32(1966):table 1; (1967, 1971–1979) Bureau of the Census, *Current Population Reports* for the respective surveys.

Much of the story of the decline in fertility from the late 1950s to the present is highlighted in the relative decrease in women expecting "large" families, which are here defined as those with four children or more. The 1960 survey, which was not conducted by the census bureau, showed that 37 percent of wives 25 to 29 years old expected more than three children. The 1979 CPS put the corresponding statistic at 9 percent. The 1960 survey found 11 percent of the wives expecting fewer than two children, compared to 18 percent in 1979. It is clear that a social norm of some considerable strength has developed around the two-child family. It is hard to see in the data of table 9–3 a clearly noteworthy increase in enthusiasm for the childless family developing among *married* women, although the one-child family may well be making gains.

To go a bit deeper into the growing convergence on the two-child family, the distribution of lifetime expected parity is shown in table 9–4 by race and by educational attainment for white wives. This analysis makes it clear that the two-child norm is observed more rigorously among the relatively more-advantaged groups. About the same percentage of white wives and black wives expect to have fewer than two children, but the proportion of wives expecting four or more children is more than twice as large among blacks as it is among whites. Among both black wives and white wives in the 25 to 29 age group in 1979, the two-child norm prevails, but by a far wider margin among white wives.

To study the relationship between educational attainment and expected parity, free of racial differences in education, the second panel of table 9–4 focuses on white wives. Those with lower attainment levels (and usually with fewer financial resources) are more likely to have larger families. The positive relationship between educational attainment and percentage of wives expecting two children or fewer during their lifetimes is clear. As attainment levels are grouped in table 9–4, the two-child norm increases in strength with each higher level of education.

Zero- and One-Parity Families

An issue of increasing interest in the study of American fertility is that of the "small" family, that is, the family with one child or no children at all. Lifetime expected parity presents an interesting preview of what young couples look forward to in this respect, and table 9–5 shows how these expectations have developed during the 1970s. This table focuses on white wives 20 to 24 years old. Although in this age group the percentage of women currently married has been decreasing over the past ten to fifteen years, they are chosen for attention because most of their lifetime childbearing still lies in the future and because changing values and social norms usually affect the youngest groups first.

Table 9–4
Expected Lifetime Parity for Wives 25 to 29 Years Old, by Race and Educational Attainment: 1979

Race and Education	Total	Less than Two Children	Two Children	Three Children	Four or More Children
Race					
White	100.0	18.0	53.0	21.2	7.8
Black	100.0	19.4	37.9	23.9	18.8
Educational attainment, white wives					
Less than high-school graduate	100.0	14.7	39.3	29.7	16.3
High-school graduate	100.0	17.5	52.6	23.2	6.7
One or more years college	100.0	19.5	57.8	16.3	6.4

Sources: Bureau of the Census, "Fertility of American Women: June 1979," *Current Population Reports,* series P-20, table 5; and unpublished tabulations from the June 1979 Current Population Survey.

During the 1971–1979 period there was a modest increase in the percentages of young white wives who expect to remain childless or have only one child. The percentage of young white wives expecting to be childless has increased by about 2 percentage points, from 4 to 6 percent, and the increase in expectations of one-child families may have been 3 or 4 percentage points. Whether or not this trend among married women will continue into the 1980s remains to be seen. The corresponding data for young black wives are of such year-to-year variability, especially in the percentage expecting one child, that no conclusions can reasonably be drawn.

The relationship of education to low fertility expectations, again with the focus on white wives, is also displayed in table 9–5. The only pattern that is clearly repeated year after year is that at each higher educational category correspondingly greater proportions of young white wives expect to remain childless throughout life. There also appears to be a pattern in the opposite direction concerning expectations of a one-child family, although the sample data show more exceptions with respect to this latter relationship.

The data shown in table 9–5 are limited in value, because a large proportion of the women 20 to 24 years old at any survey date are not yet married and it is not at all clear that the expectations of single women in the 20- to 24-year-old age group are well represented by women who are already married, especially if a substantial portion of the never-married 20- to 24-year-old women intend to remain single throughout their lives. In addi-

Table 9–5
Zero or One Lifetime Expected Parity for Wives 20 to 24 Years Old, by Race and Educational Attainment: 1971 to 1979

Race, Education, and Parity	Survey Year								
	1971	1972	1973	1974	1975	1976	1977	1978	1979
Race									
White									
No children	3.9	3.5	4.2	5.3	4.8	5.2	5.7	5.6	5.8
One child	8.2	9.2	8.3	10.9	10.9	11.8	11.8	11.9	11.4
Black									
No children	2.5	4.1	3.2	4.4	1.4	2.6	4.5	3.8	2.7
One child	10.3	13.2	19.7	23.6	10.5	12.9	16.5	14.9	9.3
Years of school completed, white wives									
Less than 12									
No children	1.5	1.5	2.6	1.8	1.9	3.6	2.8	1.7	3.5
One child	8.1	8.3	12.9	12.8	14.4	12.7	15.5	14.8	12.8
12									
No children	4.0	3.5	3.1	5.7	4.7	4.2	5.1	5.6	5.8
One child	9.2	10.7	8.3	11.8	11.5	13.0	12.6	12.6	11.3
13 or more									
No children	5.2	4.8	7.6	7.0	6.6	8.5	9.2	8.1	7.6
One child	7.0	6.5	5.1	7.9	7.4	8.7	7.6	8.6	10.5

Source: Bureau of the Census: *Current Population Reports* for the respective surveys.

Table 9–6
Completed Parity of Ever-Married White Women

	Age and Survey Date		
	50 to 59 Years, 1970 Census	*50 to 59 Years, June 1979 CPS*	*45 to 49 Years, June 1979 CPS*
Percentage with:			
No children	14.8	9.2	6.9
One child	17.9	13.1	9.9

tion, recent history provides an instructive perspective on the current levels of expected childless and one-child families. Table 9–6 shows that childlessness among selected cohorts of ever-married white women who have completed their childbearing is generally higher than that expected by today's 20- to 24-year-old wives.

Expectations of Single Women

After a modest feasibility experiment in the June 1975 CPS, all subsequent June surveys included single women 18 years old and over in the universe for the questions on childbearing to date and births expected in the future. The CPS was the first national survey of childbearing experience and intentions to include single women in a broad age range of the childbearing years.[1] The addition of single women to the survey has made it possible to obtain expected childbearing for *all* women in an age group and to assess the effects of not including them in previous surveys.

Although the record of single women in fertility surveys is relatively short, the consistency of the averages shown in table 9–7 for four surveys provides a first-level self-validation. Moreover, the average lifetime expectations of single women 18 and 19 years old, the vast majority of whom envision an eventual marriage, are similar to the average expectations of married women 18 and 19 years old (2,041 versus 2, 135 per 1,000 women in 1979). Single women 20 to 24 years old expect, on the average, about 0.3 children less than do wives of the same age, which may reflect the fact that, at each higher age group, a greater proportion of those who are still single at the survey date expect to remain so throughout their reproductive lives.

Although data on the childbearing and future expectations of single women are not detailed by race in this review, there are substantial differences between white and black women, especially in average numbers of children already born. Interested readers will find details in the respective

Table 9–7
Births to Date and Lifetime Births Expected per 1,000 Single Women:
1976 to 1979

	Survey Year			
Age of Woman and Subject	1976	1977	1978	1979
18 and 19 years				
Women (thousands)	2,036	2,184	2,201	2,196
Births to date per 1,000	84	91	80	100
Lifetime births expected per 1,000	2,072	2,067	2,013	2,041
20 to 24 years				
Women (thousands)	2,650	2,908	3,221	3,284
Births to date per 1,000	220	172	203	229
Lifetime births expected per 1,000	1,822	1,938	1,885	1,860
25 to 29 years				
Women (thousands)	907	964	1,130	1,280
Births to date per 1,000	424	420	419	463
Lifetime births expected per 1,000	1,424	1,408	1,442	1,496
30 to 34 years				
Women (thousands)	359	461	500	568
Births to date per 1,000	535	633	664	592
Lifetime births expected per 1,000	939	1,063	1,180	988

Source: Bureau of the Census, *Current Population Reports* for the respective surveys.

Current Population Reports on American fertility for the years 1976 through 1979.

The Effect of Omitting Single Women from Expectations Surveys

Prior to 1976 information about expected fertility was available on a national basis only for currently married or ever-married women. These limitations caused reasonable doubts about the reported levels of expected completed fertility, since a very crucial segment was being omitted—the young women who would marry in the near future and within a few years of the survey date bear most of the children born each year (O'Connell and

Table 9–8
Average Expected Parity, for Women of All Marital Statuses and
for Currently Married Women: 1976 to 1979

Survey Year and Age of Woman	Lifetime Births Expected per 1,000 Women		Ratio of Averages, Currently Married Women to All Women (2) ÷ (1)
	All Women (1)	Currently Married Women (2)	
1976			
20 to 24 years	2,009	2,138	1.064
25 to 29 years	2,098	2,202	1.050
30 to 34 years	2,445	2,536	1.037
1977			
20 to 24 years	2,036	2,132	1.047
25 to 29 years	2,049	2,197	1.072
30 to 34 years	2,351	2,468	1.050
1978			
20 to 24 years	2,036	2,178	1.070
25 to 29 years	2,060	2,215	1.075
30 to 34 years	2,297	2,424	1.055
1979			
20 to 24 years	2,022	2,168	1.072
25 to 29 years	2,033	2,193	1.079
30 to 34 years	2,170	2,282	1.052

Source: Bureau of the Census, *Current Population Reports* for the respective surveys.

Moore 1977). Once single women were asked about childbearing to date and all women not currently married were included in the expectations section, it became possible to assess how much earlier surveys may have overstated the expected fertility of entire age groups. The third column of table 9–8 shows at a glance how much average expected parity based on that portion of an age group which is married at the survey date exceeds that based on *all* women in the particular age group.

Generally, the overstatement is in the area of 5 to 6 percent. An interesting point is that the overstatement is no worse for the oldest age group than it is for the youngest; if anything, it is less pronounced, despite the fact that the difference in average expected parity between single women and married women of the same age is far greater at older ages than at younger ages. If this appears to be a quirk in the data, it is only apparent. The effect of including women not currently married in averages of lifetime expected parity depends both on the levels of expected parity and on the proportion not married in each age group. In the younger age groups where the proportion not married is very high, the difference in average expected parity is relatively low. Among older age groups the opposite is true—large differences in expected parity but small proportions of unmarried women.

It seems clear enough that surveys which include only currently married or ever-married women yielded expectation levels which are biased on the high side, although almost certainly by less than 10 percent. This is not unexpected and can, in fact, be adjusted for, if the use of expectations data is to predict completed cohort fertility. This kind of consideration leads to the broader issue of what predictive value expectations data do have, an issue discussed in several chapters in this book.

Birth Expectations as a Predictor

The evidence seems clear enough that questions about birth expectations have a low predictive value, if the object is to foretell what each individual respondent will do (Westoff and Ryder 1977). On the other hand, it is possible to be close to the right answer for less than the best possible reasons, and compensating errors in the aggregate seem to produce this result with birth-expectations data. Women who exceed their stated expectations are offset by others who fall short.

Although the CPS surveys have included expectations of future births since 1971, this period is still too short to see how well young women did in predicting their completed fertility. Projections were made from the 1960 GAF survey, however, which do lend themselves to comparisons of completed cohort fertility from recent surveys.

Basing their work on the expectations reported in the 1960 GAF study, Whelpton, Campbell, and Patterson (1966) adjusted the expectations reported by currently married women with their estimates of the childbearing women then single would experience in their lives (single women were not included in the 1960 GAF) to produce total cohort projections of lifetime fertility. The "most likely" series of 1960 projections are shown in table 9-9, along with completed (or almost completed) fertility as measured by the June 1976 CPS. The differences between the projections based on the 1960 data and the 1976 measures of cumulative fertility to date are extremely small, with the largest difference being about 4 percent of the projected value.

This 1966 work of Whelpton and his associates cannot be dismissed simply as a matter of luck, although it did include their *assumptions* about the fertility of women not included in the survey. Indeed, the accuracy demonstrated by this use of birth expectations affords considerable encour-

Table 9-9
Completed Fertility Projected in 1960 and Actual Lifetime Fertility as of June 1976, for Birth Cohorts from 1921-1925 to 1936-1940

Year of Birth	Age in 1960	Completed Fertility Projected in 1960 [a]	Age in 1976	Actual Lifetime Fertility as of June 1976 [b]	Ratio of Actual to Projected Lifetime Fertility
1921-1925	35-39	2,930	51-55	2,890	0.986
1926-1930	30-34	3,225	46-50	3,125	0.969
1931-1935	25-29	3,255	41-45	3,228	0.992
1936-1940	20-24	2,900	36-40	3,020	1.041

Source: Pascal K. Whelpton, Arthur A. Campbell, and John E. Patterson, *Fertility and Family Planning in the United States* (Princeton, N.J.: Princeton University Press, 1966), table 204; Bureau of the Census, special tabulations of the June 1976 Current Population Survey.

[a] Includes estimates for women marrying after 1960 who would marry by age 45 to 49 but excludes children ever born to single women who do not marry.

[b] Rates are for ever married women as of June 1976.

agement for the sophisticated use of such data for estimating future levels of completed cohort fertility.

Note

1. Studies of fertility conducted in 1971 and 1976 by Melvin Zelnik and John Kantner at The Johns Hopkins University included women of all marital statuses but were limited to women 15 to 19 years old.

References

Freedman, Ronald; Whelpton, Pascal K.; and Campbell, Arthur A. *Family Planning, Sterility and Population Growth.* New York: McGraw-Hill, 1959.

National Center for Health Statistics. *Monthly Vital Statistics Report* 27, no. 11 (1979): supplement.

O'Connell, Martin, and Moore, Maurice J. "New Evidence on the Value of Birth Expectations." *Demography* 14 (1977): 255-264.

Ryder, Norman B. "The Family in Developed Countries." *Scientific American,* September 1974, pp. 123-132.

United States Bureau of the Census. "Fertility of American Women: June 1977." *Current Population Reports,* Series P-20, no. 325 (1978).

Westoff, Charles F., and Ryder, Norman B. "The Predictive Validity of Reproductive Intentions." *Demography* 14 (1977): 431-453.

Whelpton, Pascal K.; Campbell, Arthur A.; and Patterson, John E. *Fertility and Family Planning in the United States.* Princeton, N.J.: Princeton University Press, 1966.

10

The Continuity of Birth-Expectations Data with Historical Trends in Cohort Parity Distributions: Implications for Fertility in the 1980s

George S. Masnick

In this chapter George S. Masnick examines the completed fertility of cohorts of women born since 1940 and uses birth-expectations data to complete the fertility histories of the more recently born women who have not yet reached age 35. He uses a simple, yet novel and revealing, technique: He relates the percentages of a cohort's completed families that are "large," "small," or "medium-sized" to the average (mean) size of family for the cohort. He finds that the distribution of completed families by size category has not been related in any simple way to the average size of complete family since 1940—cohorts have achieved given levels of average fertility with quite different combinations of small, medium, and large families. The youngest cohorts, whose fertility is not yet complete, expect families whose distribution would be different from that of any other recent cohort, being much more concentrated in the medium range, with a preponderance of two-child families. Yet so few of those young women have yet given birth to two children that they will have to bear second children at an unprecedented rate in order to achieve the family-size distribution they expect. Masnick believes that they are unlikely to do so and that many women will forego having the children they now consider simply "postponed." Such large scale "deficit" fertility may be a new phenomenon in American demography and society.—*Eds.*

This chapter reports on a simple exercise designed to contrast the childbearing experience of younger cohorts of U.S. women who are contributing to the recent downswing in fertility with the childbearing of older cohorts who experienced both low and high fertility in the past. Through such a comparison, we hope to gain insight into the likely future fertility of cohorts who are still in the prime of their reproductive years. At the core of the analysis are four graphs depicting the cross tabulation of cohort cumulative fertility through ages 35 to 39 by the percentage of the cohort falling into one of four categories of children ever born. Available data allow us to follow the

The author would like to thank John Pitkin, Dowell Myers, and S. Krishnamoorthy for helpful comments during the preparation of this chapter. An earlier version was presented at the annual meetings of the Population Association of America, Denver, Colorado, 11 April 1980.

actual childbearing experience of various cohorts from the beginning of this century up through 1977.[1] Cumulative fertility through ages 35 to 39 was chosen to represent a level of "almost completed fertility" in order to include as many cohorts as possible experiencing the present downswing in fertility.[2] The four parity categories we have chosen to focus on are: (1) zero children; (2) only one child; (3) two or three children; and (4) four or more children ever born. These cross tabulations were plotted separately for white and nonwhite women.

In addition, data on birth expectations from the June 1976 Current Population Survey, which for the first time included single women, allow us to calculate expected completed fertility and parity distributions when cohorts who were 30 to 34, 25 to 29, and 20 to 24 years old in 1976 reach ages 35 to 39 in 1981, 1986, and 1991 respectively.[3] These hypothetical data points for the future can be compared to the fertility pattern already established by cohorts who were 35 to 39 or older in 1977, and provide additional insight into the value of birth-expectations data as a barometer of future fertility.

Three additional graphs of the trajectories by which the younger cohorts (born after 1940) are approaching their alternative parity levels round out our descriptive analysis.

Large Families

Figure 10–1 demonstrates that there has been a very close association between total fertility and the proportion of a cohort with four or more births. Each point is labeled with the year the cohort reached ages 35 to 39, and reflects childbearing that took place before that date. With the exception of 1976 and 1977, the data points are spaced five years apart and represent nonoverlapping quinquennial cohorts, these latter two dates being included to indicate the direction of the most recent trends.

For both whites and nonwhites, 1945 was the date at which this grouping of 35- to 39-year-olds resulted in those born 1906–1910 having had the lowest total fertility, and 1970 the date when 35- to 39-year-olds (born 1931–1935) had the highest. The magnitude of the swing in total fertility for nonwhites has been greater than that for whites, but the essential pattern of the relationship between total fertility and the incidence of large families of four or more children has been almost identical for whites and nonwhites. The higher the total fertility, the greater the fraction of the cohort with four or more live births; and this relationship is almost linear, with white and nonwhite patterns exceedingly similar.

Fertility at ages 35 to 39 for cohorts who have not yet reached that age was estimated at 95 percent of the value given for average expected com-

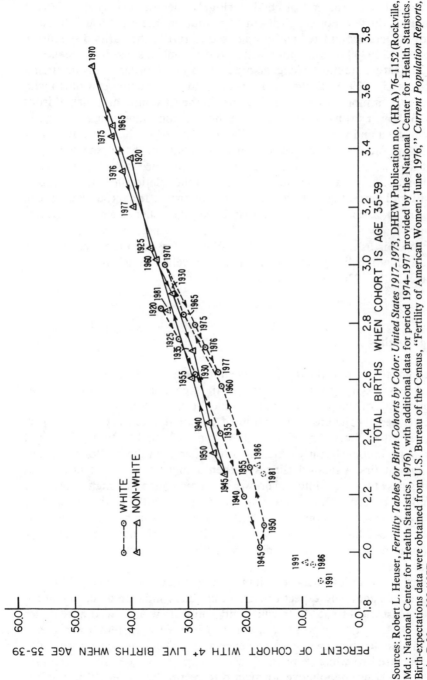

Sources: Robert L. Heuser, *Fertility Tables for Birth Cohorts by Color: United States 1917–1973*, DHEW Publication no. (HRA) 76–1152 (Rockville, Md.: National Center for Health Statistics, 1976), with additional data for period 1974–1977 provided by the National Center for Health Statistics. Birth-expectations data were obtained from U.S. Bureau of the Census, "Fertility of American Women: June 1976," *Current Population Reports*, series P-20, no. 308 (1977).

Figure 10–1. Percentage of Cohort with Four or More Live Births by Total Fertility When Cohort is Aged 35 to 39: White and Non-White Trends (Observations: 1920–1977; Expectations: 1981–1991)

pleted fertility by the end of childbearing, as determined by the Current Population Survey. For simplicity in computation, the unadjusted distribution of expected completed parity was used to reflect the parity distribution at ages 35 to 39. This assumption will introduce only a small bias because of a slightly larger fraction of higher-order than lower-order births occurring after ages 35 to 39. With these caveats in mind, the fraction of women who expect four or more births among cohorts in their twenties and early thirties in 1976 show a strong consistency with the declining family size of slightly older women and with the women who contributed to the first downswing in fertility before the post–World War II baby boom. If the expected fertility of the under-35-year-olds materializes, it will place them slightly below the trend established by historical cohorts on the relationship between total fertility and percentage with four or more live births. In fact, as can be seen in figure 10–2, cohorts born since 1945 have established themselves on trajectories that will most likely lead them to a lower percentage with four or more live births than that of the 1911 cohort, chosen to represent the historically low fertility pattern of women who went through their reproductive ages in the 1920s and 1930s.

Small Families

As straightforward as the trend has been in the association between cohort cumulative fertility and the percentage with large families, the association at the other end of the parity distribution has been much more complex. Figure 10–3 depicts the cross tabulation of cumulative fertility with the percentage of the cohort remaining childless at ages 35 to 39. During the initial downswing in total fertility there was little change in the proportion childless, with at first a small decline and then a slight rise. The level of total childlessness for both white and nonwhite women remained high at between 20 and 30 percent. During the upswing in total fertility, the percentage childless dropped substantially for both whites and nonwhites to a level near 10 percent. On the recent downswing in fertility, whites have begun to show an upturn in the percentage childless, while nonwhites have yet to exhibit a similar trend.

Birth-expectations data revealing the percentage of women still in their reproductive ages who expect to remain childless indicate a further break with the historical trend. Both white and nonwhite women who were under the age of 35 in 1976 expect to remain at or below the current low percentage childless, with nonwhite women expecting a declining percentage childless compared to white women, all while total fertility is simultaneously expected to continue to move downward to record low levels. Will the historical precedent set during the earlier period of the downswing in total fer-

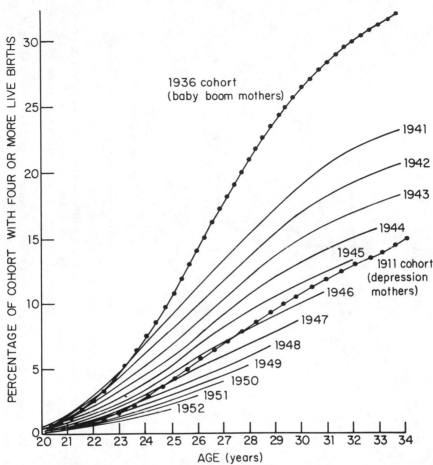

Sources: Robert L. Heuser, *Fertility Tables for Birth Cohorts by Color: United States 1917–1973*, DHEW Publication no. (HRA) 76–1152 (Rockville, Md.: National Center for Health Statistics, 1976), with additional data for period 1974–1977 provided by the National Center for Health Statistics.

Figure 10–2. Percentage of Cohorts of All U.S. Women with Four or More Live Births During Prime Reproductive Ages: Trends for Cohorts Born since 1940

tility (when the proportion childless remained constant) repeat itself, but this time at much lower levels?

In order to address this question, three interpretations can be given to the birth-expectations data appearing in figure 10–3. First, a new pattern of association between declining total fertility and constant proportion childless is indeed emerging for women born since 1940. However, as we shall see later in this chapter, other evidence suggests that the pattern for women with very small families is emerging among the younger cohorts in a manner

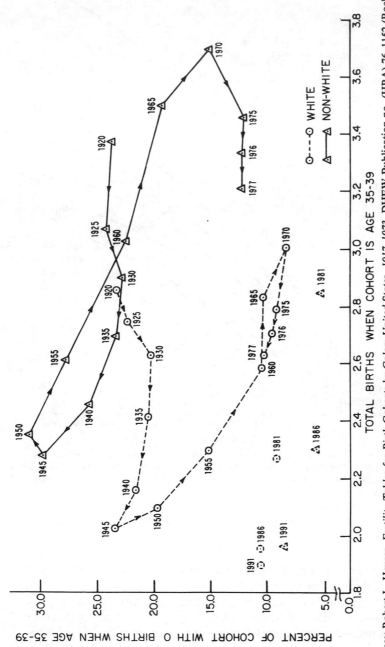

PERCENT OF COHORT WITH 0 BIRTHS WHEN AGE 35-39

TOTAL BIRTHS WHEN COHORT IS AGE 35-39

○----○ WHITE
△——△ NON-WHITE

Sources: Robert L. Heuser, *Fertility Tables for Birth Cohorts by Color: United States, 1917–1973*, DHEW Publication no. (HRA) 76-1152 (Rockville, Md.: National Center for Health Statistics, 1976, with additional data for period 1974–1977 provided by the National Center for Health Statistics. Birth-expectations data were obtained from U.S. Bureau of the Census, "Fertility of American Women: June 1976," *Current Population Reports.* series P-20. no. 308 (1977).

Figure 10–3. Percentage of Cohort With Zero Live Births by Total Fertility When Cohort Is Aged 35 to 39: White and Non-White Trends (Observations: 1920–1977; Expectations: 1981–1991)

very similar to the pattern in the older cohorts who experienced low overall fertility. This suggests the need for other interpretations of the birth-expectations data.

A second interpretation is that the birth-expectations data themselves are more a *normative* statement of what women would like to do if everything could work out as planned, with a higher fraction of these cohorts actually likely to remain childless because "everthing else" will not turn out as hoped. The very low expectations for the proportion remaining childless among nonwhites would seem especially to argue in favor of a normative influence in their response to questions about birth expectations, nonwhites being a group of women whose traditional early assumption of motherhood roles has made childlessness a deviant position.

A third interpretation recognizes that not all women reported on birth expectations, with a very high fraction of the nonrespondents being childless or having only one child at the time of the survey. The reported expectations data might therefore be approximately accurate for those who gave answers but not representative of the cohort as a whole, who actually are expecting higher proportions childless and lower total fertility, because of lower birth expectations concealed by the nonrespondents.

Similar questions about the predictive value of birth-expectations data are called forth when examining figure 10-4, where the proportion of each cohort with only one child is cross tabulated by total fertility. Here, the negative linear association between total fertility and parity is more consistent, both on the two downswing phases as well as the upswing phase of the historical trend in fertility. The similarity in the historical pattern for whites and nonwhites is striking. The closeness of this association between total fertility and only-child families would lead us to predict that an average total fertility of two children for a cohort would include between 25 and 30 percent who would have only one child, based on the proportion observed to have an only child in the historical pattern. However, when the proportions expecting to end up with one child among cohorts who will be completing their fertility in the 1980s are added to the trends in figure 10-4, a departure from the consistent historical pattern is indicated. First, white cohorts do not expect to increase their proportions having an only child while their overall fertility declines, but nonwhite women do. The levels of expected single-child parenthood, 10 to 12 percent for white women and 15 to 20 percent for nonwhite women, are both well below historical levels that were consistent in the past with a low, near-replacement level of fertility.

It is interesting that a higher proportion of nonwhite women expect to have only one child, whereas a lower fraction of nonwhite compared to white cohorts expect to remain childless. Arguing from the perspective that the nonwhite women are being more "realistic" (given the historical pattern) about their prospects of having an only child, one could speculate that

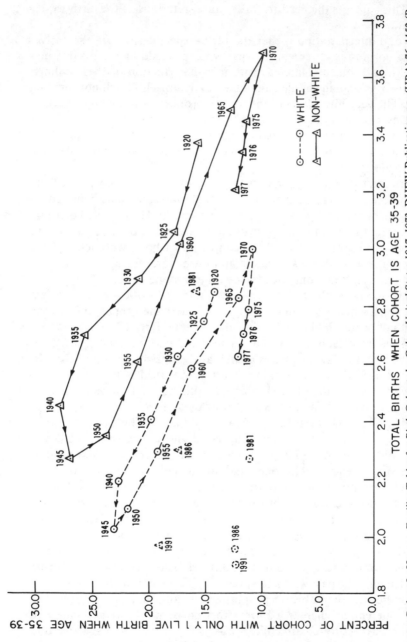

TOTAL BIRTHS WHEN COHORT IS AGE 35-39

Sources: Robert L. Heuser, *Fertility Tables for Birth Cohorts by Color: United States 1917–1973*, DHEW Publication no. (HRA) 76–1152 (Rockville, Md.: National Center for Health Statistics, 1976), with additional data for period 1974–1977 provided by the National Center for Health Statistics.

Figure 10–4. Percentage of Cohort with One Live Birth by Total Fertility When Cohort Is Aged 35 to 39: White and Non-White Trends (Observations: 1920–1977; Expectations: 1981–1991)

several factors might be important. First, nonwhite children are perhaps less likely to be raised as "only" children because of the closer proximity of same-age cousins and neighbors in nonwhite households and neighborhoods, thus making one-child expectations more normatively acceptable for nonwhites than for whites. Second, the higher labor-force participation of nonwhite mothers might make them more sensitive to the difficulties of having more than one child given the demands that children place on time and money today. Third, some of the nonwhite women who actually expect to remain childless might report that they expect to have one child as a first step toward admitting the possibility of having none. Similarly, some childless women who would like to have two or more children might report higher expectations for having one child as a compromise they realize that they may have to accept because of social and economic conditions. The lower rates at which nonwhite women have been able to get married and settle down, largely a function of economic difficulties, one suspects, might introduce a note of greater realism into the calculation of the likelihood of having only one child by nonwhite women. White women in similar circumstances might be more likely to hold on to the belief that conditions will improve for them and that their desires can be achieved. The higher rate of entering motherhood among nonwhites outside of marriage allows some women who do not expect to get married to proceed with motherhood in any case, but under such circumstances it is probably more normatively acceptable to stop at one.

It was previously noted that although the trend in the percentage with zero or one child among 35- to 39-year olds has, since 1970, indeed appeared to move away from the historical association with total fertility and in the direction of the levels indicated by birth expectations for these women, the actual emerging behavior of women under the age of 35 in 1975 places them closer to the historical observations. This conclusion is supported by the data in figure 10–5, which plots the percentage of single-year birth cohorts of all U.S. women who have zero or one child at each single year of age between 20 and 34. Each successive younger cohort in this figure has embarked on a path of transition into small completed family size that has placed them closer and closer to the high proportions childless or having only one child among women passing through the reproductive ages during the late 1920s and 1930s (as exemplified by the 1911 cohort). While there is still room for these younger cohorts to establish small differences from historical cohorts in proportions with zero or one child at the end of reproductivity, the large differences indicated by expectations data appear unlikely if not impossible departures from already established trajectories. Expectations seem to address norms about motherhood and only children more directly than likely behavior. These norms could influence both the

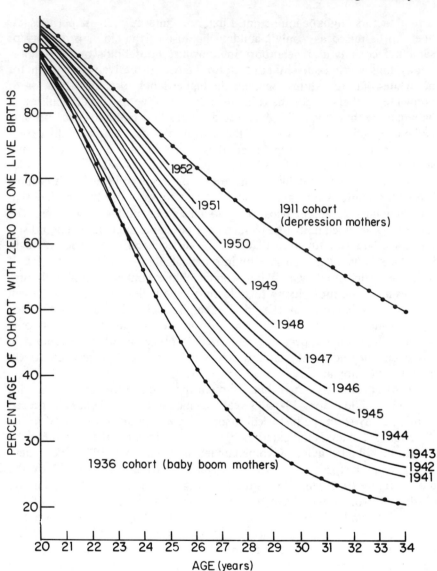

Sources: Robert L. Heuser, *Fertility Tables for Birth Cohorts by Color: United States, 1917-1973,* DHEW Publication no. (HRA) 76-1152 (Rockville, Md.: National Center for Health Statistics, 1976), with additional data for period 1974-1977 provided by the National Center for Health Statistics.

Figure 10-5. Percentage of Cohorts of All U.S. Women with Zero or One Live Birth During Prime Reproductive Ages: Trends for Cohorts Born since 1940

fraction of those who report on birth expectations and the pattern of reporting of those who do.

Medium-Sized Families

Having discussed both small and large families, including those with zero, one, and four or more children, we now consider medium-sized families, those consisting of two or three children. Figure 10-6 shows the historical trend in the percentage of women in successive cohorts who have had two or three children by ages 35 to 39. Once again, the pattern of historical change is complex, with nonwhite women having remained at between 20 and 25 percent on both the initial downswing and the post–World War II upswing in fertility, whereas white women steadily increased from 30 percent bearing two or three children to 50 percent over this same time period. On the recent downswing, nonwhite women have sharply increased their proportion with two or three children, while white women have increased their share of medium-sized families at a more moderate pace. Such a pattern indicates convergence of white and nonwhite trends, but the actual levels still are very different for white and nonwhite women.

The historical trend in the proportion of the cohort with two or three children can probably be best understood in terms of it being a residual category affected by swings in small and large families. On the initial downswing side, the decline in families with four or more children and the increase in families with only one child left the fraction with two or three relatively unchanged. On the upswing side the fraction with two or three children first increased for white women at the expense of declines in zero- or one-child families, then eventually decreased slightly as more and more who achieved two or three children went on to have four or more. For nonwhite women the upswing was marked by an almost simultaneous increase in families with zero or one, leaving the proportion with two or three relatively unchanged. During the recent downturn in fertility, the proportion with four or more fell more rapidly for nonwhites as more and more mothers stopped at two or three children. Those with zero or one have not increased their share as rapidly for cohorts who are in their late thirties. Consequently, the proportion of women with two or three children took a surge upward. In the future, cohorts who approach their mid-thirties will experience a sharp increase in the fraction in the zero- or one-child category relative to the decline in the fraction with four or more, resulting in a *decline* in the fraction with two or three.

Birth-expectations data foretell no such imminent decline in the fraction with two or three children, with the women projecting themselves at

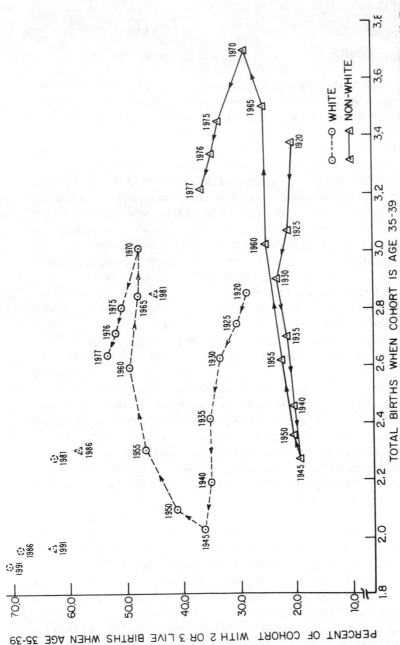

Sources: Robert L. Heuser, *Fertility Tables for Birth Cohorts by Color: United States, 1917–1973*, DHEW Publication no. (HRA) 76–1152 (Rockville, Md.: National Center for Health Statistics, 1976), with additional data for period 1974–1977 provided by the National Center for Health Statistics. Birth-expectations data were obtained from U.S. Bureau of the Census, "Fertility of American Women: June 1976," *Current Population Reports*, series P-20, no. 308 (1977).

Figure 10–6. Percentage of Cohort with Two or Three Live Births by Total Fertility When Cohort Is Aged 35 to 39: White and Nonwhite Trends (Observations: 1920–1977; Expectations: 1981–1991)

between 60 and 70 percent ultimately arriving in the medium family-size range. Anticipating that a much higher fraction of women during the 1980s will actually approach the end of their reproductive years having no children or one child, probably no more than 50 or 55 percent of the cohorts in question will have two or three children; and perhaps this figure could fall as low as 45 percent.

Figure 10-7 presents the picture of how women born since 1940 are approaching the fraction of the cohort reaching the level of two or three children. The mid-thirties represents a point in the life course where the rate at which women are entering this parity category has slowed substantially. Those who are still moving from one child to two are counterbalanced by those progressing from three children to four. In order for women in the cohorts born during the 1950s to exceed 55 percent having two or three children, given the trajectories that these cohorts have established, they will have to *raise* their rates of bearing a second child during their thirties approximately *tenfold* over present levels, while simultaneously reducing the rates at which the fourth child is being born to near zero. Such approximate calculations indicate the unreasonableness of birth expectations as indicators of future behavior for upwards of 20 to 25 percent of cohorts born in the 1950s who expect to have two or three children but who will in fact end their reproductive careers with zero or one child.

Discussion

Our examination of birth-expectations data for 1976 and of historical trends in cohort parity distributions indicates that a substantial fraction of women who are now in the first half of their reproductive ages will move from postponed to foregone fertility as they approach the end of their fecund years. We can be fairly confident, because of consistency in the cohort patterns, that foregone fertility will occur, yet we have only a rudimentary understanding of why this is so and even less of an understanding of the consequences on the lives of the women and their families of such levels of foregone fertility. Of course, if there is response bias in who reports birth expectations, and if expectations are offered as normative answers simply to satisfy the demands of the interview and thus do not accurately reflect anticipated behavior of the respondents, there may be no gap between actual expectations and behavior. If, on the other hand, the expectations data are real and representative, and foregone fertility is a phenomenon beginning to materialize for a substantial fraction of the baby-boom cohorts, it deserves our close attention. While it may be presumptuous to argue for the importance of research on a phenomenon before it actually takes place, it would be foolish to wait until the cohorts have

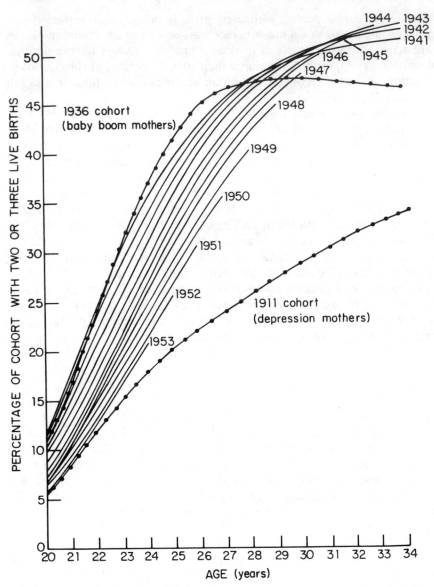

Sources: Robert L. Heuser, *Fertility Tables for Birth Cohorts by Color: United States,*
1917-1973, DHEW Publication no. (HRA) 76-1152 (Rockville, Md.: National Center for
Health Statistics, 1976), with additional data for period 1974-1977 provided by the National
Center for Health Statistics.

Figure 10-7. Percentage of Cohorts of All U.S. Women with Two or Three
Live Births During Prime Reproductive Ages: Trends for
Cohorts Born Since 1940

passed entirely through their reproductive ages and then attempt to reconstruct the events and conditions that served to cause some women, initially expecting to have two or more children, to have an only child, and others to forego parenthood altogether.

Three categories of conditions operate on women who expect to but will fail to replace themselves in the population. The first is hidden physiological problems that will prevent a couple from achieving their expected fertility. The second relates to those changes in attitudes about childbearing that make women and couples change their minds and decide to stop at none or one; these include role conflicts, concerns over costs of raising children, and the emerging importance of life styles that benefit from minimal demands of the type made by children. In these cases the decision to reduce fertility is understood at the time as a positive step taken by the women or couple, although there may be regrets at a later point in the life course when career, the acquisition of material goods, or personal freedom no longer seem so important. The third category of reasons leading to foregone fertility includes essentially uncontrollable events and circumstances that conspire for low fertility against the wishes of those who are potential parents. These include singlehood and divorce, lack of a suitable partner with whom to raise children, lack of confidence in ability to assume parenthood roles and "temporary" postponements of childbearing until the "time is right" that may lead to an inability to have children later in life for physiological or emotional reasons. It is this third category of causes that will be difficult to capture in a single survey and to reconstruct retrospectively, and that may disappear entirely from research findings (based on standard survey methods) as reasons for falling short of birth expectations.

The consequences of foregone fertility have received little attention in fertility research. One needs to be sensitive to consequences throughout the life course, with the reproductive ages, the middle years, and old age expected to provide different contexts within which to evaluate the impact of deficit fertility. Likewise, the reasons for below-replacement fertility, as listed in this chapter, will probably influence the adjustments that men and women make to being childless as well as the accommodations that only children and their parents make to life-course variables such as education, work, leisure, divorce, and old age.

Notes

1. These data are contained in Robert L. Heuser, *Fertility Tables for Birth Cohorts by Color: United States, 1917-1973*, DHEW Publication no. (HRA) 76-1152 (Rockville, Md.: National Center for Health Statistics,

1976); additional data for the period 1974–1977 were provided by the National Center for Health Statistics.

2. Among cohorts born during this century who are no longer in the reproductive ages, between 90 and 95 percent of their total fertility was completed by ages 35 to 39.

3. U.S. Bureau of the Census, "Fertility of American Women: June 1976," *Current Population Reports,* series P-20, no. 308 (1977).

11 Interstate Variations in Birth Expectations

Martin O'Connell

Chapter 9 by Moore and chapter 10 by Masnick are typical of birth-expectations studies in their emphasis on national estimates. That is, the statistics presented and analyzed are for the population of women of childbearing age in the nation as a whole. Estimates for smaller areas are seldom produced because they would not be reliable with samples of the size usually taken in expectations studies. This chapter is important, therefore, because its author, Martin O'Connell, presents estimates of birth expectations for individual states. He is able to do this with a tolerable level of variation in the estimates by combining Current Population Survey data for two years, 1977 and 1978.

The state estimates of birth expectations make available a useful new tool for population forecasting. Much of the demand for forecasting is at the state level; but in the past, as O'Connell notes, forecasts for states have had to assume that their future fertility would be some function of national birth-expectations estimates. With state estimates of expectations, state forecasts have a more realistic future-fertility target.

The state and regional estimates O'Connell provides also shed new light on fertility differentials. He notes, for instance, that although the South has higher current fertility than the non-South, expectations of lifetime births are actually lower in the South. The author concludes that the regional differential in period fertility may represent a difference in timing rather than in ultimate family size; that is, Southern women are bearing children earlier than non-Southern women, but their completed family size is expected to be smaller.—*Eds.*

Introduction

Birth-expectations data often play an integral part in the selection of target fertility levels in national population projections. The basic assumption is that women will bear children according to a fertility schedule that will result in a completed cohort fertility rate equivalent to the prevailing average number of lifetime births expected by women in the primary reproductive ages (U.S. Bureau of the Census 1977).

In the preparation of subnational population projections, most demographers use a cohort-component model that requires assumptions concerning the future time paths and levels of migration, mortality, and fertility rates. Occasionally, target fertility levels for individual states are established based on historical fertility trends pertinent to a particular area (New York

1974) or are simply held constant at their current level (Kentucky 1972). Most states, however, rely on census-bureau fertility projections that are modified to suit their particular needs. In the past, some states have directly incorporated the census-bureau fertility projections into their own population projections (Renshaw 1973). Others, however, have either (1) adopted the time trend of the census-bureau projections, assuming that the ratio of current state fertility rates to national rates remains constant or diminishes slightly over the projection period (Black and Tarver 1965; Iowa 1973) or (2) accepted the ultimate census-bureau target fertility rates, assuming the rates currently in effect for the state will converge with the national rates at some time during the projection period (California 1968; Rhode Island 1966).

The assumption of converging rates was used by the census bureau (1979) in its recent series of state population projections and is often a recommended procedure (Pittenger 1976) in the absence of substantial historical data that would indicate otherwise. This assumption may be especially appealing in light of the absence of a true or native cohort of women in a state owing to interstate migration. The blending of fertility patterns between state and nation over the projection period naturally depends not only on the magnitude of the interstate migration but on the prevailing fertility differences among the states of origin and destination.

In any case, the use of census-bureau fertility projections for any state implicitly involves the use of national birth-expectations data. In this chapter, using birth-expectations data from recent June fertility supplements to the Current Population Survey (CPS), which is a national probability sample of about 55,000 households, and new estimates of fertility rates for states for intercensal years, we will examine whether or not various underlying assumptions employed in state fertility projections are justified. The evidence for any convergence or divergence in the fertility rates for states will be analyzed for the 1940–1977 period, and the correspondence between actual and expected fertility among states for the 1977–1978 period will be examined.

Historical Trends in Period Fertility Rates

The variation in the total fertility rate (TFR)[1] among the states for the period from 1940 to 1977 is shown in table 11-1 for the United States and for its two historically dichotomous regions, the South and the non-South, the latter consisting of the Northeast, the North Central and the West census-defined geographical regions.

The relative variation in the fertility rates in the United States decreased by almost one-half during the baby-boom years between 1940 and 1960,

Table 11-1
Total Fertility Rates (TFR) and Relative Variation of Fertility Rates for the United States, and for South and Non-South Regions, 1940–1977

Year	United States		South		Non-South		Ratio of South to Non-South TFR
	TFR[a]	Relative Variation[b]	TFR	Relative Variation[b]	TFR	Relative Variation[b]	
1977	1,802	0.179	1,877	0.110	1,768	0.204	1.062
1975	1,777	0.159	1,850	0.114	1,743	0.177	1.061
1970	2,480	0.086	2,524	0.076	2,461	0.090	1.026
1960	3,654	0.090	3,652	0.071	3,651	0.093	1.000
1950[c]	3,091	0.133	3,213	0.101	2,916	0.149	1.102
1940[c]	2,119	0.163	2,372	0.127	1,992	0.182	1.191

Source: See table 11-2

[a] Rates may differ from those shown in annual volumes of *Vital Statistics of the United States* because of differences in the adjustment for under-enumeration of the population and registration of births.

[b] Standard deviation divided by the mean for individual states.

[c] Data for this table and subsequent tables exclude Alaska and Hawaii for 1940 and 1950.

remained fairly constant through 1970, but has since doubled by 1977 to a level (0.179) exceeding even that shown for 1940 (0.163). This reduction and subsequent increase in the relative variation in the state fertility rates is the result of the fact that both the greatest increase in fertility during the 1940–1960 period and the greatest decline in fertility during the 1960–1977 period occurred in the states that had the lowest fertility rates, principally the Northeast and North Central states (see table 11–2).

The range of increase during the 1940–1960 period varied from +24 percent for West Virginia to +110 percent for New Jersey; the corresponding range for the 1960–1977 period was from −20 percent for Utah to −61 percent for Massachusetts. The two latter states also had the highest and lowest total fertility rates in 1977 with the rate for Utah (3,454 per 1,000

Table 11–2
Total Fertility Rates by State, 1940 to 1977

State	1977	1975	1970	1960	1950	1940
New England						
Maine	1,817	1,814	2,603	3,892	3,206	2,397
New Hampshire	1,680	1,652	2,497	3,786	3,003	2,198
Vermont	1,683	1,694	2,592	4,018	3,352	2,647
Massachusetts	1,390	1,440	2,349	3,597	2,647	1,847
Rhode Island	1,600	1,536	2,415	3,505	2,562	1,804
Connecticut	1,421	1,444	2,340	3,561	2,506	1,738
Middle Atlantic						
New York	1,625	1,624	2,390	3,298	2,537	1,651
New Jersey	1,615	1,627	2,417	3,448	2,505	1,644
Pennsylvania	1,593	1,590	2,382	3,359	2,633	1,974
East North Central						
Ohio	1,727	1,739	2,518	3,611	3,002	1,997
Indiana	1,823	1,820	2,531	3,688	3,124	2,223
Illinois	1,866	1,845	2,528	3,693	2,838	1,833
Michigan	1,684	1,692	2,586	3,837	3,216	2,270
Wisconsin	1,733	1,732	2,537	3,838	3,159	2,234
West North Central						
Minnesota	1,732	1,716	2,530	4,203	3,487	2,378
Iowa	1,885	1,808	2,508	3,856	3,361	2,287
Missouri	1,793	1,751	2,407	3,640	2,994	1,986
North Dakota	2,191	2,163	2,727	4,399	3,952	2,736
South Dakota	2,212	2,163	2,746	4,371	3,917	2,481
Nebraska	1,936	1,894	2,488	3,965	3,333	2,144
Kansas	1,888	1,820	2,380	3,721	3,170	2,049

Table 11–2 continued

State	1977	1975	1970	1960	1950	1940
South Atlantic						
Delaware	1,642	1,624	2,490	3,865	3,033	2,019
Maryland	1,518	1,493	2,262	3,725	2,850	2,079
Dist. of Col.	1,525	1,442	2,210	3,469	2,750	1,702
Virginia	1,666	1,651	2,364	3,477	3,122	2,505
West Virginia	1,975	1,923	2,522	3,297	3,371	2,657
North Carolina	1,751	1,721	2,429	3,396	3,272	2,519
South Carolina	1,963	1,902	2,542	3,603	3,679	2,592
Georgia	1,878	1,853	2,603	3,613	3,458	2,269
Florida	1,711	1,699	2,472	3,675	3,074	1,979
East South Central						
Kentucky	1,979	1,930	2,517	3,676	3,591	2,807
Tennessee	1,795	1,750	2,368	3,336	3,163	2,159
Alabama	1,930	1,891	2,561	3,631	3,502	2,505
Mississippi	2,232	2,233	3,047	4,264	4,002	2,752
West South Central						
Arkansas	2,016	2,015	2,572	3,711	3,695	2,308
Louisiana	2,152	2,051	2,692	4,091	3,725	2,391
Oklahoma	1,913	1,903	2,370	3,419	3,120	2,284
Texas	2,037	2,041	2,669	3,811	3,444	2,238
Mountain						
Montana	2,093	2,007	2,620	4,231	3,762	2,627
Idaho	2,680	2,501	2,889	4,176	3,786	2,808
Wyoming	2,403	2,212	2,733	3,992	3,545	2,573
Colorado	1,763	1,748	2,353	3,656	3,424	2,300
New Mexico	2,203	2,167	2,875	4,566	4,351	3,414
Arizona	2,191	2,196	2,873	4,229	3,972	2,793
Utah	3,454	3,092	3,310	4,332	4,015	2,993
Nevada	1,951	1,907	2,533	3,784	3,147	2,384
Pacific						
Washington	1,785	1,684	2,352	3,708	3,210	2,023
Oregon	1,815	1,718	2,249	3,595	3,273	2,014
California	1,846	1,783	2,355	3,626	3,035	1,975
Alaska	2,356	2,340	3,084	4,881	a	a
Hawaii	2,256	2,182	2,719	3,887	a	a

Sources: Forrest E. Linder and Robert D. Grove, *Vital Statistics Rates in the United States, 1900–1940* (Washington, D.C.: U.S. Government Printing Office, 1943); Robert D. Grove and Alice M. Hetzel, *Vital Statistics Rates in the United States, 1940–1960* (Washington, D.C.: U.S. Government Printing Office, 1968); National Center for Health Statistics, *Natality*, Vital Statistics of the United States, vol. 1 (Washington, D.C.: U.S. Government Printing Office, 1975); and U.S. Bureau of the Census, unpublished estimates.

[a] Not in the birth registration area in 1940 or 1950.

women) being two and one-half times as large as the rate for Massachusetts (1,390 per 1,000 women).

Even within the two major regions, the relative variation in fertility rates among the states followed the same pattern as that of the United States, although the level of variation for the South is much less than that of the rest of the country for all the periods shown in table 11–1. The principal fertility differences that persist in the South are between the low-fertility South Atlantic states and the high-fertility South Central states. Likewise, the consistent fertility differential in the non-South is between the low-fertility Northeast states and the high-fertility Western states, especially those in the Mountain division. Overall, the difference between the South and the non-South in the TFR (table 11–1) has fallen from being 19 percent higher in the South in 1940, to essentially the same rate in 1960, to around 6 percent higher in the South again in the mid-1970s.[2]

Although the South–non-South regional fertility difference appears to be of lessening importance, figure 11–1 highlights the individual differences in state total fertility rates for 1977. If anything, the state fertility map reveals that the traditional South/non-South fertility differential may be somewhat dated. The new emerging geographical stratifier may be among coastal versus interior states. The very low fertility rates recorded by states along the East Coast and the Great Lakes area are about 0.5 children below the replacement fertility level (about 2.115 per woman), a level exceeded by only eleven states in 1977. A further analysis of the data also indicates a consistent rank ordering of interstate fertility differences for the United States as a whole and within each major region not only between successive time periods but for the entire 1940–1977 observation period (table 11–3).

As a brief summary of the historical fertility variations among the states since 1940, the following points can be made:

1. Although the differences in the level of fertility between the South and non-South regions have considerably decreased since 1940, there appears to be no indication of fertility-rate convergence among individual states either nationally or within these two regions.
2. Considerable variation remains in the rate of change in the state fertility rates over time.
3. A persistent rank-ordering of state fertility rates has existed since 1940 both nationally and within the two major regions.

These findings suggest a careful reexamination of state fertility-projection assumptions, especially those that involve the linking of state to national fertility-projection paths and levels.

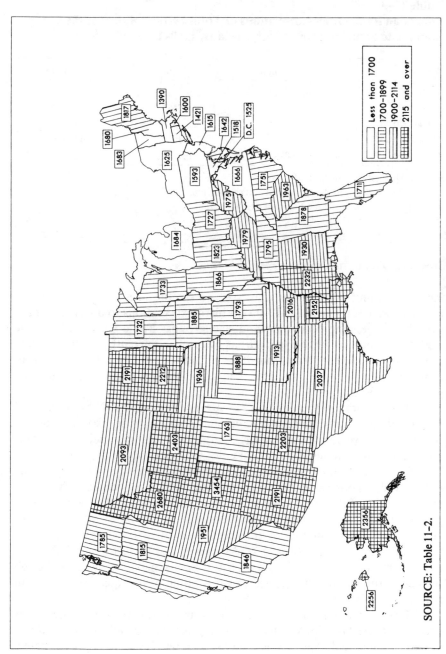

Figure 11-1. Total Fertility Rates, 1977

SOURCE: Table 11-2.

Table 11-3
Spearman Rank-Order Correlations of Total Fertility Rates for the United States, and South and Non-South Regions, 1940-1977

Period [a]	United States	South	Non-South
1940-1977	0.740*	0.621*	0.734*
1970-1977	0.773*	0.855*	0.722*
1960-1970	0.753*	0.552*	0.844*
1950-1960	0.667*	0.353	0.898*
1940-1950	0.879*	0.714*	0.923*

Source: Derived from rates in table 11-2.
[a] Correlations pertain to the fertility rates at the beginning and the end of the stated period.
* = significant at the 0.05 level for a two-tailed test.

Regional Trends in Expected Fertility

The lack of uniformity in the universe and sample sizes of various fertility surveys restricts the historical data on birth expectations to analysis of only very broad geographical units and age groups. Table 11-4 outlines the regional trends in birth-expectations data for currently married white women 18 to 39 years olds from the 1955 and 1960 Growth of American Families Surveys (GAF), the 1965 National Fertility Study (NFS) and the June 1977 CPS.

The authors of the 1955 GAF survey (Freedman, Whelpton, and Campbell 1959) indicate that the regional differences in expectations for wives 18 to 39 years old are not large enough to be statistically significant. However, among wives 18 to 24 years old, women living in the South expect fewer children on the average than those living in the non-South. On the other hand, among wives 35 to 39 years old, the authors noted that women in the South generally recorded more expected births on the average. This reversal in the regional fertility differential from the older to the younger cohorts and the continuing lower expectations of married white women in the South can be seen in the 1960 GAF survey and the 1965 NFS.[3] By 1977 the gap between the South and the non-South had narrowed, although women in the South still reported lower lifetime birth expectations than in the rest of the nation.

More recent data on birth expectations for the 1976-1979 period is shown in table 11-5 for women 18 to 29 years old for all marital statuses and races combined. Age 29 was used as an upper limit since approximately 90 percent of all lifetime births expected have already been born to women

Table 11–4
Average Number of Lifetime Births Expected by Currently Married White Women, 18 to 39 Years Old, by Region of Residence: 1955, 1960, 1965, and 1977

Region of Residence	1977	1965	1960	1955
United States	2.4	3.3	3.1	3.0
South	2.3	3.1	3.1	3.0
Non-South	2.4	3.4	3.3	3.0
Northeast	2.4	3.4	3.2	3.0
North Central	2.5	3.4	3.3	3.1
West	2.4	3.3	3.3	3.0

Sources: Ronald Freedman, Pascal K. Whelpton, and Arthur A. Campbell, *Family Planning, Sterility and Population Growth* (New York: McGraw-Hill, 1959); Norman B. Ryder and Charles F. Westoff, *Reproduction in the United States, 1965* (Princeton, N.J.: Princeton University Press, 1971); and unpublished data from the June 1977 Current Population Survey.

Table 11–5
Births to Date and Lifetime Births Expected per 1,000 Women 18 to 29 Years Old, by Region of Residence, 1976 to 1979

Region	1979	1978	1977	1976
Births to date				
Total U.S.	828	833	837	910
South	890	920	945	992
Non-South	798	790	786	871
Northeast	734	751	737	833
North Central	828	791	815	880
West	819	831	796	895
Lifetime births expected				
Total U.S.	2,033	2,044	2,050	2,059
South	1,970	2,006	2,002	2,019
Non-South	2,063	2,062	2,073	2,078
Northeast	2,026	2,060	2,051	2,062
North Central	2,090	2,062	2,112	2,105
West	2,061	2,066	2,041	2,055

Source: Unpublished data from the June Current Population Surveys.

by age 30, whereas among women 18 to 29 years old, only 40 percent of life-time expected births have been born to date. Although women in the South for these four survey dates have an average number of births to date some 10 to 20 percent higher than in the non-South, the South still shows slightly lower expected fertility.[4] Whether this higher childbearing to date in the South simply reflects a different child-spacing pattern or a real and persistent difference that will eventually raise the South's completed fertility above that of the rest of the nation will be reviewed in the final section of this chapter.

Interstate Variations in Expected Fertility

For each state the average number of lifetime births expected per 1,000 women 18 to 29 years old for 1977–1978 is shown in figure 11-2 and reported, along with the standard error for each average, in table 11-6. An average of the 1977 and 1978 rates, weighted by the numbers of women reporting on birth expectations in each state for each survey year,[5] was used to obtain a more stable fertility rate considering the often small size of the base of reporting women in some states.[6]

Although the state birth-expectations data produce a good correlation with the state fertility rates ($r = 0.595$), even when Utah is omitted from the calculations,[7] the relative variation in the average number of lifetime births expected (0.061) is less than one-half that of the total fertility rate (0.140). This is not an unexpected finding since period fertility rates, such as the total fertility rate, are traditionally more subject to variation resulting from current circumstances and timing patterns than are cohort or completed fertility rates such as the number of lifetime births expected (Campbell 1973; Ryder 1974).

The highest average number of lifetime births expected is found in Utah, 3,468 per 1,000 women, which is essentially the same as its total fertility rate of 3,454 per 1,000 women in 1977. The second highest state is Idaho, with 2,472 births per 1,000 women, which also has the second highest TFR for 1977, 2,680 births per 1,000 women. The high rates reported in both these states and in the Mountain states in general are probably indicative of the substantial Mormon influence in this area. (Spicer and Gustavus 1974) The lowest lifetime birth rate is reported for Washington, D.C., which at an average of 1.8 children per woman is still above its 1977 total fertility rate of 1.5 children per woman.

Only thirteen states record lifetime birth expectations above replacement-level fertility; out of the eleven states that have period total fertility rates for 1977 in excess of replacement-level fertility, seven states also have

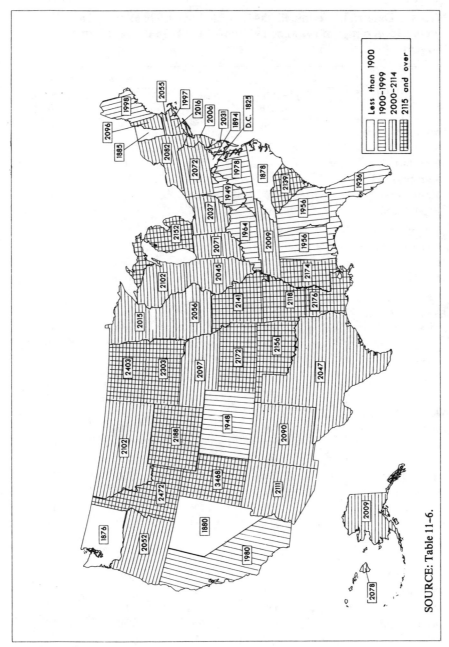

Figure 11–2. Lifetime Births Expected, 1977–1978

SOURCE: Table 11-6.

Table 11–6
Births to Date and Lifetime Births Expected per 1,000 Women 18 to 29 Years Old: Average of the June 1977 and June 1978 Current Population Surveys

State	Number of Women [a]	Births to Date	Lifetime Births Expected Rate	Lifetime Births Expected Standard Error of Rate
New England				
Maine	74	987	1,998	109
New Hampshire	73	817	2,096	123
Vermont	45	859	1,885	153
Massachusetts	455	668	2,055	49
Rhode Island	68	756	1,997	125
Connecticut	231	672	2,016	76
Middle Atlantic				
New York	1,222	748	2,082	31
New Jersey	488	721	2,006	48
Pennsylvania	946	772	2,072	34
East North Central				
Ohio	894	847	2,037	36
Indiana	463	917	2,071	49
Illinois	972	780	2,045	34
Michigan	737	825	2,152	39
Wisconsin	372	804	2,102	53
West North Central				
Minnesota	320	717	2,015	61
Iowa	237	743	2,056	67
Missouri	408	670	2,141	53
North Dakota	58	824	2,403	134
South Dakota	54	806	2,303	156
Nebraska	139	795	2,097	81
Kansas	194	852	2,172	71
South Atlantic				
Delaware	44	649	2,031	143
Maryland	337	775	1,894	58
Dist. of Col.	54	646	1,825	172
Virginia	458	777	1,978	48
West Virginia	167	1,020	1,949	80
North Carolina	495	872	1,878	41
South Carolina	236	1,079	2,139	60
Georgia	428	956	1,956	50
Florida	605	839	1,936	43

Table 11-6 continued

State	Number of Women [a]	Births to Date	Lifetime Births Expected	
			Rate	*Standard Error of Rate*
East South Central				
Kentucky	288	936	1,964	62
Tennessee	386	1,023	2,009	53
Alabama	325	994	1,956	53
Mississippi	185	1,117	2,174	85
West South Central				
Arkansas	141	1,287	2,118	83
Louisiana	333	995	2,176	62
Oklahoma	220	1,137	2,156	70
Texas	1,008	905	2,047	35
Mountain				
Montana	69	939	2,102	128
Idaho	78	927	2,472	150
Wyoming	37	850	2,188	179
Colorado	247	804	1,948	65
New Mexico	99	889	2,090	119
Arizona	177	826	2,111	84
Utah	121	1,144	3,468	150
Nevada	56	837	1,880	147
Pacific				
Washington	325	784	1,876	58
Oregon	229	872	2,052	64
California	1,806	778	1,980	26
Alaska	34	893	2,009	188
Hawaii	75	679	2,078	143

Source: Unpublished data from the June 1977 and June 1978 Current Population Surveys.
[a] Number of women in thousands. Rates based on number of women reporting on birth expectations.

their lifetime birth expectations above replacement (Utah, Idaho, Wyoming, North and South Dakota, Louisiana, and Mississippi) while the remaining four (Hawaii, Alaska, New Mexico, and Arizona) have lifetime birth expectations of at least two children per woman.

A further analysis of the birth-expectations data is presented in table 11-7, which shows the simple zero-order correlations between several socioeconomic indicators available from the CPS and the two components of the

Table 11–7
Zero-Order Correlations Between Birth Expectations Data and Socioeconomic Variables for Women 18 to 29 Years Old: Average of the June 1977 and June 1978 Current Population Surveys [a]

Socioeconomic Variables	Births to Date	Additional Births Expected	Lifetime Births Expected
College [b]	−0.595*	0.579*	0.127
Labor force [c]	−0.507*	0.303*	−0.144
Poverty [d]	0.725*	−0.605*	−0.020
Black [e]	0.165	−0.351*	−0.286*
Married [f]	0.602*	−0.239	0.330*
South [g]	0.478*	−0.584*	−0.258

Source: June 1977 and June 1978 Current Population Surveys.
* = significant at the 0.05 level for a two-tailed test.
[a] Correlations exclude Utah.
[b] Percentage of women in state having one or more years of college.
[c] Percentage of women in state in the labor force.
[d] Percentage of women in state living in areas of poverty.
[e] Percentage of women in state who are black.
[f] Percentage of women in state who are currently married.
[g] Dummy variable: non-South = 0, South = 1.

birth-expectations data, the actual number of births to date and the additional number of births expected. While the usual associations found between socioeconomic indicators and the number of births to date prevail on a state-by-state basis (for example, higher fertility in states in the South and in states with relatively few women with a college education or in the labor force), little association is found between these same variables and the average number of lifetime births expected. In fact, surprisingly little correlation ($r = 0.191$) was found between the number of births to date and the number of lifetime births expected! Of course, these correlations do not and are not meant to establish any causality among the variables. They do, however, describe the association between traditional socioeconomic indicators (which themselves are often used to project future fertility patterns) and the fertility indicators, and point out the relatively disappointing nonvariation among the majority of the states in the number of lifetime births expected.[8]

One interpretation of the results shown in table 11–7 would suggest that women in the survey first mentally fix their completed family size and then report the appropriate number of additional births expected to meet the stated number. Assuming relatively uniform responses to completed family size throughout the United States, the states with the initially higher average number of births to date would, of course, report a smaller number of additional births expected. This type of response pattern would account for the reversal of the signs of the correlation coefficients between the births to date and the additional births expected indicators ($r = -0.668$ for births to date versus additional births expected). A rather pessimistic evaluation of these expectations data, then, would be that the women in the survey are reporting an abstract family-size value instead of a realistic appraisal of their current situations.

On the other hand, a more optimistic advocate of birth-expectations data would point to the aknowledged fact that cohort-fertility indicators such as lifetime births are not nearly as sensitive to current conditions as are period-fertility indicators. The stronger association between current socioeconomic indicators and actual fertility to date than with projected fertility, therefore, may be quite reasonable. Perhaps a more cogent level of analysis would be to examine expected fertility with the lifetime outlook of women in terms of their projected educational or working plans (Waite and Stolzenberg 1976) rather than with their current situation.

Prospects for the Future

What does this comparative analysis of actual and expected fertility suggest for the future trends of fertility rates? On the regional level, data indicate that the South–non-South difference is substantially smaller than it was some thirty to forty years ago. Although the South still has higher levels of births to date and TFR, women in the South have traditionally shown an expected completed family size less than or equal to that for the rest of the nation. This anomaly can be partly explained by the differences in the timing of births in the two regions. Whereas age-specific fertility rates for women up to age 24 have been traditionally higher in the South, these same women have had lower levels of fertility past age 25 for more recent time periods (Grove and Hetzel 1968: U.S. Bureau of the Census 1979).

In addition, various fertility surveys in the past decade have shown that contraceptive sterilization operations, which are most frequently performed on women in their late twenties or thirties, are more prevalent among women in the South than in the non-South (Westoff and Ryder 1977; Westoff and McCarthy 1979). These two points lend support to the credibility of the South's lower lifetime expectations despite its higher average number of births to date.

Even Ryder and Westoff, who are not generally considered enthusiastic supporters of birth-expectations data, conclude

> ... that there is probably little intrinsic cultural quality still differentiating regions in terms significant for fertility. ... And since regions of the country are becoming more similar in education and income and increasingly more uniformly exposed to sets of national norms diffused through the mass media, the whole concept of region has become less important in differentiating not only fertility but behavior of all kinds. [Ryder and Westoff 1971, p. 89]

Whether the blending of regional fertility norms and rates is caused by the mass media, by the spread of contraceptive knowledge, or by the migration of women themselves, it seems reasonable to use similar target fertility rates for population projections for both the South and non-South regions, although it would be preferable to allow for a more rapid and earlier childbearing pattern in the South.

The assumption that one must use either national fertility trends or target fertility rates for individual states, however, can be a precarious one unless strong historical data is present. Figure 11-3 indicates, in percentage points, how much the state TFR for 1977 is above or below the average number of lifetime births expected by women 18 to 29 years old currently residing in that state for the 1977–1978 period. The unweighted mean deviation for all states is − 9 percent and ranges from a low of − 20 to − 30 percent in the Northeast to around 0 to + 10 percent in the Mountain states. A low of − 32 percent was recorded for Massachusetts and a high of + 17 percent for Alaska.

Considering the theoretical and computational differences between the period fertility rate and the average number of lifetime births expected,[9] does the apparent "backlog" of fertility for many Northeastern states, as judged by their currently low fertility rates, signify that the current cohorts of women in the prime reproductive ages in these states will fail to live up to their expectations or replacement-level fertility? An additional appraisal of these chances may be made by examining how many births women have already had to date in relation to their lifetime birth expectations. In other words, is the current tempo of childbearing commensurate with the expected number of lifetime births?

For the United States as a whole, the percent of lifetime births already born for women 18 to 29 years old for the 1977–1978 period was about 40 percent. Although the states with the highest percentages were concentrated in the South, those with the lowest percentages did not display any pronounced regional pattern. In fact, Massachusetts and Utah, the two states with the lowest and highest TFRs and lifetime births expected, both had 33 percent of lifetime expected births already born by the survey date.

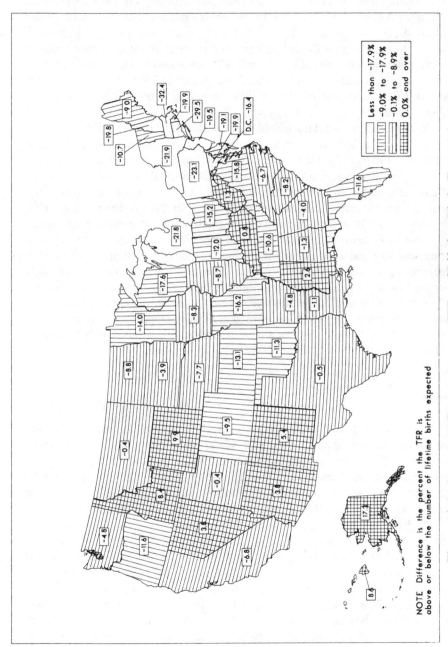

NOTE Difference is the percent the TFR is above or below the number of lifetime births expected

Figure 11–3. Percent Difference Between TFR and Lifetime Births Expected, 1977

Placing these statistics in historical perspective, the 1904–1915 birth cohort of American women completed their childbearing years with about 2.3 children per woman; in 1933, when this cohort was 18 to 29 years old, they had an average of 0.8 births per woman already born to date (Heuser 1976) or about one-third of their lifetime fertility completed. This rate compares favorably with that of Massachusetts which in 1977–1978 had an average of 2,055 lifetime births per 1,000 women and 668 births to date per 1,000 women.

This aspect of the data would seem to indicate that the birth expectations of Massachusetts women are more in line with their cumulative number of births to date than are those of women in Utah. In Utah, women of the same age expect almost one more additional birth (2.3 additional births per woman) than women in Massachusetts (1.4 additional births per woman), yet they have the same proportions of lifetime births already born; obviously, they have a lot more to accomplish in the same amount of time.

This brief examination of both state fertility rates and birth-expectations data illustrates the potential pitfalls involved in making state fertility projections. By using both sets of data together, one may better formulate current fertility projections and judge the credibility and likely persistence of the prevailing period fertility rates and cohort birth expectations. Perhaps the interstate migration of women, and with them their accompanying fertility norms, may prove to be the greatest leveler of state fertility patterns in the long run.

Notes

1. The total fertility rate (TFR) for à given year is the number of children a woman would have at the end of her reproductive life, if she experiences at each age the prevailing age-specific birth rates in effect for the specified year. Arithmetically, it is the sum of the five-year age-specific birth rates between 10 to 14 and 45 to 49 years of age, multiplied by 5. The rates in this chapter usually are expressed as births per 1,000 women.

2. Rindfuss (1978) reports that the South has had lower TFRs than the non-South since the mid-1950s. His rates, however, are indirectly estimated from "own-children" data recorded in the 1960 and 1970 censuses. An examination of the rates presented in his paper, even during census years when both state-population counts and vital-registration data on births are available, indicates an underestimation of fertility in both major regions. As he shows elsewhere (Rindfuss 1976), blacks, who proportionately are more concentrated in the South, have a greater degree of underestimation of their fertility (8.5 percent) during the period 1945–1969 than do whites

(2.5 percent). His use of own-children data, then, seems questionable as a means of establishing a difference in fertility levels between the two regions.

3. The realization of these birth expectations is suggested in recent 1970 census data (U.S. Bureau of the Census 1973, table 1) and CPS data (U.S. Bureau of the Census 1978, table 8), where the completed fertility of ever-married white women 35 to 44 years old is lower in the South than in the rest of the nation. This is true even when the data are examined according to region of birth and not just current residence (U.S. Bureau of the Census 1973, table 15).

4. This same pattern of childbearing in the South—higher average numbers of births to date but lower lifetime births than in the non-South—was also noted in the 1955 GAF survey (Freedman, Whelpton, and Campbell 1959, p. 317).

5. About 75 percent of all women 18 to 29 years old in the surveys provided a numerical response to the birth-expectations question. The likely effect of omitting nonreporting women from the calculations of lifetime birth rates seems to be minimal (Moorman, Moore, and O'Connell 1978).

6. An examination of the CPS data was made to see if the survey could be feasibly used to analyze fertility rates down to the individual state. An abbreviated general fertility rate for women 20 to 44 years old was computed for each state from the June 1977 CPS for births reported in the survey for the period July 1976 to June 1977. This rate was compared with an average of general fertility rates by state for 1976 and 1977 computed from vital-registration data and census-bureau population estimates for states. A two-year average was used to account for the CPS overlap of two calendar years. The resulting zero-order correlation for the fifty states and the District of Columbia was 0.776, and the Spearman rank-order correlation was 0.637. The unweighted mean of the general fertility rates using the vital-statistics data was 74.0 births per 1,000 women 20 to 44 years old, whereas the CPS data produced a mean of 76.3 births per 1,000 women.

7. Since the TFR and the lifetime birth rate for Utah are considerably above the general range of data for the other fifty areas and therefore seriously distort the ensuing statistical analysis, all correlations subsequent to this section omit Utah.

8. Only one-sixth (206) of the 1,225 possible comparisons of the average number of lifetime births expected among the forty-nine states (Utah excluded) and the District of Columbia were found to be significantly different at a level of two standard errors (table 11–6). Utah, however, was found to be significantly different from all the states.

9. The TFR is a hypothetical estimate of completed fertility for a synthetic cohort of women based on fertility rates for a given year, whereas the number of lifetime births expected is an estimate of completed fertility for a

true cohort of women projected to the end of their reproductive life span. In times of declining fertility, the TFR is usually below the cohort fertility rate (Ryder 1974).

References

Black, Therel R., and Tarver, James D. *Age and Sex Population Projections of Utah Counties.* Bulletin 457, Agricultural Experiment Station, Utah State University, Logan, 1965.

California, Department of Finance. *Estimated and Projected Population of California, 1960-2000.* Sacramento, 1968.

Campbell, Arthur A. "Three Generations of Parents." *Family Planning Perspectives* 5 (1973): 106–112.

Freedman, Ronald; Whelpton, Pascal K.; and Campbell, Arthur A. *Family Planning, Sterility and Population Growth.* New York: McGraw-Hill, 1959.

Grove, Robert D., and Hetzel, Alice M. *Vital Statistics Rates in the United States, 1940-1960.* Washington, D.C.: U.S. Government Printing Office, 1968.

Heuser, Robert M. *Fertility Tables for Birth Cohorts by Color: United States, 1917-73.* DHEW Publication no. (HRA) 76-1152. Washington, D.C.: U.S. Government Printing Office, 1976.

Iowa. *Population Projections by Age and Sex for State and Counties of Iowa, 1975-1990.* Agriculture and Home Economics Experimental Station, Iowa State University, 1973.

Kentucky, Program Development Office. *Kentucky Population Projections: 1975-2020,* vol. 1. Frankfort, 1972.

Linder, Forrest E., and Grove, Robert D. *Vital Statistics Rates in the United States, 1900-1940.* Washington, D.C.: U.S. Government Printing Office, 1943.

Moorman, Jeanne E.; Moore, Maurice J.; and O'Connell, Martin. "Predicting Future Births for Nonreporting Women: An Application of Discriminant Analysis." In *1978 Proceedings of the Social Statistics Section,* pp. 698–703. Washington, D.C.: American Statistical Association, 1978.

National Center for Health Statistics. *Natality.* Vital Statistics of the United States, 1970, vol. 1. Washington, D.C.: U.S. Government Printing Office, 1975.

New York, State Office of Planning Services. *Demographic Projections for New York State Counties to 2000 A.D.* Albany, 1974.

Pittenger, Donald B. *Projecting State and Local Populations.* Cambridge, Mass.: Ballinger Publishing Company, 1976.

Renshaw, Vernon. *Nebraska Population Projections: State, County, Region, and Town, 1975–2020.* Lincoln: University of Nebraska Bureau of Business Research, 1973.

Rhode Island, Statewide Comprehensive Transportion and Land Use Planning Program. *Population Projections for the State of Rhode Island and Its Municipalities, 1970–2000.* Providence, 1966.

Rindfuss, Ronald R. "Annual Fertility Rates from Census Data on Own Children: Comparisons with Vital Statistics Data for the United States." *Demography* 13 (1976): 235–249.

———. "Changing Patterns of Fertility in the South: A Social-Demographic Examination." *Social Forces* 57 (1978): 621–635.

Ryder, Norman B. "The Family in Developed Countries." *Scientific American,* September 1974, pp. 123–132.

Ryder, Norman B., and Westoff, Charles F. *Reproduction in the United States, 1965.* Princeton, N.J.: Princeton University Press, 1971.

Spicer, Judith C., and Gustavus, Susan O. "Mormon Fertility Through Half a Century: Another Test of the Americanization Hypothesis." *Social Biology* 21 (1974): 70–76.

United States Bureau of the Census. "Women by Number of Children Ever Born." *Subject Reports.* Census of Population, 1970, PC(2)-3A. Washington, D.C.: U.S. Government Printing Office, 1973.

———. "Projections of the Population of the United States: 1977 to 2050." *Current Population Reports,* series P-25, no. 704 (1977).

———. "Fertility of American Women: June 1977." *Current Population Reports,* series P-20, no. 325. (1978).

———. "Illustrative Projections of State Populations by Age, Race, and Sex: 1975 to 2000." *Current Population Reports,* series P-25, no. 796 (1979).

Waite, Linda J., and Stolzenberg, Ross M. "Intended Childbearing and Labor Force Participation of Young Women: Insights from Nonrecursive Models." *American Sociological Review* 41 (1976): 235–251.

Westoff, Charles F., and McCarthy, James. "Sterilization in the United States." *Family Planning Perspectives* 11 (1979): 147–154.

Westoff, Charles F., and Ryder, Norman B. *The Contraceptive Revolution.* Princeton, N.J.: Princeton University Press, 1977.

12

Desired Family Size of Young American Women, 1971 and 1976

Marilyn B. Hirsch,
Judith R. Seltzer, and
Melvin Zelnik

Authors of earlier chapters have noted that most expectations data are collected for married women. Only since 1976 has the Current Population Survey (CPS) asked about birth expectations of single women, and so far the CPS has limited those questions to adult women, aged 18 or older. As Moore noted in chapter 9, the omission of single women from the CPS before 1976 resulted in an overstatement of average birth expectations of about 5 percent. That is, had single women been included, as they were in later years, birth expectations would have been slightly lower. The error was larger among younger women, a larger proportion of whom were single. Since today's young women will be responsible for the bulk of fertility in the near future, it should be apparent that good information about birth expectations, both among the single and the married, is necessary for fertility forecasting.

A good beginning toward that goal has been made by the National Surveys of Young Women in 1971 and 1976, which are the basis for this chapter by Hirsch, Seltzer, and Zelnik. Those surveys included national samples of women 15 to 19 years of age, both married and single. In this chapter the authors focus on the trend in fertility desires among teenagers between 1971 and 1976, and on differences between subgroups of the teenaged population. Their work can be compared with Ryder's in chapter 7, which also examined trends in fertility orientations, but among older, married women. Ryder found that fertility desires declined between 1970 and 1975, apparently because of changing social and economic conditions. The authors of this chapter reach a similar conclusion: The fertility desires of teenaged women declined between 1971 and 1976, and the reasons were apparently financial—in 1976 both single and married teenagers (but especially the married) were coming to believe they simply could not afford the larger families desired by teenagers five years before.

It may be surprising that the fertility desires of even unmarried teenaged women should be responsive to short-term fluctuations in the economy. It bespeaks a kind of "rationality" in fertility-related behavior that, once

The 1971 and 1976 surveys on which this chapter is based were supported by grant no. HD-05255 from the National Institute of Child Health and Human Development, Department of Health, Education, and Welfare (DHEW). Assistance was also received from the Ford Foundation and the General Services Foundation. The analysis itself has been funded, at least in part, with DHEW funds under contract N01-HD-82848. The contents of this chapter do not necessarily reflect the views or policies of DHEW. The authors gratefully acknowledge the assistance of Judy Gehret and Nelva Hitt.

understood, could make prediction possible. That is not to say, of course, that all variation in fertility orientations can be understood in rational economic terms. Hirsch, Seltzer, and Zelnik demonstrate in this chapter that many characteristics of teenaged women's backgrounds, such as race and number of siblings, are closely related to their fertility desires, probably causally related; it is hard to interpret such relationships in rational terms. However, the existence of such structurally determined differences need not conflict with the interpretation of changes as economically motivated; for instance, the authors' data show that there was a substantial difference between the fertility desires of black and white teenagers in both 1971 and 1976, but that in both racial groups there was a decline in fertility desires between those dates.—*Eds.*

Introduction

Family-size preference is sometimes used to estimate future fertility for cohorts of married women. Because of the widespread use of effective contraceptives by married women in the United States, data on family-size preference are considered a fairly reliable indicator of future fertility trends. Only recently have the fertility preferences of both unmarried and ever-married adolescent women been a subject of interest in social-science research. In two National Surveys of Young Women (NSYW) conducted in 1971 and 1976, young women aged 15 to 19 were asked how many children they wanted to have. In 1971 a sample of 4,359 teenagers indicated an average desired family size of 2.68. By 1976 another sample of 2,183 teenagers had lowered their average desired family size to 2.52.[1]

The literature refers to various concepts related to the number of children or family size: ideal, desired, intended, and expected. In the 1965 National Fertility Study (NFS), comparisons were made of responses to questions on the ideal number of children as well as the number desired, intended, and expected (Ryder and Westoff 1969). *Ideal* connotes what may be ideal for the average American family rather than what individual couples may want for themselves. Ryder and Westoff found that the difference between the number of children expected and the number intended was insignificant and suggested therefore that the terms may be used synonymously. The difference between desired and intended parity was equally small for the total sample, although the distribution for the two concepts varied, that is, the most likely values for desired family size were 2 and 4, but for intended family size, 2 and 3. When desires and intentions were analyzed by race, desires exceeded intentions for whites (3.29 compared to 3.16) and intentions were greater than desires for blacks (3.79 versus 3.21). In comparing intentions and desires, Ryder and Westoff also found that 80 percent of women who "intended" to have more children gave the same responses to questions on the number desired and the number intended. They concluded that there was an apparent identity in responses to questions referring to these various concepts of family size on an aggregate level.[2]

Data on desired family size from the two NSYW surveys is compared to data on lifetime birth expectations from the Current Population Survey (CPS) in table 12–1.[3] Both sources of data show a decline in desired and expected family size between 1971 and 1976. The young women in the NSYW surveys reported somewhat higher desires than were reported in the CPS for approximately equivalent age groups regardless of whether currently married women or all women are considered.

Differences in these two sources of data may result from varying perceptions of the terms *desired family size* and *birth expectations* despite the Ryder and Westoff finding of no difference at the aggregate level. Another possible source of difference may be the percentage of the sample reporting. In both NSYW surveys, nearly 100 percent of the sample responded, while in the 1976 CPS, 84 percent of the ever-marrieds and 63 percent of the

Table 12–1
Desired Family Size and Lifetime Birth Expectations for All Women and Currently Married Women, 1971 and 1976

	1971		1976	
	All Women	Currently Married	All Women	Currently Married
Desired family size (NSYW), by age				
15–17	2.68	2.53	2.54	2.52
18–19	2.67	2.64	2.50	2.45
Lifetime birth expectations (CPS), by age				
14–17	NA	2.50	NA	2.03
18–19	NA	2.26	2.09	2.16

Sources (desired family size): National Surveys of Young Women, 1971 and 1976; lifetime birth expectations (1971): U.S. Bureau of the Census, "Fertility Histories and Birth Expectations of American Women: June 1971," Current Population Reports, series P-20, no. 263 (1974), table 68, p. 144; (1976): U.S. Bureau of the Census, "Prospects for American Fertility: June 1976 (Advance Report)," Current Population Reports, series P-20, no. 300 (1976) table 2, p. 2; and ibid., "Fertility of American Women: June 1976," Current Population Reports, series P-20, no. 308 (1977), table 6, p. 17.

NA = not available.

never-marrieds in the sample responded to this question.[4] Those not reporting either were uncertain about the number of expected births or gave a
nonnumerical response. In addition, data from the NSYW and the CPS
may be subject to different levels of sampling and nonsampling variability.

The downward trend in the average desired family size between 1971
and 1976 for the NSYW surveys was produced by slightly higher percentages of young women at the later date responding that they wanted 0, 1,
or 2 children and slightly lower percentages wanting 4 or more (see table
12-2). The shift to smaller desired family size occurred for both blacks and
whites, although a considerably higher proportion of black teenagers
wanted families with two or fewer children than did their white counterparts
in either survey year.[5] In 1971, 61.9 percent of blacks wanted two or fewer
children compared to 64.4 percent in 1976. Among white teenagers, the
shift to smaller desired family size was somewhat greater—from 50.3 percent in 1971 to 55. 6 percent in 1976. Differences in average desired family
size between the racial groups were statistically significant in both years
($p < .01$). In table 12-3, the difference in average desired family size
between 1971 and 1976 is examined and found to be highly significant for
whites and all 15 to 19 year olds ($p < .01$) and less significant for blacks
($p < .10$).

Comparison of Differences in Average Desired Family Size

In the first stage of the analysis, desired family size was examined in relation
to various background and explanatory variables for both surveys. Average
desired family size is discussed instead of percentage distributions in order
to simplify tabular presentations and to facilitate testing of differences
among the means of the categories of variables. All analysis was carried out
separately for black and white teenagers as well as for the total sample. In
other analyses of these data, the attitudes and behavior of blacks and whites
have been sufficiently different as to suggest that separate examination by
race is useful.[6]

Previous research on family-size preferences led to the conclusion that
young people form their attitudes at a relatively early age (Gustavus and
Nam 1970; Westoff and Potvin 1966). In the two NSYW surveys, teenagers
were not queried as to whether they had previously thought about family
size; but the fact that almost the entire sample of young women in both 1971
and 1976 responded to this question may indicate earlier consideration of
desired family size. Fairly low percentages of nonresponse to a succeeding
question on reasons for having a specified number of children gives additional evidence of previous thought to family-size desires.

Table 12–2
Percentage Distribution of Desired Family Size by Race, 1971 and 1976 [a]

Desired Family Size	White (%)	Black (%)	Total (%)
1971			
0	4.0	6.5	4.8
1	3.6	9.8	5.6
2	42.7	45.6	43.7
3	24.1	15.8	21.4
4	17.0	15.3	16.4
5	3.6	2.8	3.4
6 or more	5.0	4.2	4.7
Total	100.0	100.0	100.0
N	(2935)	(1424)	(4359)
Mean	2.77	2.49	2.68
S.D.	1.28	1.35	1.31
t		6.76 (0.01) [b]	
1976			
0	5.7	7.3	6.2
1	4.8	11.8	7.0
2	45.1	45.3	45.2
3	23.4	17.2	21.4
4	13.9	12.0	13.3
5	3.7	2.3	3.2
6 or more	3.3	4.0	3.5
Total	99.9	99.9	99.8
N	(1486)	(697)	(2183)
Mean	2.59	2.38	2.52
S.D.	1.26	1.33	1.28
t		3.64 (0.01)	

[a] This and all subsequent tables refer to women 15 to 19 years of age. Statistics presented in all tables are based on unweighted data. Other published articles on the 1971 and 1976 NSYW generally use weighted data to reflect the U.S. population of women.

[b] Significance level of differences among means for categories of a variable, according to a t-test, is shown in parentheses.

Age

Stratifying the respondents by age at interview showed no significant differences among stated family-size desires for black teenagers in either survey year, although in 1976 the average desired family size tended to increase

Table 12–3
Average Desired Family Size by Race, 1971 and 1976 [a]

	White		Black		Total	
	1971	1976	1971	1976	1971	1976
N	(2935)	(1486)	(1424)	(697)	(4359)	(2183)
Mean	2.77	2.59	2.49	2.38	2.68	2.52
S.D.	1.28	1.26	1.35	1.33	1.31	1.28
t	4.44 (0.01) [a]		1.77 (0.10)		4.69 (0.01)	

[a]Significance level of differences among means for categories of a variable, according to a $t \pm$-test, is shown in parentheses.

with age from 2.27 at age 15 to 2.54 at age 19. For young white women in 1976, desired family size declined with increasing age, and differences among the means were significant ($p < .05$). Whites 15 years old stated an average desired family size of 2.71 while whites 19 years old desired 2.43 children (see table 12–4).

Education of Raisers

Mean education of the parents or individuals rearing each young woman was used as a proxy of socioeconomic status (SES).[7] Table 12–4 indicates that only among black teenagers in 1971 was the level of education of the raisers relatively significant ($p < .10$). Contrary to the generally observed inverse relationship between SES (or education) and fertility for both whites and blacks in the United States, the average desired family size was actually larger with higher levels of education of the raisers for this group of black teenagers.

Family Stability

In the belief that being raised by married parents (and the integrity and stability of that family of origin over time) are important factors in the development and behavior of adolescents, a measure of family stability was developed and examined to determine what relation, if any, there might be with a young woman's desired family size. The three categories of family stability are: (1) a presumably "ideal" situation in which young women were reared by their natural (or adoptive) mothers and natural (or adoptive) fathers, lived with both parents from birth to at least age 15, and had

Table 12-4
Average Desired Family Size by Age, Mean Educational Level of Raisers, Family Stability, and Number of Siblings Lived with between Tenth and Fifteenth Birthdays, by Race, 1971 and 1976

Characteristics	1971			1976		
	White	Black	Total	White	Black	Total
Age	(NS)	(NS)	(NS)	(0.05)	(NS)	(NS)
15	2.85	2.48	2.72	2.71	2.27	2.57
16	2.80	2.45	2.69	2.69	2.20	2.54
17	2.71	2.50	2.65	2.56	2.41	2.51
18	2.76	2.54	2.69	2.57	2.47	2.53
19	2.73	2.49	2.66	2.43	2.54	2.46
Education of raisers (years)	(NS)	(0.10)	(NS)	(NS)	(NS)	(NS)
8 or less	2.78	2.44	2.61	2.55	2.24	2.41
9-11	2.82	2.41	2.66	2.59	2.30	2.49
12	2.75	2.63	2.73	2.60	2.42	2.55
13-15	2.76	2.73	2.75	2.66	2.62	2.65
16 or more	2.73	2.58*	2.70	2.53	2.43*	2.51
Family stability	(0.05)	(NS)	(0.01)	(0.01)	(NS)	(0.01)
Ideal	2.81	2.50	2.74	2.67	2.36	2.61
Less ideal	2.66	2.56	2.61	2.42	2.30	2.37
Least ideal	2.68	2.44	2.53	2.37	2.47	2.43
Number of siblings	(0.01)	(NS)	(0.05)	(0.01)	(NS)	(0.10)
0	2.66	2.47	2.58	2.52	2.44	2.49
1	2.68	2.48	2.63	2.38	2.74	2.46
2	2.65	2.58	2.63	2.47	2.23	2.41
3	2.80	2.40	2.69	2.53	2.58	2.54
4	2.81	2.50	2.70	2.80	2.27	2.61
5	3.07	2.35	2.77	3.04	2.25	2.69
6 or more	3.32	2.57	2.87	3.02	2.33	2.63

Notes: Significance level of differences among means for categories of a variable, according to an F-test, is shown in parentheses. The N for each category is at least 50 except where indicated by an asterisk (*). The asterisk indicates an N between 20 and 50.

mothers who were married only once and never divorced; (2) a less-ideal situation in which young women were reared by their natural (or adoptive) mothers and natural (or adoptive) fathers but for whom at least one of the other conditions in the ideal situation was not met; and (3) a residual category for young women who were not reared by their natural (or adoptive) mothers and their natural (or adoptive) fathers. In both survey years white teenagers reared in the ideal situation had the highest average desired family size, and white teenagers in the least-ideal category in 1976 and the less-ideal category in 1971 had the lowest desires. In both years the differences among the three categories were statistically significant ($p < .05$ in 1971 and $p < .01$ in 1976). In 1976, for example, an average of 2.67 children was desired by young white women included in the ideal category, while 2.37 children was the average desired family size of young white women in the least-ideal category (see table 12–4). For young black women there was no statistical relationship between desired family size and our measure of family stability. It is interesting to note that 75 percent of whites in 1971 and 70 percent in 1976 were included in the ideal category, in contrast to 42 percent of blacks in 1971 and 36 percent in 1976.

Number of Siblings

Several previous studies have examined the relationship between the number of children born in two successive generations and have generally found small but positive correlations. In the Indianapolis Study of Fertility, which included information on sociological siblings (children in the family, regardless of blood relationship, with whom the respondent grew up), it was found that the size of the family from which the parents came had a very slight influence on the number of children born to them (Kantner and Potter 1954). Duncan et al. (1965) explored this relationship using data from the 1955 Growth of American Families (GAF) and the 1962 CPS.[8] Seeking a "sociologically relevant measure of family size," the GAF question was: "How many brothers and sisters did you have altogether while you were growing up?" In the 1962 CPS, the question about how many brothers and sisters an individual had included the instruction: "Count those born alive but no longer living, as well as those alive now. Also include stepbrothers and sisters and children adopted by your parents" (Duncan et al. 1965). The authors found a small though significant association between fertility and the size of the family of orientation in both the GAF and the CPS data. They concluded that, "The size of the family is only one in a complex of factors determining what the child learns about how family life should be organized. Whether the child has a satisfying or an unsatisfying experience in his family of orientation will affect his tendency to recapitulate his earlier experience when he builds his own family."

Another study of young people's attitudes about fertility was conducted in 1968 and included 1,123 students in grades 6, 9, and 12 in Georgia and Florida (Gustavus and Nam 1970). The authors found that ideal family size was positively correlated with the number of siblings, although the correlation was very small.

The two NSYW surveys provided an opportunity to study the relationship between the number of siblings and desired family size. Desired family size from these data could result in a higher correlation with number of siblings, since fertility desires have not yet been influenced by actual fertility experience for about 90 percent of the sample in either year. The measure of number of siblings in the NSYW data was based on the question: "How many brothers and sisters did you live with between your 10th and 15th birthdays?" This question obviously omitted siblings who had died or who were not living in the same household during this period. Table 12–4 shows the average desired family size by the number of siblings for whites and blacks aged 15 to 19. In both 1971 and 1976, the association for whites was positive, so that as the number of siblings increased so did desired family size, although not monotonically ($p < .01$). In 1971 mean desired family size increased from 2.66 for teenagers with no siblings to 3.32 for those with six or more siblings. Among blacks aged 15 to 19 there was no discernible relationship between desired family size and number of siblings in either survey year. Adolescent women with no siblings had the lowest average desired family size in 1971. However, their counterparts in 1976 desired an average family size that exceeded the desires of young women who had one or two siblings.

Religion

Religion had until recently been observed to be an important variable in differential-fertility research (Westoff and Jones 1979). Religious affiliation, for this analysis, was divided into five groups for whites and for the total sample: "fundamentalist Protestant," "other Protestant" (including Mormon), "Catholic," "non-Christian," and "none." Because of very small numbers in certain categories, blacks were divided into only four groups with non-Christian and none classified simply as "other." For both races in the two surveys, Catholics had the highest family-size desires, although black Catholic teenagers' desires were lower than those of white Catholic teenagers (see table 12–5). In 1971, black Catholics stated a desired size of 2.85 compared to 3.08 for white Catholics, and similarly in 1976 black Catholics desired 2.50 compared to 2.87 for their white counterparts. Among blacks, fundamentalist Protestants were second highest in their desires followed by other Protestants. However, for whites, other Protestants ranked second. Composition of the fundamentalist Protestant category undoubtedly differed by race, since although blacks in general had lower desired family size, for this religious group blacks exceeded whites. In all groups the lowest desired family size was given for those teenagers with no religious affiliation. The differences among the average values for each religious group were highly significant for the white teenagers in 1971 and 1976 ($p < .01$), as well as for the black teenagers in 1971 ($p < .05$).

Table 12-5
**Average Desired Family Size by Religion, Religiosity, Marital Status, Live
Births, and Educational Aspiration, by Race, 1971 and 1976**

	1971			1976		
Characteristics	*White*	*Black*	*Total*	*White*	*Black*	*Total*
Religion	(0.01)	(0.05)	(0.01)	(0.01)	(NS)	(0.01)
Fundamentalist Protestant	2.54	2.62	2.57	2.38	2.45	2.41
Other Protestant	2.69	2.46	2.59	2.50	2.37	2.45
Catholic	3.08	2.85	3.06	2.87	2.50*	2.85
Non-Christian	2.62⎱	2.32	2.57	2.32*⎱	2.36	2.41*
None	2.26⎰		2.30	2.24⎰		2.27
Religiosity	(0.01)	(NS)	(0.01)	(0.01)	(NS)	(0.01)
High	2.93	2.44	2.72	2.88	2.42	2.70
Medium	2.82	2.55	2.74	2.56	2.38	2.50
Low	2.53	2.56	2.53	2.39	2.31	2.37
Marital status	(0.05)	(NS)	(NS)	(0.05)	(NS)	(NS)
Never-married	2.79	2.48	2.69	2.62	2.38	2.54
Ever-married	2.61	2.58	2.61	2.44	2.38*	2.43
Live Births	(0.01)	(0.05)	(0.01)	(NS)	(0.05)	(0.01)
0	2.79	2.52	2.71	2.61	2.38	2.54
1	2.40	2.28	2.32	2.39	2.22	2.30
2 or more	2.68*	2.77*	2.74	2.94 [a]	2.84*	2.87
Educational aspiration (years)	(NS)	(0.01)	(0.01)	(0.05)	(NS)	(0.01)
11 or less	2.69	2.17	2.49	2.36	2.33*	2.35
12	2.80	2.36	2.64	2.51	2.24	2.43
13-15	2.87	2.61	2.79	2.66	2.40	2.58
16 or more	2.72	2.68	2.71	2.68	2.50	2.62

Notes: Significance level of differences among means for categories of a variable, according to
an *F*-test, is shown in parentheses. The *N* for each category is at least 50 except where indicated
by an asterisk (*). The asterisk indicates an *N* between 20 and 50.
[a] $N = 17$.

Religiosity

An index of religiosity was created from several variables including fre-
quency of attendance at a religious service (stratified by religious affiliation)
and the importance of religion to the respondent and in the life of her
family of orientation. The index, which ranged from a low of 0 to a high of

6, was grouped into three categories: low (0–2), middle (3–4) and high (5–6). The degree of religiosity was positively related to desired family size for whites in 1971 and 1976. Young white women with a low religiosity score desired an average family size of 2.53 in 1971 compared to 2.93 desired by their high-religiosity counterparts. The same relationship existed in 1976, with desired family size of 2.39 for low- and 2.88 for high-religiosity white teenagers. The relationship between religiosity and desired family size was highly significant for whites in 1971 as well as 1976 ($p < .01$) but not significant for blacks in either year (see table 12–5).

Marital Status and Premarital Sex

Several variables were studied that reflected more recent behavior of young women to further differentiate teenagers with regard to their desired family size. The young women were grouped according to whether they had ever or never been married. White teenagers who had never been married desired, on the average, larger families than those who had ever been married. In 1971 never-married whites wanted 2.79 children and ever-marrieds 2.61 ($p < .05$) (see table 12–5). Among young black women there were no significant differences based on marital status in the average family size desired in 1971 or 1976.

Both ever- and never-married teenagers were queried as to whether or not they had engaged in premarital sexual intercourse. There was no significant difference in average family-size desires for young black women who had premarital sex and for those who did not have premarital sex (not shown in table). Among young white women in 1971 only, those with premarital sexual experience desired significantly smaller families on the average than those without such experience ($p < .01$); sexually experienced white teenagers desired 2.66 children compared to 2.81 for those sexually inexperienced. This finding might in part be explained by relating more traditional attitudes of higher family size to the more traditional behavior of the sexually inexperienced young women.

Number of Live Births

Since marital status was associated (at least for whites) with diminished family-size desires, it was interesting to examine whether the actual fertility experience of sexually active teenagers was related to family-size desires. Fertility experience was measured by total number of live births. The small numbers for certain categories of this variable were a problem, but more so for white teenagers than for black teenagers. In 1971, 18.2 percent of blacks and only 5.4 percent of whites had at least one live birth; and in 1976, 20.7 percent of blacks and 9.0 percent of whites had ever experienced a live birth. Despite these small numbers, the association with desired family size was significant for blacks and the total sample in both survey years and for whites in 1971. The general pattern for all groups was that young women who had had no live births wanted more children on the average than those who had had one, but generally fewer children than those who had had two or more births. For example, all women in 1976 who had had one live birth wanted an average of only 2.30 children compared to 2.54 for nulliparous women and 2.87 for those with two or more live births (see table 12–5). Some experience with childbirth and childrearing might understandably have altered family-size desires. If a women had had more than one birth while still a teenager she might have felt very committed or even tied to her role as a mother.

Educational Aspiration

Because of the young age of the teenagers in the sample, many were still enrolled in school at the date of interview. The young women were asked about the highest grade of school or year of college they planned to complete. For those who had no aspiration for additional education, responses to a question about the highest level of school already completed were used. Over 36 percent of teenagers in both survey years aspired to be college graduates. For black women in 1971 and white women in 1976 the relationship between desired family size and aspired education was positive (see table 12–5). For example, black teenagers in 1971 who aspired to less than twelve years of school had a desired family size of 2.17, while those who hoped to complete at least their college education wanted 2.68 children. This result was quite unexpected if aspired education were a true surrogate of the ultimate level of completed education, because educational attainment is usually inversely related to fertility.[9] However, this association compares aspirations and desires; it is likely that actual future behavior may develop somewhat differently in either or both respects. The relationship between aspired education and desired family size was significant for blacks in 1971 ($p < .01$) and for whites in 1976 ($p < .05$).

Multiple-Classification Analysis

The second stage of this analysis involved the use of a multivariate procedure, multiple-classification analysis (MCA), to predict the effect of significant (from the previous section) and other important variables on desired family size.[10] Ten predictor variables were included in the model: race, age, mean educational level of raisers, family stability, number of siblings, religion, religiosity, marital status, total number of live births, and educational aspiration.[11] The values of desired family size ranged from 0 to 6, and MCA generated unadjusted and adjusted means as well as unadjusted and adjusted deviations from the sample mean. These deviations facilitated an understanding of changes in the categories of each variable resulting from the adjustment procedure. A series of these dummy-variable multiple regressions was carried out separately for blacks, whites, and total sample in 1971 and in 1976. When all the predictor variables were included in the model, a small but significant proportion of the variance in desired family size (R^2) was explained ($p < .01$) for all groups except blacks in 1976 (see tables 12–6, 12–7, and 12–8).

Table 12–6
Unadjusted and Adjusted Deviations from Mean Desired Family Size for Various Predictor Variables, Young Women of All Races, 1971 and 1976

	1971		1976	
Predictor Variables	*Unadjusted*	*Adjusted*	*Unadjusted*	*Adjusted*
Race	(0.01)		(0.01)	
White	0.087	0.073	0.074	0.074
Black	−0.189	−0.158	−0.168	−0.166
Number of siblings	(0.01)		(0.05)	
0	−0.101	−0.059	−0.076	−0.011
1	−0.047	−0.085	−0.075	−0.095
2	−0.042	−0.049	−0.100	−0.127
3	0.004	−0.017	0.031	0.003
4	0.009	0.003	0.095	0.079
5	0.111	0.128	0.123	0.160
6 or more	0.174	0.245	0.117	0.168
Religion	(0.01)		(0.01)	
Fundamentalist Protestant	−0.091	−0.095	−0.139	−0.121
Other Protestant	−0.091	−0.073	−0.078	−0.074
Catholic	0.365	0.293	0.321	0.244
Non-Christian	0.012	0.034	−0.189	−0.156*
None	−0.375	−0.274	−0.259	−0.082
Religiosity	(0.01)		(0.01)	
High	0.040	0.064	0.180	0.191
Medium	0.058	0.043	−0.019	−0.031
Low	−0.161	−0.181	−0.175	−0.173

Table 12–6 continued

Predictor Variables	1971		1976	
	Unadjusted	*Adjusted*	*Unadjusted*	*Adjusted*
Number of live births	(0.01)		(0.05)	
0	0.031	0.021	0.020	−0.005
1	−0.360	−0.256	−0.255	−0.074
2 or more	0.068	0.146	0.329	0.513*
Educational aspiration (years) [a]			(0.10)	
11 or less			−0.154	−0.055
12			−0.102	−0.096
13–15			0.063	0.050
16 or more			0.089	0.075
Grand mean	2.696		2.522	
R^2	0.045		0.057	
Significance level	(0.01)		(0.01)	

Notes: Significance levels of the increment to R^2 added by a variable according to an F-test, are shown in parentheses. The N for each category is at least 50 except where indicated by an asterisk (*). The asterisk indicates an N between 20 and 50.

[a] Educational aspiration was not statistically significant for the total sample in 1971.

The following section reviews the results of the MCA analyses of desired family size for the total sample, whites, and blacks. Only those predictor variables for which average desired family size (from the first section) and/or the predictive value in the MCA was statistically significant are discussed.[12] The effect of adjustment on the deviations from the sample mean is discussed, and tables of the unadjusted and adjusted deviations for the significant predictors are included.

Race was a variable only when the total was analyzed. In both 1971 and 1976, differences by race in average desired family size were shown to be statistically significant. After adjustment, race was a highly significant predictor of desired family size in both survey years ($p < .01$). The adjustment process reduced the size of the deviations for all groups except whites in 1976, although they all remained relatively large. The adjusted deviations for blacks fell below the sample mean in both years, while the adjusted deviations for whites were above the mean (see table 12–6).

Age was a moderately significant predictor of desired family size only among white teenagers in 1976 ($p < .10$). Adjustment increased the deviations for 17-year-olds but diminished the deviations for the other ages (see table 12–7). Average desired family size by mean education of the parents or raisers of young women in the two surveys was statistically significant only for blacks in 1971. Adjustment for all predictor variables essentially eliminated differences among the means, and this variable was insignificant as a

Table 12-7
Unadjusted and Adjusted Deviations from Mean Desired Family Size for Various Predictor Variables, White Young Women, 1971 and 1976

Predictor Variables	1971		1976	
	Unadjusted	Adjusted	Unadjusted	Adjusted
Age[a]			(0.10)	
15			0.141	0.131
16			0.102	0.087
17			−0.029	−0.039
18			−0.027	−0.004
19			−0.198	−0.185
Number of siblings	(0.01)		(0.01)	
0	−0.105	−0.076	−0.093	−0.020
1	−0.095	−0.087	−0.212	−0.180
2	−0.110	−0.079	−0.133	−0.132
3	0.015	0.013	−0.059	−0.051
4	0.026	0.001	0.196	0.154
5	0.295	0.263	0.443	0.420
6 or more	0.527	0.419	0.471	0.382
Religion	(0.01)		(0.01)	
Fundamentalist Protestant	−0.243	−0.285	−0.190	−0.185
Other Protestant	−0.087	−0.073	−0.098	−0.082
Catholic	0.301	0.240	0.276	0.196
Non-Christian	−0.075	0.109	−0.188	0.008*
Other	−0.481	−0.298	−0.354	−0.137
Religiosity	(0.01)		(0.01)	
High	0.145	0.143	0.294	0.267
Medium	0.052	0.035	−0.017	−0.043
Low	−0.250	−0.224	−0.230	−0.178
Number of live births[b]	(0.05)			
0	0.019	0.019		
1	−0.383	−0.376		
2 or more	−0.033	−0.060*		
Grand mean	2.783		2.597	
R^2	0.059		0.088	
Significance level	(0.01)		(0.01)	

Notes: Significance levels of the increment to R^2 added by a variable according to an F-test, are shown in parentheses. The N for each category is at least 50 except where indicated by an asterisk (*). The asterisk indicates an N between 20 and 50.

[a] Age was not statistically significant for the white sample in 1971.

[b] Number of live births was not statistically significant for the white sample in 1976.

Table 12–8
Unadjusted and Adjusted Deviations from Mean Desired Family Size for Various Predictor Variables, Black Young Women, 1971 and 1976

	1971		1976	
Predictor Variables	*Unadjusted*	*Adjusted*	*Unadjusted*	*Adjusted*
Religion [a]	(0.10)			
Fundamentalist Protestant	0.201	0.209		
Other Protestant	−0.043	−0.037		
Catholic	0.337	0.233		
Other	−0.148	−0.123		
Number of live births	(0.10)		(0.10)	
0	0.031	0.020	0.008	0.009
1	−0.214	−0.168	−0.191	−0.181
2 or more	0.264	0.340*	0.446	0.409*
Educational aspiration (years)[a]	(0.01)			
11 or less	−0.307	−0.339		
12	−0.143	−0.120		
13–15	0.120	0.112		
16 or more	0.189	0.172		
Grand mean	2.507		2.354	
R^2	0.036		0.048	
Significance level	(0.01)		(NS)	

Notes: Significance levels of the increment to R^2 added by a variable according to an F-test, are shown in parentheses. The N for each category is at least 50 except where indicated by an asterisk (*). The asterisk indicates an N between 20 and 50.

[a] Neither religion nor educational aspiration were statistically significant for the black sample in 1976.

predictor of desired family size. Family stability exhibited statistically significant differences in the average desired family size for whites in 1971 and 1976, as well as for both races combined. After adjustment, family stability was not an important predictor of desired family size for any group in 1971 or 1976.

Number of siblings remained a highly significant predictor of desired family size for whites in both 1971 and 1976 ($p < .01$) although adjustment diminished the deviations from the sample mean for every category. Young white teenagers with two or fewer siblings in 1971 or with three or fewer siblings in 1976 wanted, on the average, smaller families than was indicated by the entire sample mean. For example, in 1976 the deviation of the group of teenagers who had one sibling fell .180 below the sample mean. Among young white women in either year who had at least five siblings, the deviations were considerably above the mean (see table 12–7).

The analysis of the total sample reflected a slightly different pattern. For the young women who had up to three siblings in 1971 and up to two siblings in 1976, the deviations fell below the sample mean. Conversely, for young women from families with at least four siblings in 1971, or at least three siblings in 1976, the deviations exceeded the sample mean desired family size. Number of siblings was significant for the total sample ($p < .01$ in 1971 and $p < .05$ in 1976) (see table 12–6).

As has been noted elsewhere in this chapter, highly significant differences existed among religious groups in the average desired family size for each race in 1971 and for whites in 1976, as well as for the totals in both years. Adjustment reduced the deviations from the sample mean for most groups, although the deviations increased in 1971 for black, white, and total fundamentalist Protestants, and for white and total non-Christians. Table 12–8 shows that for blacks in 1971, the adjusted deviations for Catholics and fundamentalist Protestants were positive and above the sample mean by 0.233 and 0.209 respectively. The two remaining categories for blacks, other Protestants and other (including non-Christian and none) had negative deviations. For young white women in both 1971 and 1976, Catholics and non-Christians had adjusted deviations above the mean. The adjusted deviations for the three other religious groups among whites were below the sample mean—rather substantially below for fundamentalist Protestants and for those white teenagers categorized as none in both survey years. Religion was a highly significant predictor of desired family size for whites and the total sample in both years ($p < .01$) and somewhat less significant for blacks in 1971 ($p < .10$) (see tables 12–6, 12–7, and 12–8).

Religiosity was a very significant predictor of desired family size among young white women and total women in 1971 and 1976 ($p < .01$). This was not surprising, given differences among the unadjusted means previously discussed. For young white women, controlling for all other variables decreased the deviations from the sample mean for all categories except "medium" religiosity in 1976. Even so, the adjusted deviations remained fairly large for both the high- and low-religiosity categories. For the total sample in both years, adjustment slightly increased the deviations of the high-religiosity group (see tables 12–6 and 12–7).

Among whites there was a statistically significant difference in the average desired family size by marital status in both survey years. Controlling for other predictor variables eliminated differences between ever- and never-marrieds and caused marital status to be an insignificant predictor of desired family size.

Total number of live births was a statistically significant predictor of desired family size for all MCA analyses except for whites in 1976. For the category of two or more live births, the adjusted deviations increased except for 1976 blacks. For blacks and the total sample in both survey years, the adjusted deviations for young women with one live birth fell below the sample mean, and the adjusted deviations for those who had two or more live births exceeded the sample mean. For whites in 1971, the deviations fell below the mean for the categories of one and two or more live births. After adjustment, this variable had modest predictive value for blacks in both years ($p < .10$), was fairly significant for whites in 1971 and for total in 1976 ($p < .05$), and was highly significant for the total sample of teenagers in 1971 ($p < .01$) (see tables 12-6, 12-7, and 12-8).

Significant differences by educational aspiration were found in the previous section among the means of desired family size for blacks in 1971, for whites in 1976, and for the total sample in each survey year. Table 12-8 indicates that the adjusted deviations in 1971 remained large for all categories of educational aspiration among young black women. The adjusted deviations for black teenagers who aspired to twelve or fewer years of school were below the sample mean, while the deviations exceeded the sample mean for black teenagers who wanted at least some college education. This pattern was also observed for the total sample in 1976, although the adjusted deviations were not as large (see tables 12-6 and 12-8). After adjustment for all variables, educational aspiration remained a highly significant predictor ($p < .01$) for blacks in 1971. In contrast, educational aspiration for whites in 1976 was not a significant predictor of desired family size when other variables were controlled. When both races were analyzed together, adjustment diminished the deviations in the educational aspiration categories in 1971 and 1976. In the former year, educational aspiration was no longer a significant variable, while in 1976 it had a moderate predictive value ($p < .10$).

In summary, when the significance of each predictor was examined after adjustment for all other variables, race, religion, religiosity, number of siblings, and total number of live births were highly significant for the total sample in 1971. In the later survey of young women, the same variables were again statistically significant as predictors of desired family size; and educational aspiration, although only moderately important, was added to the list. When the analyses were carried out separately for the two racial groups, differences emerged in terms of which variables were significant. For whites in 1971, three variables—religion, religiosity, and number of siblings—were highly significant predictors, and total number of live births was quite significant. Among blacks, however, only aspired education was highly significant, while total number of live births and religion were of modest predictive value. In 1976, for whites the same three variables (religion, religiosity, and number of siblings) were highly significant; and one other variable, age, was somewhat less significant. For the 1976 sample of blacks, only one variable, total number of births, was even moderately significant.

Reasons for Desired Family Size

In addition to asking adolescent women about desired family size, the 1971 and 1976 national surveys included an open-ended question about why the young women wanted a particular number of children. The responses to this question may clarify the factors that teenagers consider important in selecting a given family size. Differentials in reasons stated by race, age, mean educational level of raisers, marital status, and specific desired family sizes were also examined.

Open-ended questions pose particular problems for categorizing the responses. While many different reasons were cited in both surveys, these have been grouped into ten categories, including a residual category of "other." Most of the categories are self-descriptive, but some are not. "Good number" includes: "It is an optimum number," "A number not too large or too small," "A good number," "I always wanted that number," "That's enough," "I just like that number," "I want twins." "Sex distribution" refers to such responses as: "I have always wanted to have two boys and two girls," "I'd like one of each: a boy and a girl." "Financial" incorporates: "Nowadays it's hard to afford more," "The cost of living is so high and that's all I could support." "Number can manage" refers to: "That's all I could handle," "I feel I can probably take care of (that number), and more would be too much." "Siblings are helpful" includes: "Children provide companionship for each other," "One child would be lonely or get spoiled," "I don't want just one."

In both survey years about 92 percent of the sample responded to this question with a codable answer.[13] Only about 5 percent of teenagers in 1971 and slightly more than 6 percent in 1976 wanted no (more) children. For young women not wanting any (more) children in 1971 and 1976, the more frequently given reasons were: "I don't like or want children," "Children are too much trouble," and "They tie you down or interfere with having a career." Some respondents already had children and didn't want more, while others did not plan to marry or remarry.

Table 12-9 shows the percentage distribution of reasons for desired family size for all women who wanted at least one (more) child in both survey years. In 1971 approximately equal numbers of teenagers indicated "good number" or "sex distribution" as their reason for a specific-sized family. Other major reasons included "number can manage" and "siblings

Table 12–9
Percentage Distribution of Reasons for Desired Family Size and Average Desired Family Size by Reason for All Young Women, 1971 and 1976[a]

	1971		1976	
Reason	*Percentage*	*Average Desired Family Size*	*Percentage*	*Average Desired Family Size*
Good number	18.3	2.98	13.1	2.74
Sex distribution	18.4	2.88	10.2	2.55
Financial	8.3	2.41	18.8	2.26
Number can manage	13.8	2.22	7.1	2.02
Siblings are helpful	11.4	2.82	17.5	2.82
Likes children	7.3	4.20	10.8	4.14
Population explosion	6.7	2.09	4.1	2.06
Wants small family	3.2	2.20	4.9	2.18
Wants large family	3.0	5.33	0.8	4.65[a]
Other	9.5	2.70	12.7	2.64
Total	99.9		100.0	
N	(4,039)		(2,016)	

Notes: Figures are for all young women who want at least one (more) child. Denominators (*N*s) for average desired family size range from 83 to 743 except where otherwise indicated.
[a] *N* = 17.

are helpful.'' By 1976, "financial" had moved to the fore as the most important reason, followed by "siblings are helpful," "good number," "likes children," and "sex distribution."

Much interest has been focused on the sex preference for children in the United States and in some developing countries (Williamson 1978). In both NSYW studies, sex distribution ranked fairly high as a reason for desired family size. In most cases, the sex distribution indicated by these young women implied at least one child of each sex. The enhanced importance of financial reasons was hardly surprising given the fairly high level of inflation in the United States during the 1970s. Despite considerable attention given to population-growth problems in the media and by population educators in the United States, very few teenagers cited concern with the population explosion as a reason for desired family size. Even if young women didn't perceive that desires were or should have been directly affected by such a consideration, the observed downward trend in desired family size was evidence of changing values and norms in favor of reducing population pressures. For example, almost equivalent (although small) per-

Table 12–10
Percentage Distribution of the Three Most Frequently Cited Reasons for Desired Family Size and Average Desired Family Size by Reason for White and Black Young Women, 1971 and 1976 [a]

	1971			1976	
Reason	Percentage	Average Desired Family Size		Percentage	Average Desired Family Size
White					
Good number	17.5	3.07	Siblings are helpful	19.2	2.84
Sex distribution	16.7	2.88	Financial	18.8	2.33
Siblings are helpful	12.8	2.91	Likes children	11.6	4.12
Black					
Sex distribution	22.0	2.89	Financial	18.8	2.13
Number can manage	20.9	2.12	Good number	18.4	2.63
Good number	20.0	2.82	Siblings are helpful	13.6	2.76

[a] *N*s range from 626 to 2,761.

centages indicated that they wanted a small or a large family in 1971. By 1976 almost none of the sample wanted a large family, while the percentage who wanted a small family had increased.

Average desired family size is also shown for each of the ten reasons in table 12–9. The smallest average in 1971 was 2.09 given by teenagers citing "population explosion" as their reason for a specified family size, while in 1976 those citing "number can manage" had the smallest average. The largest average applied to those teenagers who say they want large families, 5.33 in 1971 and 4.65 in 1976.

When only the three most frequently cited reasons were examined by race, two of the three reasons given by blacks and whites in 1971 were the same, "good number" and "sex distribution," although a higher percentage of blacks cited them than whites (see table 12–10). In 1976 equal percentages of whites and blacks cited "financial" reasons as among the more important reasons, although the most frequent response for whites was "siblings are helpful," and this reason ranked third for blacks.

Analysis by age at interview showed no unique pattern with increasing age. For each group in both years the two most important reasons correspond to the most important reasons overall. Reasons were also examined in relation to the level of education of the raisers. The main reasons given for desired family size were, for the most part, uniform for all levels of education and were generally similar by race. The one exception was that "population explosion" appeared for the first time among the top-ranking reasons for the total sample of teenagers in 1971 whose parents or raisers had at least some college education and for those young women in 1976 whose raisers were college graduates.

When the samples of women were analyzed for differences by marital status, the most striking change was that ever-marrieds were much more inclined to state "financial" reasons than were never-married women; 18.4 percent of the ever-married white teenagers cited financial reasons in 1971 while for never-marrieds it did not even appear among the most important reasons. For blacks in 1971, financial reasons were not among the more important reasons regardless of marital status. By 1976 there was a sizable difference for blacks as well as whites between the never- and ever-married teenagers, although the number of observations was quite small. It may be presumed that a married woman was more likely to be aware of her family's financial needs than she was as a dependent in her parents' or raisers' household, and hence financial considerations generally predominated in the decision to have a specific-sized family (see table 12–11).

Finally, reasons were analyzed by each level of desired family size. Because of relatively similar distributions and small numbers, particularly in 1976, reasons were considered for the total samples rather than separately by race. The major difference between the two surveys was the importance of financial considerations (see table 12–12). It is quite obvious that teenagers in 1976 were more concerned about the cost of raising a family than were 15 to 19 year olds in 1971. While those wanting only one child in 1971 did cite financial reasons among the three most important factors, those wanting two children responded most frequently with reasons such as "sex distribution," "number can manage," and "good number." By 1976 financial considerations were the primary factors for teenagers wanting one or two children, and were even given as one of the more important reasons for those young women wanting three children. Another difference between the two surveys was that "sex distribution" was the predominant reason for teenagers wanting two and four children in 1971. Teenagers at that point in time were apparently attracted by the idea of having children of both sexes and in equal numbers. At the later survey, however, "sex distribution" was only the third most important reason among those wanting two offspring.

Conclusion

By 1975 the U.S. census bureau had adopted a new population-projection series, in part to reflect lower levels of fertility among American women. The assumptions of average number of lifetime births range from a high of

Table 12–11
Percentage Distribution of the Three Most Frequently Cited Reasons for Desired Family Size by Marital Status and Race for All Young Women, 1971 and 1976 [a]

	Never-Married Percentage		Ever-Married Percentage
1971			
White			
Good number	17.8	Financial	18.4
Sex distribution	16.8	Sex distribution	16.2
Siblings are helpful	12.5	Siblings are helpful	15.8
Black			
Sex distribution	22.1	Good number	25.0
Number can manage	21.1	Sex distribution	20.8
Good number	19.7	Siblings are helpful } Number can manage }	16.7
1976			
White			
Siblings are helpful	19.0	Financial	24.3
Financial	17.6	Siblings are helpful	20.2
Good number	11.5	Likes children	13.0
Black			
Good number	18.1	Financial	35.0
Financial	17.8	Good number	22.5
Siblings are helpful	14.0	Number can manage	12.5

[a] Ns range from 40 to 2,489.

2.7 to 1.7 (U.S. Bureau of the Census 1975). Data from the National Surveys of Young Women show that average desired family size declined from 2.68 to 2.52 between 1971 and 1976. As has been discussed, the CPS indicated somewhat lower average lifetime birth expectations of 2.09 for all 18- to 19-year-old women. Nevertheless, the values from both the 1976 NSYW and the 1976 CPS still exceeded actual fertility of American women, which was only 1.77 in that year (National Center for Health Statistics 1978). Lacking longitudinal data, we can only speculate as to whether or not the desires of these young women will be borne out. We have found that marriage (for whites) and childbearing (for both races) were associated with lower desires, and that by 1976 financial considerations were a primary reason for choosing a particular family size. Therefore, it seems likely that as

Table 12–12
Percentage Distribution of the Three Most Frequently Cited Reasons for Desired Family Size by Desired Family Size for All Young Women, 1971 and 1976 [a]

Desired Family Size		1971 Percentage		1976 Percentage
One	Number can manage	38.6	Financial	27.2
	Financial	10.7	Number can manage	17.2
	Good number	8.6	Good number	10.6
Two	Sex distribution	19.7	Financial	23.6
	Number can manage	18.0	Siblings are helpful	19.0
	Good number	12.9	Sex distribution	13.3
Three	Good number	28.8	Good number	19.5
	Siblings are helpful	14.0	Siblings are helpful	18.2
	Sex distribution	13.6	Financial	16.7
Four	Sex distribution	29.6	Likes children	22.7
	Good number	26.0	Siblings are helpful	21.0
	Likes children	11.8	Good number	16.4
Five	Likes children	30.6	Likes children	52.9
	Good number	17.4	Siblings are helpful	17.1
	Wants large family	16.0	Good number	11.4
Six or more	Likes children	37.2	Likes children	60.5
	Wants large family	33.8	Siblings are helpful	15.8
	Sex distribution	8.3	Wants large family	6.6

[a] Ns range from 70 to 1,864.

these young women mature, their desires will be tempered by their experiences and circumstances.

Notes

1. Of a total sample of 4,392 in 1971, 99.2 percent responded to the question about desired family size. In 1976, 99.5 percent of a total sample of 2,193 responded.

2. The 1971 NSYW included questions on both desired and intended family size; 94 percent of the respondents gave the same answer to questions on both concepts.

3. To obtain data on lifetime birth expectations, women 14 to 39 years old who were currently married and women 18 to 34 who were not currently

married (including women widowed, divorced, separated, and never married) were asked the following question: "Looking ahead, do you expect to have any (more) children?" If the answer to this question was positive, women were then asked, "How many (more) do you expect to have?" For ever-married women, lifetime births referred to the sum of reported births to date and additional births expected.

4. Percentage of nonresponses was not indicated for the 1971 CPS.

5. *Whites* in both NSYW surveys refers to whites and other non-blacks.

6. Because of the large sample size, small differences in mean desired family size may be statistically significant. The means reported in this paper should therefore be viewed in this context.

7. An average of the number of years of completed education of the male and female raisers was computed. There has been a long-term upward trend in the level of completed education in the United States. In cases where the respondent was raised by grandparents, an adjustment was made to take account of generational differences in education so that these respondents would not be penalized in terms of SES. The adjustment, carried out separately for each race and sex, consisted of adding to a grandparent's years of completed education the difference between the average years of completed education for all grandparents and the average years of completed education for all other raisers (essentially the parental generation).

8. The 1955 data pertained to a sample of currently married women aged 18 to 39, and included information on number of live births to date as well as the most likely expected number the woman would have by the end of her childbearing period. The 1962 CPS included two samples of currently married women, one aged 27 to 46 and the other aged 47 to 61, who were asked their total number of children ever born.

9. While the direct relationship between educational aspirations and desired family size for blacks in 1971 was unexpected, it did correspond with the direct relationship observed between mean education of raisers and desired family size for this same group.

10. In applying MCA, cases with missing data for the dependent and any of the predictor variables were excluded. MCA is a dummy-variable multiple-regression technique used to accommodate nominal variables. Since continuous variables cannot be used as such in MCA, some information is lost by treating the continuous predictor variables as discrete variables. In addition, the categories of the predictor variables used in MCA should include at least fifty observations to avoid larger sampling errors. In the present analysis several variables did contain categories with fewer than fifty observations, and the results for these categories should be interpreted with some caution. (Andrews, Morgan, and Sonquist 1969).

11. Race was deleted from the analyses carried out for blacks and whites.

12. Since MCA and ordinary least squares regression give approximately the same R^2, the latter method was used to determine the statistical significance of the individual predictors. The unadjusted R^2 of the full model was compared to the unadjusted R^2 of a reduced regression model for each variable, and an F statistic was calculated to determine the level of statistical significance.

13. Young women who responded "Don't know," or gave no answer or no reason were excluded as were those who gave a nonnumerical response or no answer to desired family size.

References

Andrews, Frank M.; Morgan, James N.; and Sonquist, John A. *Multiple Classification Analysis.* Survey Research Center, Institute for Survey Research, University of Michigan, Ann Arbor, November 1969.

Duncan, Otis Dudley; Freedman, Ronald; Coble, J. Michael; and Slesinger, Doris P. "Marital Fertility and Size of Family of Orientation." *Demography* 2 (1965): 508–515.

Gustavus, Susan O., and Nam, Charles B. "The Formation and Stability of Ideal Family Size among Young People." *Demography* 7 (1970): 43–51.

Kantner, John F., and Potter, Robert G., Jr. "The Relationship of Family Size in Two Successive Generations." *Milbank Memorial Fund Quarterly* 32 (1954): 294–311.

National Center for Health Statistics. "Advance Report: Final Natality Statistics, 1976." *Monthly Vital Statistics Report* 26 (1978): supplement.

Ryder, Norman B., and Westoff, Charles F. "Relationships among Intended, Expected, Desired and Ideal Family Size: United States, 1965." *Population Research.* Bethesda, Md.: Center for Population Research, U.S. Department of Health, Education, and Welfare, 1969.

United States Bureau of the Census. "Fertility Histories and Birth Expectations of American Women: June 1971." *Current Population Reports,* series P-20, no. 263 (1974).

————. "Projections of the Population of the United States: 1975 to 2050." *Current Population Reports,* series P-25, no. 601 (1975).

————. "Prospects for American Fertility: June 1976 (Advance Report)." *Current Population Reports,* series P-20, no. 300 (1976).

————. "Fertility of American Women: June 1976." *Current Population Reports,* series P-20, no. 308 (1977).

Westoff, Charles F., and Jones, Elise F. "The End of 'Catholic' Fertility." *Demography* 16 (1979): 209–217.

Westoff, Charles F., and Potvin, Raymond H. "Higher Education, Religion and Women's Family-Size Orientations." *American Sociological Review* 31 (1966): 489–496.

Williamson, Nancy E. "Boys or Girls? Parents' Preferences and Sex Control." *Population Bulletin* 33 (1978): 1–36.

13

The Childlessness Option: Recent American Views of Nonparenthood

Judith Blake and
Jorge H. del Pinal

In chapter 9 Moore noted that the decline in birth expectations in the late 1970s largely resulted from a decline in the proportions of women expecting large families of four children or more, but he also noted some increase in the proportions of women expecting to remain childless throughout life. In chapter 12 it was noted by Hirsh, Seltzer, and Zelnik that the decline in desired fertility among teenagers between 1971 and 1976 included an increase in the relative number desiring no children, although that proportion remained quite small. In this chapter Blake and del Pinal examine the small but apparently growing group of Americans who prefer to remain childless. Do they represent a new alternative lifestyle, perhaps viable, but destined to remain very small? Or do they indicate a groundswell of anti-natalist sentiment, destined to reduce fertility to even lower levels?

The data for this investigation are questions asked of a national sample of adults, men and women, as part of a Gallup Poll in 1978. Blake and del Pinal sought to determine how Americans perceived both the costs and the benefits of having children, and how the cost-benefit equation differed for parents and nonparents. They found that the major perceived costs of children are the direct costs of parents' time, money, and effort; the major perceived benefits of children are as a social investment—giving their parents a more recognized and secure social role—and the intrinsic rewards of interacting directly with children. Although nonparents saw fewer benefits and more costs than parents, they did not give strong support to childlessness—a majority of nonparents thought the benefits of children were equal to or greater than their costs. Thus, even to the limited extent that it exists in America today, the preference for childlessness does not appear rooted in strong antinatalist sentiment.

Furthermore, the authors speculate that some well-established social trends, such as more egalitarian relationships between sexes, may be paradoxically antithetical to nonparenthood. Women's suspicion that they will be saddled with a disproportionate share of the direct costs of parenthood in a traditional marriage has been a strong disincentive to childbearing in the past. To the extent that this suspicion is allayed by the social trend toward egalitarian marriage, the cost-benefit ratio of childbearing will become less favorable to nonparenthood.—*Eds.*

Since the late 1960s Americans have reacted strongly against the family behavior of the 1950s. Not only have actual and desired family size decreased, but people—young and not so young—have begun to claim for

themselves a wider variety of options in the areas of the family and reproduction. Marriages have taken place at older ages; couples increasingly have
resided together without benefit of marriage; women with young children
have entered the labor force in unprecedented numbers; divorce has risen to
a new high in our statistical history; and abortions have become not only
legal but, compared with the past, prevalent. Have young Americans also
developed an intense aversion to having any children at all? If so, does this
view find widespread support in the general population? Are the advocates
of nonparenthood merely a vocal minority, or are they a burgeoning van-
guard? With respect to a variety of costs and benefits related to reproduction, are there systematic differences among people in their views of the
desirability of the childlessness option? Taking a variety of costs and benefits of children, where do people come out on balance in their views of the
pluses and minuses?

Questions such as these are important to demographers because it is
unclear how American fertility will be configured during the remainder of
the century. To be sure, a major baby boom—say, a rise in family size to an
average of three children per woman—is unlikely. But finely tuned predictions of variability around a very low level of fertility are incredibly
demanding. In this effort, the proportion of women who will remain childless is an important element.

What issues are involved? First we may note that both actual and
expected childlessness among American wives have definitely risen in recent
years. Actual childlessness among ever-married women aged 20 to 24 has
risen from 35.9 percent in 1970 to 40.9 percent in 1978, and, among ever-
married women aged 25 to 29, from 15.8 to 25.2 percent (U.S. Bureau of
the Census 1979, p. 34). As for expectations, the figures are small but the
increases are large. In 1967, less than 0.5 percent of wives aged 20 to 21
expected to be childless; but by 1978, 5.2 percent intended to be perma-
nently without children. Analogous figures for wives aged 22 to 24 are 1.7
percent in 1967 and 5.5 percent in 1978 (U.S. Bureau of the Census 1976,
p. 5; 1979, p. 26). Among young single women in 1978 (aged 18 to 24), 18.1
percent expected to be childless throughout their lives (U.S. Bureau of the
Census 1979, p. 28).

Second, we must remember that the youthful decision to be a non-
parent is not necessarily irreversible. A decision that seemed appropriate at
20 may become unpalatable at 32 or even at 38. Thus neither statistics on
youthful family-size expectations, nor figures on youthful behavior that
seem to presage an elevation in nonparenthood, can be taken as ironclad
guarantees that equivalent numbers of American women will be perma-
nently childless. This consideration is far from academic, as has been illustrated during the past few years by trends in age-specific fertility by birth
order. Since 1976 the fertility rate and the birth rate have been rising. From
a low of 65.8 in 1976, the number of births per 1,000 women aged 15 to 44

(the fertility rate) had risen to a seasonally adjusted level of 67.6 by October 1979 (U.S. Department of Health, Education, and Welfare 1980, p. 1). Detailed statistics show that whereas the 1977 fertility rate was 3 percent above the 1976 rate, the rise for women aged 25 to 29 was 5 percent; and for those aged 30 to 34, it was 5.5 percent. Among women in these age groups, first-order births rose 8.3 percent and 11.2 percent respectively (U.S. Department of Health, Education, and Welfare 1979). In effect, delayed first births—a retreat from nonparenthood—have been an important feature of reproductive trends during recent years.

Third, not everyone will do an about-face, nor will everyone necessarily have the option of reversing the childlessness decision. Some women will have delayed the decision to have children beyond the point of physiologically satisfactory childbearing—they will have difficulty getting pregnant, staying pregnant, or having a live birth.

How many women will change their minds? How many will be biologically precluded from childbearing because of having delayed the decision too long? Such questions are impossible to answer accurately. However, in assessing the likelihood that women will or will not change their minds, or that they will wait a long time to do so, it seems useful to have some assessment of how prevalent is support for nonparenthood among us. Is our population, as Michael Novak has suggested, fixated on personal fulfillment to the extent that children increasingly represent an opportunity cost? What proportion of young people believe that life is more satisfying and exciting without a family, that the costs of children outweigh the benefits, that having children is not an important way of investing one's time and energy? Is the figure 60 percent, 40 percent, or what?

Here we report on the results of a national survey conducted in July 1978, in which we commissioned questions on attitudes toward childlessness. The questions focused on five major issues:

1. perceptions of children as involving a direct cost—actual outlays and demands;
2. perceptions of children as involving opportunity costs—foregone advantages and opportunities;
3. perceptions of children as involving long-run economic or financial return for the individual;
4. perceptions of children as involving long-run *non*economic return for the individual;
5. perceptions of children as an interaction good—an end in itself from which satisfaction is gained, purely because of the quality of interaction and companionship involved.

The questions, presented in appendix 13A, were used to measure the direct and opportunity costs of children, children as economic investments, children as noneconomic investments, and children as providers of companion-ship or interaction benefits.

The distinction between noneconomic investment and interaction bene-fits is worth some elaboration. The point is to differentiate the gain or bene-fit individuals derive from the interactional facet of childbearing—the con-sumption aspect of reproduction, as against the other noneconomic rewards from offspring such as those of gaining parental status, acquiring a voca-tion or goal in life, being regarded as an adult because of having attained parenthood, or trying for "immortality." Both noneconomic investment and interactional motivation involve "psychic income" (subjective satisfac-tion); but, as will be seen, there is a difference between wanting children because one enjoys their company, likes interacting with them, or finds them intriguing and stimulating; and having children (regardless of whether one enjoys them) because one does not want to go through life without becoming a parent, or because one would feel aimless or empty without a family, or because having children is a rite of passage in the attainment of adult status. In the latter cases, children are a noneconomic investment for the individual—an investment in a new social status, a means of attaining deference from others, or some similar end. The children are not solely ends in themselves, but are instrumental to the achievement of other ends—in this case, status and prestige. If children are not desired at all for interac-tional reasons, then they may be solely instrumentalities for the parents—a classic example being the case of people who loathe children but may have one or more simply to attain the status of being parents.

The Balance of Costs and Benefits

Taking all the measured costs and benefits together—direct and indirect costs, economic investment, social investment, and interaction—how do respondents view the desirability of having a family as compared with remaining childless? On balance, as may be seen from table 13-1, most people perceive the benefits of children as exceeding the costs—55 percent of men and 56 percent of women fall into this category. Somewhat less than one-third of each sex see the cost-benefit relation as a toss-up (typically a pattern of high costs and high benefits), and a small minority, about 15 per-cent, see costs as exceeding benefits. These results substantiate those from a previous survey on attitudes toward childlessness conducted in 1977 (Blake 1979). There appears to be little widespread support for nonparenthood.

What characteristics distinguish the relatively rare respondents who believe that costs exceed benefits from those who believe that benefits exceed costs? Taking basic background variables alone, we see from table

Table 13–1
Having Children: The Balance of Costs and Benefits, Gallup Survey, United States, July 1978, by Selected Characteristics

	Men					Women				
	(1)	(2)	(3)	(4)	N	(1)	(2)	(3)	(4)	N
Total U.S.	15%	31%	55%	101%	(769)	16%	28%	56%	100%	(786)
Age										
18–29	20	35	45	100	(210)	22	31	47	100	(213)
30–34	20	30	50	100	(200)	19	26	55	100	(206)
45–54	6	34	60	100	(114)	14	29	57	100	(113)
55+	10	25	65	100	(239)	9	26	65	100	(245)
Race										
White	15	30	55	100	(654)	16	27	57	100	(682)
Black	14	36	50	100	(107)	16	35	48	99	(97)
Religion										
Protestant	10	26	64	100	(428)	16	25	60	101	(480)
Catholic	18	34	48	100	(212)	14	31	55	100	(237)
Jewish	33	29	38	100	(21)	15	45	40	100	(20)
None	23	42	35	100	(98)	32	37	32	101	(41)
Education										
Grade school	9	31	60	100	(105)	7	28	66	101	(87)
High school (incomplete)	11	33	56	100	(125)	10	36	55	101	(126)
High school (complete)	13	28	59	100	(282)	16	26	58	100	(337)
College (incomplete)	21	32	47	100	(130)	22	25	53	100	(128)
College (4+)	22	31	48	101	(124)	23	30	47	100	(106)
Marital status										
Single	25	39	36	100	(165)	22	38	40	100	(112)
Married	12	29	59	100	(539)	14	27	59	100	(500)
Divorced and Separated	7	32	61	100	(41)	25	27	47	99	(59)
Widowed	13	17	70	100	(23)	12	23	65	100	(114)
Parental status										
A parent	10	27	63	100	(547)	11	27	62	100	(609)
Not parent	26	38	36	100	(216)	31	32	37	100	(172)

Note: Column heads indicate the following categories: (1) costs greater than benefits; (2) costs equal to benefits; (3) costs less than benefits; (4) total.

13–2 that the results differ for men and women. Among men, parental status, age, community size, religion, marital status, and education (in order of importance) explain 18.1 percent of the variance. Among women, parental status, marital status, work status, religion, education, community size, and age (in order of importance) explain 13.4 percent of the variance. Although being a parent or not is relatively the most important predictor for both sexes—42 percent of male and 48 percent of female nonparents believed that costs exceeded benefits—the next most important predictors differ by sex.

Among men, the next most antinatalist value appears among those aged 25 to 44—approximately one-third believe that costs exceed benefits. By contrast, among those under age 25, only 4 percent share this belief. Men who live in large cities are also markedly more likely to perceive costs as exceeding benefits, as are Jews and those having no religion. In effect,

Table 13–2
Adjusted Proportions Saying That the Costs of Children Exceed the Benefits, Gallup Survey, United States, July 1978, by Sex

Predictors	Adjusted Proportions Saying Costs Exceed Benefits [a]				(Ranked) Beta Coefficients			
	Women		Men		Women		Men	
Age					0.07	(7)	0.25	(2)
Under 25	0.23	(80)	0.04	(79)				
25–34	0.21	(126)	0.34	(109)				
35–44	0.28	(93)	0.31	(89)				
45–54	0.23	(80)	0.16	(75)				
55–64	0.18	(80)	0.20	(69)				
65 +	0.20	(108)	0.17	(113)				
Religion					0.10	(4)	0.15	(4)
Protestant	0.23	(361)	0.17	(318)				
Catholic	0.18	(164)	0.26	(140)				
Jewish	0.25	(11)	0.34	(15)				
None	0.39	(26)	0.29	(57)				
Education					0.10	(5)	0.08	(6)
Grade school	0.15	(65)	0.19	(72)				
High school (1–3)	0.16	(81)	0.25	(84)				
High school (complete)	0.23	(251)	0.18	(203)				
College (1–3)	0.26	(96)	0.24	(88)				
College (4 +)	0.26	(74)	0.24	(86)				

Table 13–2 continued

Predictors	Adjusted Proportions Saying Costs Exceed Benefits [a]				(Ranked) Beta Coefficients			
	Women		Men		Women		Men	
Community size					0.09	(6)	0.16	(3)
Under 10,000	0.19	(173)	0.15	(165)				
10,000–99,000	0.25	(104)	0.18	(96)				
100,000–999,999	0.20	(186)	0.22	(183)				
1,000.000 +	0.28	(104)	0.34	(90)				
Marital status					0.17	(2)	0.09	(5)
Married	0.23.	(366)	0.22	(385)				
Widowed	0.26	(88)	0.24	(19)				
Separated	0.27	(17)	0.00	(9)				
Divorced	0.39	(26)	0.13	(19)				
Single	0.05	(70)	0.22	(101)				
Present/expected work status (women)					0.16	(3)	—	
Not employed/ not employed	0.17	(225)	—	—				
Not employed/ full time	0.13	(34)	—	—				
Part time/ part time	0.29	(52)	—	—				
Part time/ full time	0.44	(25)	—	—				
Full time/ full time	0.27	(127)	—	—				
Other combinations	0.22	(104)	—	—				
Parental status					0.33	(1)	0.32	(1)
Parent (biological only)	0.16	(408)	0.13	(354)				
Parent (biological and/or adoptive or stepchildren)	0.13	(39)	0.25	(44)				
Not a parent	0.48	(120)	0.42	(136)				
R^2	0.134		0.181					

Note: Respondents in this multiple-classification analysis are those who thought that the costs of children exceeded the benefits and those who thought that the benefits exceeded the costs.

[a] The proportions in this table have been adjusted for the effects of the other variables shown in the table. Race and family income were excluded from this regression because they had no explanatory power.

among men there is the suggestion that support for nonparenthood comes from the highly urbanized and secularized—hardly a surprising finding. What *is* surprising is that very young men seemed to have turned about—their views differ radically from those aged 25 to 34. Whether such a finding presages a continuing decline in support for nonparenthood remains to be seen.

Among women there is a strong suggestion that attitudes toward non-parenthood relate to sex roles and anticipated sex roles. For example, not only is it true that almost half of nonparents see the costs of children as exceeding the benefits, but approximately 40 percent of divorced women do so. By contrast, only 5 percent of single women take an unfavorable view of parenthood. Unfavorable views of parenthood characterize larger percentages of employed than unemployed women; and 44 percent of those who are employed part-time, but intend to become full-time employees, see the costs of children as exceeding the benefits. Age is not an important variable among women, and this fact creates an interesting disparity between men and women, because of the marked age-cohort effects among men. Twenty-three percent of young women see costs as exceeding benefits, but only 4 percent of young men do so. On the other hand, in the age group from 25 to 34, the shoe is on the other foot—men are more antinatalist than women, the figures being 34 and 21 percent respectively.

These results suggest that, in a period of rapid social change, men and women may be "out of sync" regarding reproduction. For example, it is possible that the younger generation of men may be more family oriented than is the younger generation of women. This might occur if male support for nonparenthood has had different causes from female support. If men have supported nonparenthood as part of an antiestablishment ideology bound up with opposition to the Vietnam War, support for civil rights, and concern for population growth and the environment, while women have supported it because of feminism, it may be that younger men are politically more conservative than the next older cohort, while young women continue to become more feminist. This speculation will require further research.

Components of the Perceived Costs and Benefits of Children

The rough balance of perceived costs and benefits discussed in the previous section provides a summary picture of respondents' views of reproduction and nonreproduction. However, it conceals a wealth of detail concerning responses about the direct and indirect costs of children, children as a financial and social investment, and children as an interaction good. Let us now turn to these components.

As may be seen from table 13–3, respondents perceived reproduction as involving major direct costs—especially "burdensome demands" and inability to "organize time." Conversely, there is a strong rejection of the notion that children entail significant opportunity costs—that childless couples are more intimate, lead more varied lives, or that a women incurs a major loss if she gives up working to become a mother. In this sense, nonparenthood does not seem to have a glamorous image. There is no widespread perception of the child-free life as providing highly desirable options that are unavailable to those with children.

For this reason, the balance of costs and benefits discussed in the previous section is heavily influenced by perceptions of the *direct* costs of children, not by the notion that nonparenthood involves one in uniquely advantageous life-style options. Indeed, if the direct costs of children are removed from the calculus of costs and benefits, as has been done in table 13-4, the result is a substantially enhanced perception of benefits as exceeding costs. When opportunity costs alone are balanced against benefits, 68 percent of the men and 65 percent of the women regard the benefits of children as exceeding the costs. This compares with 55 percent of the men and 56 percent of the women seeing benefits exceeding costs when both direct and indirect costs are under consideration (table 13-1).

Direct and Indirect Costs

Do respondents vary significantly according to major social and demographic characteristics in their perception of the costs of children? Briefly, the answer is no. Whatever may influence variability in perceptions of such costs, age, race, religion, education, marital status, family income, community size, and parental status do not seem to be important candidates. For example, when the questions on direct costs were combined into an index, a multivariate analysis using social and demographic predictors resulted in little explained variance (see table 13-5). The scoring for all the indexes in tables 13-5 through 13-11 attaches a low value to an antinatalist view and high value to a pronatalist one. Thus, with regard to costs, respondents who believe that children exact high costs have low scores, and respondents who think that children have low costs receive high scores.

Table 13-5 provides examples of some theoretically key relationships. As can be seen, for both men and women there is little difference by age in the index, although persons aged 55 and over do have somewhat higher values. Religious differences are also unimportant, as are those by education. The greatest variability within a major grouping is between those who are and are not parents—a difference that doubtless would be larger still were it possible to distinguish between voluntary and involuntary nonparenthood. Even so, nonparents are not strikingly distinct from parents in their views of the direct costs of children.

Table 13–3
Attitudes Toward Childlessness, Gallup Survey, United States, July 1978, by Sex

	Percentage of Total Respondents				Percentage of Women				Percentage of Men			
	(1)	(2)	(3)	(4)	(1)	(2)	(3)	(4)	(1)	(2)	(3)	(4)
Direct costs of children												
Tied down	49	6	45	100	46	6	49	100	52	6	41	100
Organize time	62	7	31	100	61	7	32	100	63	8	29	100
Burdensome demands	66	5	30	100	62	5	34	100	69	4	26	100
Lose individuality	27	6	67	100	28	6	67	100	26	6	67	100
Opportunitity costs of children												
Intimacy	23	17	60	100	23	17	60	100	22	17	60	100
Varied lives	24	12	64	100	22	12	66	100	26	12	62	100
Job chances	30	12	58	100	30	9	60	100	31	14	55	100
Children as an economic investment												
Financial	55	13	32	100	53	12	35	100	58	14	28	100
Children as a social investment												
Lonely	73	6	20	100	73	6	21	100	73	7	20	100
Goal	73	8	19	100	70	9	21	100	75	8	17	100
More adult	66	9	25	100	63	9	28	100	70	8	22	100
Divorce	36	14	50	100	30	13	57	100	42	15	43	100
Children as an interaction good												
Love and companion-ship	59	11	30	100	56	10	34	100	62	11	26	100
Stimulation and fun	82	7	10	100	83	6	11	100	82	8	10	100

Note: Column heads indicate the following categories: (1) agree; (2) undecided; (3) disagree; (4) total.

Table 13–4
Having Children: The Balance of Costs and Benefits Without Direct Costs, Gallup Survey, United States, July 1978, by Selected Characteristics, by Sex

	Men					Women				
	(1)	(2)	(3)	(4)	(N)	(1)	(2)	(3)	(4)	(N)
Total										
United States	10%	22%	68%	100%	(769)	12%	23%	65%	100%	(786)
Age										
18–29	12	29	59	100	(210)	17	24	59	100	(213)
30–34	15	24	62	101	(200)	13	25	62	100	(206)
45–54	4	19	77	100	(114)	9	24	67	100	(113)
55 +	7	14	79	100	(239)	8	20	72	100	(245)
Race										
White	10	20	70	100	(654)	11	23	66	100	(682)
Black	10	33	57	100	(107)	15	27	58	100	(97)
Religion										
Protestant	6	15	79	100	(428)	12	20	68	100	(480)
Catholic	11	30	59	100	(212)	10	26	64	100	(237)
Jewish	33	10	57	100	(21)	15	25	60	100	(20)
None	18	34	48	100	(98)	24	34	42	100	(41)
Education										
Grade school	7	16	77	100	(105)	6	17	77	100	(87)
High school (incomplete)	8	21	71	100	(125)	6	24	70	100	(126)
High school (complete)	7	21	72	100	(282)	12	23	66	101	(337)
College (incomplete)	18	28	55	101	(130)	18	23	59	100	(128)
College (4 +)	14	23	64	101	(124)	17	28	55	100	(106)
Marital status										
Single	17	35	49	101	(165)	20	26	54	100	(112)
Married	8	17	75	100	(539)	10	23	67	100	(500)
Divorced and separated	7	29	64	100	(41)	19	25	56	100	(59)
Widowed	9	17	74	100	(23)	11	19	70	100	(114)
Parental status										
A parent	7	17	77	101	(547)	8	21	71	100	(609)
Not a parent	18	34	48	100	(216)	26	30	44	100	(172)

Note: Column heads: (1) costs greater than benefits; (2) costs equal to benefits; (3) costs less than benefits; (4) total.

Table 13-5
Relation of Age, Religion, Education, and Parental Status with Indexes of the Costs of Children, Gallup Survey, United States, July 1978, by Sex

| | Adjusted Means [a] | | | |
| | Direct Costs | | Indirect Costs | |
Predictors	Men	Women	Men	Women
Age				
Under 30	2.88 (210)	2.95 (213)	3.38 (210)	3.42 (213)
30-44	2.82 (200)	2.89 (206)	3.30 (200)	3.40 (206)
45-54	2.85 (114)	2.91 (113)	3.35 (114)	3.36 (113)
55+	2.93 (239)	3.06 (245)	3.41 (239)	3.43 (245)
Religion				
Catholic	2.86 (212)	2.98 (237)	3.27 (212)	3.41 (237)
Protestant	2.91 (428)	2.98 (480)	3.44 (428)	3.42 (480)
Jewish	2.72 (21)	2.87 (20)	3.49 (21)	3.41 (20)
None	2.85 (98)	2.72 (41)	3.23 (98)	3.35 (41)
Education				
Grade school	2.90 (105)	2.93 (87)	3.34 (105)	3.36 (87)
High school (incomplete)	2.91 (125)	2.98 (126)	3.30 (125)	3.43 (126)
High school (complete)	2.85 (282)	2.95 (337)	3.41 (282)	3.41 (337)
College (incomplete)	2.84 (130)	2.94 (128)	3.32 (130)	3.48 (127)
College (4+)	2.91 (124)	3.05 (106)	3.39 (124)	3.36 (106)
Parental status				
Parent (biological only)	2.92 (483)	3.02 (557)	3.42 (483)	3.47 (557)
Parent (biological and/ or adoptive or stepchildren)	2.94 (64)	3.02 (52)	3.38 (64)	3.59 (52)
Not a parent	2.76 (216)	2.77 (172)	3.23 (216)	3.19 (172)
Grand mean	2.88 (769)	2.97 (786)	3.37 (769)	3.41 (786)
Standard deviation	0.71	0.74	0.69	0.72
R^2 (adjusted for degrees of freedom)	0.015	0.016	0.013	0.082

[a]Adjusting for all variables appearing in the table, plus residence, marital status, region, family income, and race.

As for indirect (opportunity) costs, an index was formed for these as well, and a multivariate analysis undertaken (table 13-5). Looking at the same relationships as for direct costs, among women we see little variation by age and education, and essentially none by religion. More divergence is evident according to whether women are parents or not, but it does not even approach one standard deviation. Among men, age differences are also small, as are those by education. Although religious distinctions are not large, it is of some interest that Catholic men are just about as antinatalist as are men with no religion. For both sexes, being childless is not an important predictor of views of the opportunity costs of children, although compared with other predictors this attribute is relatively impressive.

We will now consider the benefits of children—economic investments, noneconomic investments, and interaction goods. The marginal values for these variables have been shown in table 13-3.

Economic Investments

Are children primarily consumption goods? Is their value to Americans principally in the arena of immediate interaction benefits, or are they also viewed as a means to economic and social ends? In answer, we can say that the results of this survey suggest strongly that children are still viewed in our society, however modern and nonfamilistic it may be, as involving major investment components—both economic and social.

As may be seen from table 13-3, over one-half of respondents regard children as economic investments of a sort, and only one-third would deny outright that offspring play this role. Moreover, the major background variables we have used in this study tap little of the variability that exists among respondents (table 13-6). Table 13-6 shows the adjusted coefficients for four theoretically key variables—age, religious affiliation, educational level, and parental status. The variable that is most interesting is education among women. There is a definite tendency for belief in the financial importance of having children to vary inversely with educational level. No such effect is evident for men. This result suggests that less-advantaged women are disproportionately likely to look to offspring as a financial-insurance mechanism. It is also evident from this table that people who are not parents are less likely to set store by the long-run financial importance of parenthood.

Social Investments

What about social investments? Here we see (table 13-3) that two-thirds to three-fourths of respondents view children as a hedge against loneliness in

Table 13–6
Relation Between Selected Predictor Variables and Opinion That Children Are a Financial Investment, Gallup Survey, United States, July 1978, by Sex

| | Percentage Agreeing That Children Are a Financial Investment | | | |
| | Women | | Men | |
Predictor	Number	Adjusted Percentage[a]	Number	Adjusted Percentage[a]
Age				
Under 30	213	58	210	52
30–44	206	51	200	54
45–54	113	45	114	63
55 +	245	54	239	62
Religion				
Protestant	480	54	428	61
Catholic	237	49	212	54
Jewish	20	82	21	38
None	41	46	98	49
Education				
Grade school	87	69	105	57
High school (1–3)	126	62	125	59
High school	337	52	282	55
College (1–3)	128	41	130	61
College (4 +)	106	45	124	58
Parental status				
Parent (biological only)	557	56	483	62
Parent (biological and/or adoptive or stepchildren)	52	60	64	59
Not a parent	172	42	216	49
R^2 (all background variables)	0.032		0.054	

[a]The values are adjusted for all other predictor categories appearing in this table, plus race, family income, region, and community size. The R^2 shown in this table have been adjusted for degrees of freedom.

old age, as offering a goal in life, and as providing a sense of having achieved adulthood. On no other set of questions is such consensus elicited. Interestingly, a question on children as "marital cement" drew much less popular assent than did the other three. This idea was particularly objected to by women, whereas men were almost evenly divided in their confidence that children cement marriages. When the social-investment index was formed, this question was excluded, both because of its low interitem correlation with the others in the index, and because of the interaction by sex. The high degree of consensus on this index is far from vitiated by taking background variables into account. However, there is some important variation; and, among both men and women, background variables and parental status explain a much higher proportion of the variance on the social-investment index than on any other. Among men, these factors explain 10 percent of the variance and among women, 17 percent. As may be seen from tables 13-7 and 13-8, there is an interaction among age, education, and religion. The greatest reliance on children as a social investment is among older (45 and over) men having a high-school education or less (table 13-7). However, being older apparently keeps the score relatively high even if men have a college education (category 2). Conversely, being younger (under age 45) does not compensate for relatively modest education (categories 3, 4, and 5). The score will drop only when the income level is elevated (category 6). Finally, being young and college-educated serves to reduce the score, particularly for Jewish respondents. It is also clear that parenthood affects the scores for men.

Among the women (table 13-8) the story is very similar although the exact categories differ somewhat. The most reliance on children as a social investment comes from the least educated, regardless of age (category 1). The next-highest score goes to those who have completed high school (with an exception to be discussed later in this chapter) or who are age 45 and over and have some college education (category 2). An interesting exception, as with men, are high-school-educated women having family incomes of $10,000 or more who are Catholic or who have no religious affiliation (category 3). Among respondents under age 45 who have some college education, there is, for Protestants and Catholics, considerable difference between the northeastern and mid-Atlantic regions and the rest of the country (categories 4 and 5). People on the eastern seaboard are more likely to view children as a social investment than are those in other parts of the country. Finally, young, educated Jews and those having no religious affiliation (category 6) are the least likely to see children as a social investment. For women, as for men, parental status is an important explanatory factor.

In sum, as we have suggested elsewhere, people are most likely to see reproduction as being socially instrumental when their alternative means for achieving social goals are the most limited (Blake 1968, 1973, 1979). This finding helps to explain why those who are economically deprived do not tailor their family sizes, or their family-size goals, to their pocketbooks. Moreover, we must also recognize that the social-investment value of children is widely shared among Americans. It is a sentiment that removes children from pure competition with other consumer goods and, we believe,

Table 13-7

Relation Between Selected Predictor Variables and Opinion That Children Are a Social Investment, Gallup Survey, United States, July 1978, Men

Predictors	Number	Adjusted Mean [a]
Interaction term:		
Age 45 +		
1. High school complete or less	285	3.83
2. College incomplete or more	74	3.72
Under age 45		
3. High school incomplete or less	68	3.76
4-6. High school complete		
4. Protestant or Jewish	83	3.76
5. Catholic or none, with less than $10,000 income	18	3.84
6. Catholic or none, with $10,000 + income	58	3.40
7-8. College incomplete or more		
7. Protestant or Catholic	139	3.52
8. Jewish or none	44	3.11
Parental status		
Parent (biological only)	483	3.77
Parent (biological and/or adoptive or stepchildren)	64	3.76
Not a parent	216	3.43
Grand mean		3.67
Standard deviation		0.75
R^2 (all background variables)		0.105

[a]The variables are adjusted for all other predictor categories appearing in this table, plus race, family income, region, and community size. The R^2 shown in this table have been adjusted for degrees of freedom.

provides more ballast to reproductive motivation than would generally exist if children were valued solely as economic instruments or interaction goods.

Interaction Goods

Turning to children as interaction goods, it is evident (table 13-3) that offspring are perceived somewhat more as sources of stimulation and fun than of love and companionship. In both cases, however, the proportions assenting are high; and there can be little doubt that children are, indeed, interaction goods. The high level of consensus on this index does not vary much

Table 13–8
Relation Between Selected Predictor Variables and Opinion That Children Are a Social Investment, Gallup Survey, United States, July 1978, Women

Predictors	Number	Adjusted Mean [a]
Interaction term:		
1. High school incomplete or less	135	3.92
2. High school complete (except category 3) and college incomplete +, aged 45 +	440	3.72
3. High school complete, Catholic and none, $10,000 + income	59	3.32
4–6. College incomplete +, under age 45		
4–5. Protestant or Catholic		
4. All except northeastern and and mid-Atlantic regions	91	3.08
5. Northeast and mid-Atlantic	37	3.57
6. Jewish or none	24	2.66
Parental status		
Parent (biological only)	557	3.68
Parent (biological and/or adoptive and stepchildren)	52	3.70
Not a parent	172	3.36
Grand mean		3.61
Standard deviation		0.83
R^2 (all background variables)		0.170

[a] The values are adjusted for all other predictor categories appearing in this table, plus race, family income, region, and community size. The R^2 shown in this table have been adjusted for degrees of freedom.

according to the background variables considered in this chapter. Background factors explain 0.053 percent of the variance among men and 0.012 percent among women. Table 13–9 shows that there is a definite inverse relationship for women by educational level (although none for men) and, for both sexes, a lesser conviction among nonparents than parents that children are desirable interaction goods. These results suggest that, even as consumer goods, children may be more important to the disadvantaged than the advantaged.

Attitudinal Predictors of Respondents' Views about the Costs and Benefits of Childlessness

Although background factors play some role in explaining which respondents will view the overall costs of children as exceeding the benefits, with

Table 13–9
Relation Between Selected Predictor Variables and Opinion That Children Are Valuable Interaction Goods, Gallup Survey, United States, July 1978, by Sex

Predictor	Women		Men	
	Number	Adjusted Mean[a]	Number	Adjusted Mean[a]
Age				
Under 30	213	3.53	210	3.68
30–44	206	3.45	200	3.49
45–54	113	3.57	114	3.62
55 +	245	3.59	239	3.59
Religion				
Protestant	480	3.53	428	3.64
Catholic	237	3.55	212	3.61
Jewish	20	3.64	21	3.18
None	41	3.30	98	3.46
Education				
Grade school	87	3.65	105	3.57
High school (1–3)	126	3.62	125	3.55
High school	337	3.53	282	3.53
College (1–3)	128	3.42	130	3.49
College (4 +)	106	3.46	124	3.52
Parental status				
Parent (biological only)	557	3.60	483	3.74
Parent (biological and/ or adoptive or stepchildren)	52	3.78	64	3.71
Not a parent	172	3.24	216	3.24
Grand mean		3.53		3.59
Standard deviation		0.85		0.85
R^2 (all background variables)		0.012		0.053

[a] The values are adjusted for all other predictor categories appearing in this table, plus race, family income, region, and community size. The R^2 shown in this table have been adjusted for degrees of freedom.

the exception of the social-investment factor, such factors do not explain much of the variance in the components of the overall balance. Since this result was not completely unexpected, we built into our interview schedule four questions on attitudes toward sex roles in relation to parenthood. The first two of these questions are presented below. The possible responses were "strongly agree," "agree," "undecided," "disagree," and "strongly disagree."

Housework: No matter what a man might say before marriage, a woman would be unwise to believe that her husband will actually share equally in the work around the house (such as cleaning, doing dishes, and so forth) even if she is working full time.

Childrearing: Also, no matter what her husband says before they have children, she would be unwise to believe that he will actually share equally in the tasks of childrearing—even if she works full time while the children are young.

These questions were designed to measure whether respondents believe that, regardless of intentions, men and women will end up playing traditionally differentiated sex roles once they marry and/or have children. In particular, the questions were designed to elicit whether respondents believe that such intrafamilial roles will be played regardless of whether the wife works or not. Hence, we had anticipated that these questions would differentiate respondents according to whether they see marriage, and particularly childbearing, as a conventionalized trap for women in which they are caught regardless of whether they might wish to break out of traditional sex-role expectations.

A second set of questions relates to respondents' evaluations of the desirability of being a working mother.

Secure Relationship: A working mother can establish as warm and secure a relationship with her children as a mother who does not work.

Happier at Home: Women are much happier if they stay home and take care of their children.

We expected respondents who saw marriage and childbearing as generating a conventionalized division of labor between the sexes (regardless of initial intent) to be more antinatalist than those who believed that couples would share household and childrearing tasks if that was what they had originally set out to do. We also expected respondents who disagreed that mothers are happier at home rather than working, and who agreed with the idea that working mothers can establish warm and secure relations with their children, to be more antinatalist.

In considering the effect of these variables, we will first examine those respondents who see total costs as greater than total benefits, as against those who see total benefits as greater than total costs. Although "secure relationship" and "housework" do not have much effect, we find that, holding background factors constant, "happier" and "childrearing" raise the R^2 to 21 percent for men and 16 percent for women (table not shown). It will be remembered that background factors alone produced an R^2 of 18 percent for men and 13 percent for women.

For both sexes, it is clear that people who disagree that women are happier at home instead of working are markedly more inclined to see costs as exceeding benefits than are respondents who believe that women are happier at home. This relationship is particularly sharp for men. As for "child-

Table 13–10
Expectations of Sex-Role Differentiation in Marriage and Parenthood in Relation to Attitudes Toward the Costs of Children, Gallup Survey, United States, July 1978, by Sex

Predictor	Women		Men	
	Number	Adjusted Mean [a]	Number	Adjusted Mean
Direct costs:				
Childrearing				
Strongly agree	47	2.67	[b]	
Agree	306	2.76		
Undecided	96	3.06		
Disagree	305	3.17		
Strongly disagree	32	3.18		
Grand mean		2.97		
Standard deviation		0.74		
R^2		0.088		
R^2 (background only)		0.008		
Indirect costs:				
Housework				
Strongly agree	[b]		31	3.18
Agree			318	3.35
Undecided			103	3.39
Disagree			290	3.37
Strongly disagree			27	3.61
Childrearing				
Strongly agree	47	3.11	17	3.29
Agree	306	3.30	286	3.25
Undecided	96	3.42	109	3.29
Disagree	305	3.55	335	3.48
Strongly disagree	32	3.68	22	3.56

Table 13–10 continued

Predictor	Women		Men	
	Number	Adjusted Mean [a]	Number	Adjusted Mean
Happier at home [b]				
Strongly disagree			38	3.19
Disagree			253	3.30
Undecided			194	3.35
Agree			245	3.42
Strongly agree			39	3.72
Grand mean		3.41		2.97
Standard deviation		0.72		0.74
R^2		0.117		0.151
R^2 (background only)		0.063		0.100

[a] The values are adjusted for all background predictors plus other attitudinal variables in the models shown. Thus the coefficients for indirect costs for men are adjusted for background factors plus two attitudinal variables.
[b] No explanation added by this variable.

rearing," although this result is in the expected direction for both sexes, the relationship is more marked for women, as anticipated. Women who believe that childbearing inevitably thrusts one into conventionalized roles are more likely to see the cost of children as higher than the benefits.

In sum, therefore, with respect to the balance of costs and benefits, the five principal variables explaining men's disposition to see costs as exceeding benefits, are parental status, age, "happier," community size, and religion. Among women, the five principal variables are parental status, marital status, "happier," present and expected work status, and "childrearing." It is abundantly clear that the variables of importance for women are all those measuring actual and normative (or expected) social roles.

Turning to attitudinal influences on the components of the perceived costs and benefits of children, we find that the effects of just one or two questions are quite dramatic (table 13–10).

Direct and Indirect Costs

Among women, the one question on "childrearing" increases the R^2 on direct costs from less than 1 percent (background factors only) to almost 9 percent. This same question increases the R^2 on indirect costs from 6 percent (background only) to almost 12 percent. Among men, no effect of the attitudinal questions is evident with regard to direct costs; but results of the three questions, "happier at home," "housework," and "childrearing," boost the R^2 for indirect costs from 10 to 15 percent.

In effect, respondents' beliefs, particularly those of female respondents, that motherhood consigns women to conventionalized maternal-role obligations regardless of the intent of either parent, seem to be an important factor in the view that parenthood has high costs. Interestingly, although "happier at home" does not affect women's views of the indirect costs of children, it does affect those of men. Men who believe that women are happier at home taking care of the children than out working, are markedly less likely to think that children involved the indirect costs measured here. We can only surmise that the notion that women are happier at home serves as a rationalization for men in helping them overlook the indirect costs of reproduction.

Social Investments and Interaction Goods

Attitudes toward sex roles in relation to parenthood also have marked effects on respondents' views of the benefits of reproduction. With regard to the social-investment index, "happier at home" and "secure relationship" raise the R^2 for women from 17 to 23 percent (table 13-11). "Happier at home" boosts men's R^2 from 10.5 to 14.4 percent. With regard to children as interaction goods, "happier at home" raises the R^2 for women from 1 to 8 percent and, for men, from 5.3 to 11.8 percent.

In sum, as may be seen from the adjusted means, respondents who take a highly conventionalized view of the mothering role as being properly and most felicitously at home with the children, are most likely to believe that offspring are a noneconomic investment and an enjoyable interaction good.

Conclusion

The 1970s have witnessed a noteworthy increase in the proportion of young women who intend to remain childless. By 1978, 18 percent of single women aged 18 to 24 stated this intention when queried by the Bureau of the Census. We have also seen that actual childlessness among young married women is rising. Thus, young women of today will probably experience higher rates of permanent childlessness than did those who reproduced during the baby boom.

Table 13-11
Evaluations of the Working Mother in Relation to Attitudes Toward the Benefits of Children, Gallup Survey, United States, July 1978 , by Sex

Predictor	Women		Men	
	Number	Adjusted Mean[a]	Number	Adjusted Mean[a]
Social investments:				
Happier at home				
Strongly disagree	59	3.47	38	3.40
Disagree	317	3.44	253	3.55
Undecided	165	3.68	194	3.71
Agree	200	3.81	245	3.78
Strongly agree	45	3.90	39	3.96
Secure relationship				
Strongly agree	77	3.57		[b]
Agree	383	3.58		
Undecided	57	3.51		
Disagree	242	3.66		
Strongly disagree	27	3.92		
Grand mean		3.61		3.67
Standard deviation		0.83		0.75
R^2		0.229		0.144
R^2(background only)		0.170		0.105
Interaction goods:				
Happier at home				
Strongly disagree	59	3.10	38	3.13
Disagree	317	3.44	253	3.56
Undecided	165	3.51	194	3.67
Agree	200	3.71	245	4.21
Strongly agree	45	3.95	39	
Grand mean		3.53		3.59
Standard deviation		0.85		0.85
R^2		0.083		0.118
R^2 (background only)		0.012		0.053

[a]The values are adjusted for all background predictors plus other attitudinal variables in the models shown. Thus the coefficients for happier at home among women are adjusted for secure relationship and vice versa, as well as for background variables.
[b]No explanation was added by this variable.

However, it is unclear whether nonparenthood has become a widely supported goal in the United States or, rather, whether it is being established as a legitimate option by a relatively select few in our population. In the former case, we might expect not only lifetime childlessness by those who express this intention at a very youthful age, but an increase in new recruits to this lifestyle. If, on the other hand, it is simply an emerging option supported by a small minority, we would hardly anticipate an epidemic of permanent nonparenthood.

Here we attempt to illuminate these issues through an analysis of questions addressed to a national sample of voting-aged adults in the United States, on the perceived costs and benefits of being childless and of having children. This survey was conducted in July 1978, and the questions focused on five major issues:

1. perceptions of children as involving a direct cost—actual outlays and demands;
2. perceptions of children as involving opportunity costs—foregone advantages and opportunities;
3. perceptions of children as involving long-run economic or financial return for the individual;
4. perceptions of children as involving long-run *non*economic return for the individual;
5. perceptions of children as an interaction good—an end in itself from which satisfaction is gained, purely because of the quality of interaction and companionship involved.

The questions, presented in appendix 13A, were used to measure the direct and opportunity costs of children, children as economic investments, children as noneconomic investments, and children as providers of companionship or interaction benefits.

Taking all the measured costs and benefits together, most people—55 percent of men and 56 percent of women—see the benefits of children as exceeding the costs. Somewhat less than one-third of each sex see the cost-benefit equation as a toss-up (typically a pattern of high costs and high benefits). Only about 15 percent view costs as exceeding benefits. In effect, there appears to be little support for nonparenthood. The most important characteristic distinguishing those who see costs as exceeding benefits from those who see benefits as exceeding costs is actual parental status. Nonparents are heavily represented among those who emphasize the costs of parenthood. Beyond that, the results differ by sex. An interesting finding is that 23 percent of young women, but only 4 percent of young men see costs as exceeding benefits. On the other hand, in the age group 25 to 44, men are more antinatalist than women. Since other characteristics lead us to believe that young women are influenced in their view of nonparenthood by a concern for sex roles, it is possible that a share of young men and women may be currently out of step in their view of reproduction. Men may have espoused a nonparenthood ethic as part of the political ideology of the late 1960s and early 1970s. Women's views, however, may be based more enduringly on a commitment to changed sex roles.

Does the balance of costs and benefits reflect, on the side of costs, a notion that children entail major opportunity costs—that nonparenthood allows a more interesting, glamorous, and personally satisfying existence? From our data, the answer is emphatically negative. The costs of children are seen, by respondents, to be primarily direct ones—burdensome demands and inability to organize time. There is an explicit rejection of the notion that childless couples are more intimate or lead more varied lives, or that a woman incurs a major loss if she gives up working to become a mother. If direct costs are dropped from the cost-benefit equation, 68 percent of men and 65 percent of women regard the benefits of children as exceeding the costs. Only 10 percent of men and 12 percent of women see costs as exceeding benefits.

Viewing the components of the cost-benefit equation separately, respondents were found to differ very little (according to major background characteristics) in their views of children as direct and indirect costs. There is, in sum, a relatively high degree of consensus that children entail heavy direct costs, but unimportant indirect ones.

Are children primarily consumption goods? In effect, is the perceived benefit of children in modern society, as some economists have suggested, one that competes alongside that of other items of consumption? Our results indicate that the role of children in people's lives is more complex and in particular that people view offspring as being major investments as well as consumer items. A little over half of respondents see children as economic investments—only one-third would deny that children have this role. Although variability in this response is not generally explained by major social and economic cleavages, it is of interest that less-educated women are particularly prone to this view. This result may help explain why lower-income families typically want and have more children than do families with high incomes.

There is a high degree of consensus that children are a social investment—an investment in adult status, in providing a goal in life, and against loneliness in old age. Between two-thirds and three-quarters of respondents subscribe to this view. Although consensus is high on this issue, respondents do differ about it, especially by age and educational level. Commitment to children as a social investment is highest among those who are older and have relatively low educational levels and is least among those who are both young and highly educated.

Finally, high proportions of respondents see children as sources of stimulation and fun—as major interaction (consumer) goods. This sentiment differs little by social and economic categories.

We expected that respondents' views of parenthood might be conditioned by their beliefs concerning sex roles and reproduction. Hence we inserted four questions on this topic into the survey. Two related to whether respondents saw marriage and parenthood as leading to conventionally structured sex roles, regardless of the couple's original intent. In effect, are marriage and parenthood a sex-role trap for women despite good intentions? Two other questions related to respondents' view of the desirability of being a full-time, as opposed to a working, mother. Taking the cost-benefit equation, we find that those who disagree that women are happier at home than working are markedly more likely to see the costs of children as exceeding the benefits. This is particularly true among men. Among women, those who see reproduction as leading to conventionally differentiated sex roles are noticeably more likely to see the costs of parenthood as exceeding the benefits. Taking the components of the equation separately— direct and indirect costs, financial investments, social investments, and interaction goods—the attitudinal questions on sex roles have a dramatic effect in explaining variability among respondents.

In sum, it seems that insofar as antinatalist views exist in our population, they are related to a suspicion by both men and women that parenthood is a potent force inducing conventional sex roles in marriage. Additionally, respondents who do not perceive full-time mothers as happier than working mothers are less likely to regard parenthood as having benefits. Whether these sex-role responses can be interpreted literally, or as simply indicative of underlying views about conventional family behavior, cannot be ascertained at this time. They do suggest, however, that assessment of the costs and benefits of parenthood are more closely related to sex-role attitudes and anxieties than to any single traditional background characteristic. Since most respondents believe that children provide major investment benefits as well as consumption opportunities, and relatively few respondents aver that life is more interesting and glamorous without offspring, it is the sheer wear and tear of reproduction that appears to be the major drawback of parenthood. This direct cost is less likely to be emphasized by women who think that the husband will share significantly in childbearing, than it is among those who are convinced that parenthood is a classic sex-role trap for mothers. It seems probable, therefore, that an increase in nonparenthood may be checked by greater egalitarianism between marital partners, insofar as this continues to take place. This egalitarianism would help to mitigate the one strike that reproduction seems to have against it—a perception that it entails heavy direct costs, particularly for women.

References

Blake, Judith. "Are Babies Consumer Durables? A Critique of the Economic Theory of Reproductive Motivation." *Population Studies* 22 (1968): 5-25.

———. "Fertility Control and the Problem of Voluntarism." In *Scientists and World Affairs,* edited by Pugwash Committee, pp. 279-288. Proceedings of the Twenty-Second Pugwash Conference on Science and World Affairs, London 1973.

———. "Is Zero Preferred? American Attitudes Toward Childlessness in the 1970s." *Journal of Marriage and the Family* 41 (1979): 245-257.

United States Bureau of the Census. "Fertility History and Prospects of American Women: June 1975." *Current Population Reports,* series P-20, no. 288 (1976).

———. "Fertility of American Women: June 1978." *Current Population Reports,* Series P-20, no. 341 (1979).

United States Department of Health, Education, and Welfare, National Center for Health Statistics. *Final Natality Statistics, 1977* 27 (1979).

———. *Monthly Vital Statistics Report* 28 (1980).

Appendix 13A:
Text of Questions on Attitudes toward Childlessness: Gallup Survey, United States, July 1978

(The identifying words to the left are used in the tables in this paper. The responses were "strongly agree," "agree," "undecided," "disagree," or "strongly disagree").

Lonely

1. People who have had children are less likely to be lonely in their older years than persons who are childless.

Tied Down

2. Having children ties you down and makes it very difficult to do things, as a couple, spontaneously and on the spur of the moment.

More Adult

3. Becoming a parent makes a person feel more adult and mature than he or she did before having a child.

Intimacy

4. Assuming that couples with and without children are about the same age, those who have not had children tend to be emotionally closer to each other and to share a greater intimacy than do those with children.

Goal

5. Becoming a parent gives one a goal in life with more meaning than one would have otherwise.

Love and Companionship

6. When a couple decides to remain without children, they deprive themselves of one of the most important sources of love and companionship in life.

Organize Time

7. One big advantage of remaining without children is that you can organize your time and activities more efficiently than when you have to plan around young children.

Divorce

8. A couple is less likely to get a divorce if they have had children than if they have remained without a family.

Burdensome Demands

9. Becoming a parent involves a person in a lot of burdensome responsibilities and demands.

Stimulation and Fun

10. Having children gives a couple a major source of stimulation, variety, and fun in life.

Lose Individuality

11. When you become a parent you sort of lose your individuality because your life is no longer your own.

Financial

12. If you have children, you are more likely than a person without children to have someone to turn to if you need financial help when you are older.

Varied Lives

13. Assuming that couples with and without children are approximately the same age, those who have not had kids tend to lead more interesting and varied lives than those with youngsters.

Job Chances

14. A young woman pays a heavy price when she gives up her job chances to stay home and have a family.

14 Comparative Analysis of Fertility Orientations: World Fertility Survey Findings

Lee-Jay Cho and
Louise Kantrow

The last chapter of part III, like the last chapter of part II, describes fertility desires in developing countries. The authors, Lee-Jay Cho and Louise Kantrow, use data from World Fertility Study reports on eight different Asian countries. While they stress the diversity of those countries, they also note important similarities in their fertility and fertility orientations. They identify similarities that set them apart from more-developed countries such as the United States, the subject of most of the chapters in this book.

In contrast to that of the United States, the populations described by Cho and Kantrow bear far more children than they desire. Despite this apparently widespread motivation to terminate childbearing, a majority of women in need do not practice efficient contraception. In part this may reflect the inaccessibility of family-planning services—Cho and Kantrow note that the family-planning programs in some of these countries, although vigorously pursued, are relatively new and poorly funded.

But the apparent inconsistency between motivation and behavior also may reflect our failure to measure motivation adequately, or perhaps our failure to understand how fertility motivations relate to fertility behavior in a developing society. The measurement problem is confronted by Cho and Kantrow, who find that many women in these Asian nations gave different and apparently inconsistent indications of their fertility orientations. In chapter 8 Pullum demonstrated several techniques for maximizing the usefulness of these questionable data. The necessity for such techniques reminds us, as we commented in our introduction to chapter 8, that there may exist fundamentally different regimens of interrelationship between fertility orientations and future fertility. The "rational" relationships of which we found evidence in the papers by Hirsch, Seltzer, and Zelnik (chapter 12) and Blake and del Pinal (chapter 13) may not be duplicated in the third world.—*Eds.*

Introduction

The levels, patterns, and trends of fertility are influenced by a variety of factors, many of which are intricately interrelated. Reliable information on these factors has rarely been available for developing countries. Consequently, little is known of the ways in which reproductive behavior in these countries is affected by social, cultural, and demographic factors or by the unique structure of their interrelationship. The World Fertility Survey (WFS) is an international research program in which developing and developed countries are participating, carrying out scientifically designed sample surveys of fertility behavior, which are nationally representative and internationally comparable. The WFS is administered by the International Statistical Institute in collaboration with the International Union for the Scientific Study of Population. The WFS provides the first opportunity to determine levels of fertility and analyze the factors affecting fertility and fertility preferences of married women in developing countries. This chapter presents a cross-cultural analysis of these preferences, as documented in the First Country Reports for Korea, Malaysia, Nepal, Pakistan, Thailand, Fiji, Indonesia, and Sri Lanka.

The First Country Reports are first-stage analyses prepared by the national-survey staffs according to guidelines provided by WFS as to the statistical tables that should be prepared (World Fertility Survey 1977). The Core Questionnaire (World Fertility Survey 1975) was designed to be used in interviewing ever-married women in the childbearing years residing in households. It contains seven sections, including a detailed maternity history and marriage history as well as segments on contraceptive knowledge and use and on fertility preferences. Data from these published reports are analyzed here in an attempt to illuminate the measurement and analysis of fertility preferences.

While it is common practice to speak of Asia as an entity, it is essential to keep in mind—as we examine and compare the fertility aspirations and family-planning practices of the millions of couples of childbearing age who live in these Asian countries—that history, culture, religions, socioeconomic development, and the very terrain these nations occupy have resulted in the development of vastly different peoples. Their religious affiliations highlight their differences. They are Buddhist, Confucianist, Taoist, Hindu, Moslem, animist, and Christian. Some—in Nepal, for example— live in virtually total isolation from each other because of the towering mountains that separate one village from another; others, as in Malaysia, live in small, compact areas where it is almost impossible to avoid contact with one's fellow citizens. At least two of these countries—Korea and Malaysia—are well along in their social, economic, and family-planning-program development efforts; others, such as Nepal and Pakistan, have made little headway.

However, several striking similarities also exist. The vast majority of people in these eight countries live in nonurban areas, most are poor, many cannot read and write, many report having more children than they want. In all these countries, the governments have attempted to ameliorate the harsh conditions under which most people live by investing in industrial and agricultural development, and in education and public health. All have come to understand that their efforts at improvement are often frustrated by the rapidity with which their populations are growing, and have for various lengths of time supported family-planning programs.

Development and Demographic Data

Table 14-1 presents information on a variety of indicators of social and economic development. Where development is more advanced, and where there are more-effective programs, crude birth and death rates are lowest, as in Korea, Malaysia, and Fiji; the converse is also true, with the highest birth and death rates in Nepal and Pakistan. Korea and Sri Lanka have the lowest rate of natural increase (17 and 18 people per 1,000 per year, respectively). Because some of its high fertility is offset by high mortality, Nepal has one of the lowest rates of population increase, 21 to 23 per 1,000. Thailand's low mortality and moderately high fertility rates make its rate of increase (28) higher than Nepal's.

Life expectancy and infant mortality highlight the differences in development among the eight nations studied. A Nepalese woman's life expectancy is only 43—twenty-seven years less than that of a Malaysian woman. This discrepancy is, in part, a reflection of infant mortality, which is almost five times higher in Nepal (200 infant deaths per 1,000 live births) than in peninsular Malaysia (41 deaths per 1,000 live births). The lack of medical care in less-developed lands helps explain high infant mortality and short life expectancy. In Nepal, for example, there are 38,700 people for every physician. In Korea there are 1,600 people per doctor.

Literacy rates also vary with the extent of development. Four percent of women in Nepal and 17 percent of women in Pakistan are literate, whereas in Sri Lanka, Thailand, and Korea the proportion who are literate ranges from 71 to 84 percent.

While the majority of the population is rural in all eight countries, the proportion that is urban ranges from just 5 percent in Nepal to 48 percent in Korea.

Finally, table 14-1 shows the median age at first marriage for women in the eight countries, as derived from the WFS data. Marriage takes place much later in the more developed countries—Korea (23 years of age) and Malaysia (21)—than in Pakistan, Fiji, Indonesia (16) or Nepal (15). Thailand (with an average age at marriage of 19) again falls in between the most- and least-developed countries in the sample. Many factors other than cultural differences are involved in the relationship between development and rising age at marriage, among them provision of education for women (which alters their attitudes toward work, marriage, and children) and increased employment opportunities for women.

Table 14–1
Selected Demographic Data for Eight Asian Nations, 1975–1977

Measure	Korea	Malaysia[a]	Nepal	Pakistan	Thailand	Fiji	Indonesia	Sri Lanka
Estimated population (millions)	36	13	13	72	43	0.6	135	13.8
Crude birth rate[b]	24	30	42–44	40–45	37	29	37–40	27
Crude death rate[b]	7	6	20–22	15	9	7	15–18	9
Rate of natural increase	17	24	21–23	25–30	28	22	20–25	18
Life expectancy (female at birth)	67	70	43	50	64	72	49	66
Infant mortality rate[c]	60	41	200	136	80	22	140	50
Population per M.D. (in thousands)	1.6	4.4	38.7	4.1	7.9	2.4	21.7	4.2
GDP per capita (U.S. dollars)	504	602	101	128	323	999	127	235
Percentage literate[d]								
Male	94	90	24	17	89 }	85	71	85
Female	84	62	4	17	75 }		49	71
Percentage urban	48	29	5	27	20	36	19	24
Median age of women at first marriage	23	21	15	16	19	16	16	17

Sources: D. Nortman and E. Hofstatter, "Population and Family Planning Programs: A Factbook," *Reports on Population/Family Planning*, 1976, 1978; Population Reference Bureau, *1977 World Population Estimates* (Washington, D.C.: 1977).

[a] Except for total population, all data are for peninsular Malaysia only.

[b] Per 1,000 population.

[c] Per 1,000 live births.

[d] For Malaysia, Pakistan, Thailand, Indonesia, and Sri Lanka the percentage literate is of people aged 10 and over; for Korea and Nepal, aged 6 and over; for Fiji, aged 15 and over.

Government Family-Planning Programs

All the countries included in this analysis have government-supported as well as private family-planning programs. The countries vary in the length of time these programs have existed, in the amount of funding they receive, and in their ability to deliver services.

As can be seen in table 14-2, Pakistan has the oldest government-supported family-planning program, while Thailand's national program is the newest, begun only in 1970. The table also shows the amount each government allocated for family planning in a recent year, to what extent this amount was supplemented by other sources, and how much was spent.

Expressed in U.S. cents per capita, Malaysia spends the most money on family-planning programs—40¢ per person in government funds alone. Pakistan is second (with 34 cents per capita from all funding sources), followed by Korea (22 cents), Indonesia (15 cents), Nepal and Sri Lanka (12 cents), and Thailand (9 cents). By themselves these data do not give a total picture of a country's program. While Thailand spends only 9 cents per person on family planning and has had a program only since 1970, an estimated 24 percent of all married women are enrolled in the government program. In contrast, Pakistan spends almost four times as much per person (and has had a government program for eighteen years), but only an estimated 5 percent of all married women of reproductive age are using a contraceptive method. One explanation given for the low rate of contraceptive use is that Pakistan has spent a great deal of money on activities related to motivation rather than on provision of services. Data from the Pakistan WFS indicate that while almost all women have heard about methods of family planning, only about one-third know of any place where they can obtain a method of contraception.

With 35 percent of the women of reproductive age enrolled in its program, Fiji seems to have the most effective program. The programs in Korea, Malaysia, and Thailand are about equally effective, with 22 to 24 percent enrolled. Although no official estimate of women enrolled is available for Nepal, WFS data show that only 2 percent of married women are protected against unplanned pregnancy.

The government programs in all these countries include the major modern methods of contraception: the birth-control pill, the intrauterine device (IUD), male and female sterilization, and condoms. Injectable contraceptives are also offered in Thailand, and the Korean program includes menstrual regulation. For the most part, all methods are distributed without cost to the client. All methods are free in Malaysia and Nepal. In Korea there is a charge for pills—10 cents per cycle—and female sterilization is not free but is subsidized by the government. In Pakistan, IUD insertion costs 5 cents. In Thailand all methods are free to those unable to pay.

Table 14-2
Government Family-Planning Programs in Eight Asian Nations, Selected Variables, 1975–1977

Variable	Korea	Malaysia	Nepal	Pakistan	Thailand	Fiji	Indonesia	Sri Lanka
Year started	1962	1966	1965	1960	1970	1962	1968	1965
Program funds (in thousands of U.S. dollars)								
Government	6,105	4,508	1,138	8,000	935	NA	20,722	NA
All sources	7,619	NA	1,440	24,000	3,686	NA	NA	6,247
Funds per capita (in U.S. dollars)								
Government	17	40	9	11	2	NA	15	NA
All sources	22	NA	12	34	9	NA	NA	12
Women enrolled								
Total (in thousands)	1,059	332	NA	NA	1,281	32	3,701	NA
Percentage of married women 15–44	22	24	NA	NA	24	35	18	NA

Sources: International Planned Parenthood Federation, *Family Planning in Five Continents* (London: International Planned Parenthood Federation, 1976); and D. Nortman and E. Hofstatter, "Population and Family Planning Programs: A Factbook," *Reports on Population/Family Planning*, 1976, 1978.

Note: NA = not available

In response to the shortage of medical personnel in developing countries, family-planning programs have trained nonprofessionals to provide services and have instituted a variety of innovative plans to make contraceptives more accessible. One such plan, community-based distribution of a variety of methods, has been instituted in all the countries analyzed here.

Abortion laws vary among the eight countries. Korea permits abortion for a variety of indications, including the mother's mental health. At the other extreme, Pakistan and Malaysia permit abortion only to save the woman's life.

Measuring Fertility Preferences: Issues and Findings

It should be stated at the outset that there is no wholly satisfactory way to measure from sample surveys the number of children wanted by married women who have already embarked on their childbearing careers. Since the early 1960s there has been considerable research interest in fertility preferences in relation to knowledge and use of contraception among women in developing countries, because of the assumed usefulness of such information to those concerned with altering rates of population growth by reducing fertility. It is believed by many of those who advocate family planning that, based on findings of fertility surveys, family-size desires in developing countries are low. If this is so, motivational problems are minimal and popultaion growth could be reduced by preventing the pregnancies that respondents claim were unwanted. Others maintain that family-size desires are still high in most developing countries. Although this group favors providing contraceptive services, it is argued that family-size desires are resistant to change and can be reduced only through basic change in social and economic institutions (United Nations n.d.).

Considerable effort has been devoted to the measurement of fertility preferences of women from sample surveys, the goal being to gain knowledge of women's attitudes toward future childbearing, desired completed family size, and use of contraception. The underlying assumption was that expressed attitudes on any of these variables related to future childbearing would determine actual behavior. However, with some exceptions, the record has not supported this assumption (Freedman, Hermalin, and Chang 1979). Most research relating fertility attitudes to behavior has shown that attitudes contribute little to determining behavior. Many researchers have begun to question the predictive value of statements regarding future childbearing and, indeed, to question whether such responses have any meaning at all (Hauser 1967).

Important methodological issues have emerged surrounding the reliability of the measurement instrument (Coombs 1978). Each of the various dimensions of this issue has important implications. First, do the attitude questions elicit a consistent response at a single testing, or in a test-retest situation (Knodel and Piampiti 1977)? Second, is it possible to gauge levels of intensity for any given attitude? Finally, what factors account for the gap between an expressed attitude and subsequent behavior that, from the researcher's vantage point, is inconsistent?

Fertility preferences are measured by two sets of questions in the World Fertility Surveys. This provides a unique opportunity to analyze fertility preferences from more than one perspective and to investigate the issue of consistency of attitudes at a single testing. In the Core Questionnaire women were asked one question concerning their desire for more children and another question concerning the total number of children desired.

Particular attention is frequently focused on the group of women who reported they did not want more children. This is an important group of women because they are presumably *potential* candidates for family planning. Reports based on results from the WFS support the view that there is a large unmet need for family-planning services based on the evidence that a large proportion of respondents report they want no more children (Westoff 1978). An important issue to be considered is whether this proportion reporting they do not want more children accurately reflects a desire or intent to cease childbearing. Previous investigations in this area have shown that inconsistencies in results from the same data set cast doubt on the meaning of the responses of women to questions on the desire for more children (Knodel and Prachuabmoh 1973). What follows is an examination of WFS results in these Asian countries to the two questions designed to probe fertility preferences. There are considerable data for both sets of questions according to such variables as current age, number of living children, number of living sons, education of the woman, and urban or rural residence. This is followed by an investigation into cross-national differences in unwanted fertility as estimated from the surveys.

The fact that a woman states that she does not want another child does not guarantee that she will use family planning, nor does her response necessarily mean that her husband, mother, or other relatives who may influence her behavior agree. Nonetheless, the responses do indicate the magnitude of one aspect of demand.

The percentage of currently married fecund women who do not want more children is given in table 14–3. There is no doubt that the desire for no more children as presented here is surprisingly high. For all women it ranges from 30 percent in Nepal to 72 percent in Korea. Even in Pakistan, where provision of family-planning services has been minimal and the vast majority of women have remained outside the mainstream of development efforts, almost one-half of those sampled said they wanted no more children. A calculation (based on the data displayed in the table) shows that in all the countries except Nepal, more than half of the women aged 20 and over do not want more children. In Nepal this proportion does not reach a majority until age 30. In sum, these findings show that according to this measure many married women at relatively younger ages have attained their fertility desires.

Table 14–3 also displays the proportion wanting no more children according to number of living children. In each country, the proportion wanting no more children rises sharply with the number living. At zero parity, with the exception of Korea, negligible proportions say they want no more children. However, after two living children have been achieved, two-thirds of the women in Korea and almost one-half in Thailand say they want no more. Even in Pakistan almost one of every three women wants no more by the time she has two living children. In all countries, despite their differing levels of development and differing cultures, more than half the women want no more than four living children. Indeed, just under 70 percent of Pakistani women appear to be ready to stop having children after they have four who are living.

Finally, table 14–3 shows how fertility preferences change depending on the number of living sons. Son preference is most dramatic among Korean women—after they have two living sons, 94 percent of mothers want no more children. Although son preference is also strong elsewhere, with a majority in all countries wanting no more children after two living sons have been achieved, the preference is not as striking as in Korea.

As can be seen from table 14–4, age and education appear to effect fertility aspirations. In Korea, Nepal, and Pakistan, among women younger than 25 (who are most likely to have benefited from improvements in the educational systems), the more education a women has, the more likely she is not to want additional children. Although this relationship appears to be especially striking in Nepal and Pakistan, it should be noted that relatively few women in these countries have had more than a primary education. In Malaysia and Thailand, however, there appears to be an inverse relationship between education and the proportion who want no more children. Thus in Malaysia, although about 14 percent of women younger than 25 who have no education want no more children, only about half that proportion with a secondary or higher education want no more children. In part, this finding may be related to the fact that women with more education usually come from more economically advantaged families, marry later, and postpone childbearing, while their less-educated contemporaries marry and initiate childbearing at younger ages. However, even when controls for age and parity are introduced, the relationship between education and desire for more children is not consistently positive (this is not shown in table).

Table 14-3
Percentage of Currently Married Fecund Women Who Want No More Children, by Selected Characteristics

Characteristic	Korea	Malaysia	Nepal	Pakistan	Thailand	Fiji	Indonesia	Sri Lanka
Total	72	43	30	49	57	50	39	61
Current age								
20 or under	6	4	2	4	16	18	6	14
20–24	24	11	11	18	34		16	30
25–29	54	27	27	39	49	39	33	47
30–34	84	48	41	61	68	59	51	68
40–44	97	78	66	84	86	86	74	87
45–49	97	79	71	93	90		84	94
Number of living children								
0	12	0	1	2	5	3	4	2
1	13	4	5	7	19	10	9	14
2	66	21	23	30	46	33	29	50
3	86	31	39	48	64	54	45	73
4	92	52	58	69	81	62	57	87
5	95		66	78	90		68	
6	96		80	90	91		78	
7	99	78	88		97	72	87	93
8	100		89	94	94		84	
9+	100		93		99		94	
Number of living sons								
0	23	7	4	6	21	10	15	20
1	64	27	26	32	48	39	36	55
2	94	52	54	71	73	64	52	79
3	98	74	70	90	89	79	65	90
4+	100		78				79	

Table 14-4
Percentage of Currently Married Women Who Want No More Children by Current Age and Level of Education

Age and Education	Korea[a]	Malaysia[b]	Nepal	Pakistan	Thailand[c]	Sri Lanka[d]
Less than 25						
No school	—	13.5	7.7	11	33.8	38.5
Primary	21.0	10.1	8.8	13	29.6	26.1
Secondary	25.8	7.1 }	25.0	22	21.9	24.5
Higher	—	—			22.2	—
25–34						
No school	77.6	42.5	32.3	49	65.4	64.1
Primary	70.3	37.9	45.8	60	59.6	63.8
Secondary	63.5	27.3 }	62.5	49	33.9	50.1
Higher	63.4	27.9	—		12.8	29.6
35–44						
No school	94.1	67.2	59.3	80	76.1	86.0
Primary	93.9	72.2	69.2	65	84.1	86.8
Secondary	94.5	76.2 }	—	83	60.0	77.3
Higher	97.0	90.9	—		45.5	72.3

Source: First Country Reports, table 3.1.3A for all countries except Pakistan (table 3.13) and Thailand (table 3.1.2A).
[a] Middle school and high school are combined into secondary category.
[b] Primary = < 7 years; secondary = 7–12 years; and higher = > 12 years.
[c] Primary = 1–4 years; secondary = 5–10 years; and higher = > 11 years.
[d] Primary = 1–5 years; secondary = 6–11 years; and higher = > 11 years.

Note: — = N < 50.

Table 14–4 shows that among women between the ages of 25 and 34, far larger proportions of those with no education than of comparable younger women want no more children; in Korea, Malaysia, and Thailand, the more education among women aged 25 to 34, the smaller the proportions who want no more children. In Pakistan, almost half the women in that age category who have had no education want no more children; this proportion rises to 60 percent among those with a primary education and falls to about 50 percent again when secondary or higher education is achieved.

In the oldest age group, 35 to 44, the level of education makes almost no difference among Korean women, with well over 90 percent wanting no more children regardless of educational level. Thai women are again the exception, with substantially fewer who have achieved more than a primary education wanting no more children than those with no schooling or only a primary education (Cho et al. 1980; Frisch 1975). In Malaysia greater education is associated with an increase in the proportion wanting no more children. Too few Nepalese women in this age group had a higher education to permit analyses. As stated previously, in the WFS questionnaire fertility preferences were probed with two questions. All currently married women were also asked the question: "If you could choose exactly the number of children to have in your whole life how many children would that be?" The answers to this question according to number of living children, age, wife's level of education, and urban or rural residence are given in tables 14–5 through 14–8. In every country, desired family size increases with number of living children. In part, this might reflect a decline in family-size preferences and might to some extent reflect a bias that achieved fertility influences desired family size. If younger women, who are in the early stages of their reproductive careers, express a desired family size smaller than that expressed by women at the end of their reproductive careers, this could be supporting evidence that fertility norms are declining. However, it could also be the case that women with large families may rationalize unwanted fertility. Inquiry into rationalization of stated desired family size has been limited (but see chapter 8). Using data from Thailand, Knodel and Prachuabmoh (1973) suggest that if rationalization of the existing number of children is a factor influencing the choice of the desired number, then the probability of giving a particular number as the desired family size should be greater for women with that particular number of living children than for women with either more or less than that number. The authors calculate and compare these two sets of probabilities and conclude that the differences in probabilities by parities are not large. As can be seen from table 14–5, with the exception of Korea, women with 0 to 4 living children consistently report an average desired family size that exceeds achieved family size. Desired family size for all currently married women (table 14–5) ranges from a low of 3.2 in Korea to 4.4 in Malaysia. In Fiji, Indonesia,

Table 14-5
Average Number of Children Desired by Currently Married Women, by Number of Living Children

Number of Living Children	Korea	Malaysia	Nepal	Pakistan	Thailand	Fiji	Indonesia	Sri Lanka
0	2.6	3.7	3.5	3.9	2.9	2.6	2.9	2.5
1	2.6	3.7	3.6	3.9	2.8	2.7	3.2	2.4
2	2.8	3.8	3.6	4.0	3.2	3.0	3.5	2.7
3	3.1	4.2	3.9	4.1	3.6	3.6	4.0	3.3
4	3.5	4.6	4.4	4.3	4.0	4.2	4.8	3.9
5	3.7		4.8	4.5	4.3		5.6	
6	4.0	4.9	5.2	4.4	4.6	6.1	6.0	5.5
7+	4.1		5.7	4.8	4.8		7.0	
Total	3.2	4.4	4.0	4.2	3.7	4.2	4.2	3.8

Table 14-6
Average Number of Living Children Achieved and Average Number of Children Desired by Currently Married Women, by Current Age

Age	Korea	Malaysia	Nepal	Pakistan	Thailand	Fiji	Indonesia	Sri Lanka
15–19								
Actual	0.4	0.8	0.3	0.5	0.6	0.5	0.5	0.7
Desired	2.8	3.9	3.6	4.1	2.9	2.7	3.3	2.5
20–24								
Actual	1.0	1.6	1.1	1.5	1.4	1.4	1.4	1.6
Desired	2.8	4.0	3.7	4.0	3.1	3.1	3.7	2.8
25–29								
Actual	1.9	1.9	2.2	2.7	2.4	2.6	2.4	2.6
Desired	2.8	4.2	3.9	4.2	3.4	3.6	4.0	3.2
30–34								
Actual	3.1	4.0	3.1	3.9	3.4	4.0	3.3	3.9
Desired	3.1	4.4	4.2	4.2	3.8	4.5	4.3	3.7
35–39								
Actual	4.0	5.0	3.7	4.8	4.3	4.9	3.9	4.9
Desired	3.4	4.6	4.2	4.3	4.0	5.0	4.8	4.3
40–44								
Actual	4.4	5.5	3.9	4.9	5.1	5.7	4.1	4.6
Desired	3.6	4.6	4.3	4.4	4.1	5.6	5.0	4.4
40–49								
Actual	4.7	5.4	4.0	4.9	5.6	6.0	3.8	6.3
Desired	3.8	4.7	4.3	4.3	4.6	5.9	5.0	4.7

Table 14-7

Average Number of Children Desired by Currently Married Women, by Number of Living Children and Level of Education

Level of Education / Number of Living Children	Korea	Malaysia	Nepal	Pakistan	Thailand	Fiji	Indonesia	Sri Lanka
No education								
0 living children	3.1	4.1	3.5	4.0	2.8	2.6	2.7	2.5
1	3.3	4.0	3.6	4.0	3.0	2.6	3.1	2.4
2	3.4	4.1	3.6	4.1	3.6	2.9	3.3	2.7
3	3.2	4.4	3.9	4.2	3.8	3.4	4.1	3.3
4	3.7	4.7	4.4	4.3	4.0	4.2	4.9	4.0
5	3.9 }		4.8	4.6	4.3 }		5.7 }	
6+	4.1 }	5.1	5.3	4.6	4.7 }	6.2	6.5 }	5.0
Primary								
0 living children	2.8	3.7	3.1	3.3	3.0	2.7	3.0	2.5
1	2.7	3.7	3.1	3.4	2.8	2.9	3.2	2.5
2	2.9	3.9	3.2	3.6	3.1	3.0	3.6	2.8
3	3.2	4.2	3.6	3.7	3.6	3.6	3.9	3.3
4	3.4	4.6	4.3	3.8	4.1	4.2	4.6	3.8
5	3.7 }		NA	4.0	4.3 }		5.5 }	
6+	3.9 }	4.8	NA	4.0	4.7 }	6.1	6.4 }	5.2
More than primary								
0	2.3	3.1	NA	3.4	2.9	2.5	3.3	2.5
1	2.4	3.3	NA	3.2	2.7	2.7	3.2	2.3
2	2.6	3.4	NA	3.0	3.1	3.0	3.2	2.6
3	3.0	3.9	NA	3.0	2.9	3.5	3.7	3.2
4	3.2	3.9	NA	3.5	3.4	4.1	4.3 }	
5	3.1 }		NA	3.3	4.1 }		5.1 }	
6+	3.6 }	4.3	NA	3.5	NA }	5.9	NA	5.2

Note: NA = not available

Table 14-8
Average Number of Children Desired by Currently Married Women by Number of Living Children and Place of Residence

Place of Residence Living Children	Korea	Malaysia	Nepal	Pakistan	Thailand	Fiji	Indonesia	Sri Lanka
Urban								
0	2.3	3.2	NA	3.5	2.0	2.5	3.0	2.5
1	2.4	3.2	NA	3.7	2.7	2.6	3.1	2.1
2	2.7	3.3	NA	3.7	3.1	2.8	3.5	2.6
3	3.0	3.9	NA	3.8	3.3	3.4	4.0	3.2
4	3.3	4.0	NA	4.0	3.8	4.0	4.5	3.7
5	3.4 }	4.4 }	NA	4.0	4.4 }	5.9 }	5.3 }	5.1 }
6+	3.7		NA	4.2	4.9		6.5	
Rural								
0	2.9	3.8	NA	4.1	3.0	2.6	2.9	2.5
1	2.9	3.8	NA	3.9	2.8	2.8	3.2	2.5
2	3.0	4.0	NA	4.1	3.2	3.1	3.5	2.7
3	3.3	4.4	NA	4.2	3.6	3.7	4.0	3.4
4	3.7	4.7	NA	4.4	4.1	4.3	4.8	4.0
5	3.8 }	5.0 }	NA	4.7	4.3 }	6.2 }	5.7 }	5.6 }
6+	4.2		NA	4.8	4.8		6.7	

Note: NA = not available.

Malaysia, Nepal, and Pakistan, currently married women desire an average of 4 or more children.

In both table 14–5 and 14–6, desired family size increases with age and parity in every country except Pakistan. This phenomenon is more marked in Korea, Thailand, Fiji, Indonesia, and Sri Lanka, where desired family size increases by more than one child between the youngest and oldest women. In the remaining countries, fertility preferences are more similar and do not change by more than one child among all age groups. In addition to rationalization of children already born, this phenomenon may also reflect declining fertility preferences. Korean women in every age group report wanting fewer children than women in the other countries. Korean women's fertility preferences have undergone a major reduction since the early 1960s—attributable in part to the strong national family-planning program that has been in effect for almost two decades. In Korea, Thailand, and Sri Lanka, women under age 30 desire strikingly fewer children than older women, probably because of the family-planning programs and recent socioeconomic advances in these countries. In Nepal and Indonesia, where program activity is more recent, accessibility is a problem, and knowledge that fertility can be controlled is limited, the number of children desired is greater than the number living at every age.

When desired family size according to number of living children and background variables is investigated (see tables 14–7 and 14–8), it is possible to observe which socioeconomic categories of women have surpassed their fertility desires. If the average number of children desired exceeds the number of living children, women have not yet reached desired parity; otherwise, their actual fertility has equaled or exceeded their fertility desires. Again, in Korea, where fertility decline has been most pronounced, desired family size is also lowest regardless of number of living children. Fertility has shown little decline in Pakistan and Nepal, and in these countries desired family size is high and differences are associated with number of living children or level of education or place of residence. Women who are beginning their reproductive careers in Nepal and Pakistan desire almost as many children as women who have already had five or more. A similar but less-pronounced pattern exists in Malaysia, where the crude birth rate has declined by 26 percent since 1965. An interesting pattern, which exists for all countries, is that regardless of the average desired family size, fertility preferences of childless women or of those with one living child are almost identical.

In addition to information from the direct question on the desire for more children, it is possible to measure the desire to cease childbearing indirectly, by using the question on total number of children desired. A comparison of these two variables provides an indication of the degree of consistency between the two measures of fertility preferences. The proportion of women whose actual number of children is equal to or greater than their desired number should be the same as the proportion of women who want no more children. The results, classified by number of living children, are presented in table 14-9. In three countries—Fiji, Indonesia, and Sri Lanka—the measures are close for all women. In the remaining countries the difference in the two measures of the desire to cease childbearing is most pronounced for women with no more than three living children. In Korea, for women who have two living children, the proportion not wanting any more (as measured from the question on desired versus actual) is 38 percent, compared with 66 percent as measured from the direct question. In Malaysia and Pakistan these differences are 21 versus 13 percent and 30 versus 15 percent, respectively. An unusually high proportion of zero-parity women in Korea (12 percent) and Thailand (5 percent) say they want no more children. This potential level of childlessness would be high even in countries where fertility has declined to very low levels. However as seen in table 14-9, 99 percent of these same zero-parity women indicate they have had less than the number of children they desire.

Similar differences in measuring fertility preferences are also evident when you compare estimates for unwanted fertility from WFS results. Interest in measuring the extent of unwanted fertility stems from the notion that it is one indication of the demand for family-planning services, and that it provides an estimate of what the level of fertility would be if women had only the number of children they wanted. From WFS it is possible to measure unwanted fertility by several methods. Two measures are presented in table 14-10. The first is the difference between the average number of children desired and the total fertility rate for ever-married women, that is, the number of children each ever-married woman would have in her lifetime if current age-specific fertility rates were to persist. The second measure is the weighted mean of the difference between the average number of children desired for ever-married women according to current age in those age groups for which achieved parity exceeds desired parity. The essential difference between these measures is that the latter takes into account the effect of infant mortality, while the former does not. As can be seen in table 14-10, there is considerable difference in the two measures of unwanted fertility. Any measure of unwanted fertility is a hypothetical construct and therefore subject to bias. The second measure may underestimate excess fertility to the extent that desired family size is influenced by achieved parity and the first measure is biased by the failure to account for the difference between children ever born and actual living children.

In developing countries, women who do not want more children constitute an important group. Presumably, they may be candidates for family-planning services. Precisely because it is such a significant group, it becomes important to define this group carefully. From the preceding analysis it is clear that further investigation into the meaning of fertility preferences from survey responses is necessary. There is still ambiguity con-

Table 14-9
Measures of Desire for More Children from the World Fertility Survey

Number Living Children	Korea		Malaysia		Nepal		Pakistan		Thailand		Fiji		Indonesia		Sri Lanka	
	Percentage	Desired Versus Actual	Percentage	Desired Versus Actual	Percentage	Desired Versus Actual	Percentage	Desired Versus Actual	Percentage	Desired Versus Actual	Percentage	Desired Versus Actual	Percentage	Desired Versus Actual	Actual Percentage	Desired Versus Actual
0	12	1	0	8	1	0	2	0	5	0	2	2	4	0	2	0
1	13	3	4	1	5	3	7	1	19	3	7	7	9	8	14	10
2	66	38	21	13	23	26	30	15	46	34	34	30	29	26	50	46
3	86	73	31	16	39	48	48	29	64	59	49	47	45	39	73	65
4	92	90	52	60	58	70	69	69	81	83	67	70	57	52	87	82
5	95	97		70	66	81	78	82	90	90			68	57		86
6	96	97	78	88	80	89	90	93	91	96	83	86	78	69	93	90
7	99	99		88	88	90	94	89	97	95			87	77		92
8+	100	98		96	89	90			94	96			84	73		90

Table 14–10
Measures of Unwanted Fertility from the World Fertility Survey

	Unwanted Fertility	
Country	Total Marital Fertility Rate Versus Desired	Desired Versus Achieved
Korea	1.5	0.8
Malaysia	1.2	0.7
Nepal	4.6	0.0
Pakistan	2.8	0.6
Thailand	1.2	0.8
Fiji	0.9	0.1
Indonesia	0.0	0.0
Sri Lanka	0.8	0.8

cerning who the women are who want no more children and, more importantly, what the relationship is between a stated desire to cease child-bearing and actual future behavior. Insufficient attention has been focused on the issue of why women who may express a desire to cease childbearing are *not* candidates for family-planning services. Such crucial determinants of future childbearing as husband's attitudes and extended family or peer pressure have yet to be assessed and included in the equation.

Contraceptive Practices

As noted previously, many women of childbearing age in these eight developing countries report that they have more children than they want and desire no additional children. Table 14–11 provides some insight into the contraceptive practices of these women. In Thailand, Indonesia, Korea, and Malaysia, the countries with the most active family-planning programs, the largest proportions of women who want no more children are attempting to control their fertility—and the largest proportions are using the most-effective methods. In Thailand and Malaysia, 20 percent of women who have all the children they want are using the birth-control pill, and almost that proportion in Thailand report that they or their husbands have been sterilized for contraceptive purposes; just over 10 percent of Malaysian women rely on sterilization. In Sri Lanka sterilization is the most-preferred method among women who want no more children. In Korea, more than 25 percent of women who want no more children are using the pill and the IUD, while about 9 percent rely on sterilization. In Indonesia 27 percent rely on the

Table 14–11
Percentage Distribution of Exposed Women Who Want No More Children, According to Pattern of Current Contraceptive Use, by Method

Method	Korea	Malaysia	Nepal	Pakistan	Thailand	Indonesia	Sri Lanka
Efficient: total	43.5	37.4	8.6	7.4	51.5	47.2	33.8
Pill	13.1	20.1	1.2	2.8	20.2	26.8	2.2
Injectable	0.4		0.1		2.8		0.5
IUD	13.1	1.4	0.2	1.8	9.5	13.7	7.5
Sterilization	8.9	10.6	6.8	3.2	18.4		20.7
Condom	7.6	4.9	0.3	2.4	0.5	4.1	1.5
Other scientific[a]	0.4	0.4	0.0	0.4	0.1	1.6	1.4
Inefficient: total	12.2	15.1	0.0	4.2	4.1		19.7
Withdrawal	4.1	3.5	0.0	0.2			2.1
Rhythm	7.1	5.2	0.0	0.2	3.6	4.3	11.5
Abstinence	0.6	3.9	0.0	3.4			6.0
Other folk method	0.4	2.5	0.0	0.4	0.5	2.9	0.1
No method	44.3	47.5	91.4	88.4	44.4	46.6	46.5
Total	100.0	100.0	100.0	100.0	100.0	100.0	100.0

Source: First Country Reports—Korea, table 5.2.1; Malaysia, tables 5.2.3 and 4.4.1; Nepal, table 5.2.3; Pakistan, table 5.2.3; Thailand, table 5.2.1; Sri Lanka, table 5.2.3; Indonesia, table 4.5.4.
Note: Includes sterilized women in both the numerator and denominator.
[a]Includes diaphragm and spermicides.

birth-control pill. The situation in Nepal, Pakistan, and Fiji presents a sharp contrast to this picture. In Nepal 21.3 percent of ever-married women know of any method of contraception; however, 91 percent of women who want no more children are using no method, while among those using contraception, sterilization is the most common method. Pakistani women are least likely to use efficient methods to attain their fertility desires. Only 7 percent of those who want no more children are using any efficient method, and knowledge of contraception is extremely high (75 percent of ever-married women report knowing any method of contraception).

While about 55 percent of women who want no more children are using contraception in Korea, Malaysia, Indonesia, Sri Lanka, and Thailand, the proportions using efficient methods differ substantially, ranging from 51 percent in Thailand to 34 percent in Sri Lanka. It should be noted that there remains a substantial proportion of women in all eight countries who, despite their desire to have no more children, are using no method.

It is of some interest to examine the use and nonuse of contraception by currently married, fecund women who report that they have more children than they want (table 14-12). In Korea 33 percent of such women have more children than they want; in Malaysia, 25 percent; in Pakistan, 23 percent; and in Thailand, 20 percent. As table 14-12 shows, in Korea just over half of these women (or their husbands) are using an efficient method. In Malaysia, of the 25 percent who say they have more children than they want, 40 percent are users of efficient methods. In Thailand 20 percent of women have more children than they want, but just 35 percent of them are users. As might be expected, Pakistan has the smallest proportion of women who want no more children who are users of efficient methods (13

Table 14-12
Percentage Distribution of Currently Married Fecund Women Who Have More Children Than They Want, by Use and Nonuse of Efficient Contraceptive Methods

User Status	Korea	Malaysia	Pakistan	Thailand	Indonesia
User	51	40	13	35	36
Nonuser	49	60	87	65	64
Total	100	100	100	100	100

Source: First Country Reports—Korea, Thailand, table 5.2.1; Malaysia, Nepal, and Pakistan, table 5.2.3; Indonesia, table 4.5.3.

Note: "Fecund women" includes those contraceptively sterilized and those currently pregnant. "Efficient contraceptive methods" are the pill, injectable contraceptives, the IUD, sterilization, the condom, and diaphragm with spermicide.

percent), although almost one-quarter say they have more children than they want.

References

Cho, Lee-Jay; Suharto, S.; McNicoll, G.; and Made Mamas, S.G. *Growth of Indonesian Population,* chapter 4. Honolulu: University Press of Hawaii, 1980.

Coombs, Lolagene C. "How Many Children Do Couples Really Want?" *Family Planning Perspectives* 10(1978):303–308.

Freedman, Ronald; Hermalin, A.I.; and Chang, M.C. "Do Intentions Predict Fertility? The Experience in Taiwan, 1967–74." *Studies in Family Planning* 10(1979):75–95.

Frisch, R.E. "Demographic Implications of the Biological Determinants of Female Fecundity." *Social Biology* 22(1975):17–22.

Hauser, Philip M. "Family Planning and Population Programs." *Demography* 4(1967):397–414.

International Planned Parenthood Federation. *Family Planning in Five Continents.* London: International Planned Parenthood Federation, 1976.

Knodel, John, and Piampiti, Sauvaluck. "Response Reliability in a Longitudinal Survey in Thailand." *Studies in Family Planning* 8(1977): 55–66.

Knodel, John, and Prachuabmoh, Visid. "Desired Family Size in Thailand: Are the Responses Meaningful?" *Demography* 10(1973):619–637.

Nortman, D., and Hofstatter, E. "Population and Family Planning Programs: A Factbook." *Reports on Population/Family Planning,* 1976, 1978.

Population Reference Bureau. *1977 World Population Estimates.* Washington, D.C., 1977.

United Nations. *Measures, Policies and Programmes Affecting Fertility, with Particular Reference to National Family Planning Programmes.* United Nations Publication, Sales no. E.72.XIII-2, pp. 1–16.

Westoff, C.F. "The Unmet Need for Birth Control in Five Asian Countries." *International Family Planning Perspectives* 4(1978):97.

World Fertility Survey. "Core Questionnaires." *Basic Documentation.* London, 1975.

World Fertility Survey. "Guidelines for Country Report No. 1." *Basic Documentation.* London, 1977.

**Part IV
Predicting Fertility: A
Synthetic Exposition**

15 Needed Research on Birth Expectations

Arthur A. Campbell

In this section a summing up is attempted. Arthur A. Campbell, himself an important actor in the history of the birth-expectations research he briefly reviews, indicates the specific issues toward which future research on that subject should be directed. In the final chapter we will identify and discuss some of the themes, explicit and implicit, that relate the papers in the book.—*Eds.*

The use of questions on birth expectations began over twenty-five years ago, following the failure to predict the strong resurgence of fertility in the late 1940s and early 1950s. Such questions were first used in the Interim Economic Survey of the Survey Research Center of the University of Michigan in October 1954. The following year they were used in the Detroit Area Survey of the University of Michigan and on a national sample in the Growth of American Families (GAF) Study. Since 1955 comparable questions have been used in nationwide fertility surveys in the United States in 1960, 1965, 1970, 1973, 1975, and 1976 and in the census bureau's Current Population Surveys (CPS) for 1967 and for each year from 1971 through 1979. In addition, questions on birth expectations have been used in special U.S. studies such as the 1964–1966, 1967–1969, 1972, and 1980 National Natality Surveys (NNS) and in many other countries.

On the basis of this broad experience, questions on birth expectations as well as other questions regarding the orientation of couples toward past and future childbearing have been shown to be of great value in interpreting data on other variables included in fertility surveys. For example, questions concerning whether or not a birth was wanted in interpregnancy intervals may be used to distinguish those couples who wanted additional children from those who did not. Surveys have shown that the two groups behave differently; those who do not want more children are more likely to use contraception and less likely to have accidental pregnancies (Westoff and Ryder 1977a). These relationships hold true not only with the use of retrospective questions in cross-sectional surveys, but also with the use of prospective questions in longitudinal surveys (Westoff, Potter, and Sagi 1963). Therefore, questions regarding the orientation of couples toward their future childbearing (whether asked in terms of desired, expected, or intended births) are of undoubted worth in fertility surveys and should continue to be used. However, the various chapters of this book are concerned with birth expectations as dependent variables with presumed predictive power, rather than as independent variables with proven explanatory power. The research that is needed, therefore, should address the general problem of the predictability of birth expectations. This problem may be further divided into two researchable issues: the reliability of short-term and long-term birth expectations.

Short-Term Birth Expectations

As several of the chapters in this book have shown, the use of birth expectations to predict fertility within five-year periods is questionable. In numerous instances actual fertility is above or below the level expected. On the basis of a careful analysis of the predictive validity of reproductive intentions gathered in the longitudinal portion of the National Fertility Studies (NFS) for 1970 and 1975, Westoff and Ryder summarize their findings as follows:

> It would have been encouraging to find clues from our survey at the end of 1970 which would suggest, at least for this select group, that fertility was likely to decline in the next five years. It is our impression, to the contrary, that reproductive intentions are tailored to conditions at time of interview and, thus, share the same possibilities of misinterpretation as other period indices. In brief, we are skeptical of the usefulness of reproductive intentions, as least for short-range population projection purposes. They seem little better than conventional period indices, although their validity as predictors of completed cohort fertility may be better. On the other hand, their validity at the level of individual prediction is considerable in comparison with most other demographic and social indicators [Westoff and Ryder 1977b, p. 434]

One reason that short-term birth expectations are not good predictors is that period fertility rates (that is, fertility rates observed for the entire population of women of childbearing age over a brief span of time) are highly variable in comparison with completed fertility rates for cohorts of women. Period fertility rates depend not only on the level of completed fertility to be attained by cohorts in the reproductive years of life, but also on the maternal ages at which their births occur. A trend toward later maternal ages will tend initially to depress period rates and later to inflate them. A trend toward younger maternal ages will have the opposite effects. To use birth expectations as predictors in this situation is comparable to aiming at a rapidly moving target.

Another problem with using birth expectations to predict fertility over relatively short periods of time arises from the fact that questions on expectations have generally been limited to currently married women who will have fewer than half of all births occurring in the five years following the interview. However, since 1976 the census bureau has been asking all women, including those never married, not only the total number of births they expect but also the number they expect in the next five years. (This practice has been followed in the four years 1976 through 1979, but the question on short-term birth expectations has been omitted from the 1980 survey.) Although the census bureau has not yet published the short-term birth expectations for all women, it is planning to do so. Accordingly, if the June 1981 CPS contains the questions needed to elicit numbers of births during the preceding five years, it will be possible to compare five-year birth expectations collected in 1976 with the number of children born between 1976 and 1981. The improvement in coverage from currently married women to all women may or may not improve the accuracy of five-year birth expectations. The addition of unmarried women to those reporting short-term birth expectations represents the addition of a group whose future childbearing decisions are surely less well defined than those of currently married women. Consequently, the results may provide a no-more-reliable basis for predicting short-term fertility rates than the expectations of currently married women. Fortunately, we should not have to wait long for the results of such comparisons.

In considering the usefulness of short-term birth expectations for predicting fertility, we should compare not only actual and expected fertility for specific cohorts, but also the fertility forecasts based on these expectations with fertility forecasts based on the use of analytical techniques that do not employ data on short-term birth expectations. For example, if the sciences of social and economic demography develop a theory relating short-term fertility fluctuations to socioceonomic change, it may be possible to use this theory to forecast fertility over short periods of time solely with the use of data on probable socioeconomic change and recent trends in cohort fertility rates. In any case, we should regard short-term birth expectations as only one basis for making short-term fertility forecasts and not necessarily as the best available predictor of period fertility rates.

In summary, these considerations lead to the following recommendations for research on short-term expectations:

1. Comparisons should continue to be made between short-term birth expectations of currently married women and their subsequent fertility. Although we know that short-term birth expectations cannot be regarded as highly accurate predictors of fertility, additional comparisons between expected and actual fertility should provide estimates of the error variance inherent in these predictions, so that we will have a better idea than we now do about the probable magnitude of the difference between expected and actual fertility.

2. Comparisons between expected and actual fertility should be made for various subgroups of the population in order to gain some idea of the

sources of deviation of actual fertility rates from expected rates. Longitudinal studies are especially helpful for this purpose, since they enable the investigator to compare the expected and actual fertility of individual women. Among the explanatory variables to be included in such analyses should be the degree of certainty with which expectations were expressed. As suggested by Oakley in chapter 2, the degree of uncertainty may provide some measure of the predictive validity of birth expectations.

3. It would be more useful to focus on birth expectations over five-year intervals rather than one- or two-year intervals. In general, shorter time intervals may show wider variations in period fertility rates than longer time intervals. Also, the time involved in collecting data; preparing for analysis; and carrying out the processes of analysis, projection, and publication would render one- or two-year projections out of date by the time they were published.

4. When the data become available for the period 1976–1981, comparisons should be made between expected and actual fertility for all women, as well as for currently married women.

5. Alternative methods of forecasting fertility over short periods of time should be developed and the results compared with those based on short-term birth expectations.

Long-Term Birth Expectations

Because of the greater stability of cohort completed fertility rates than of period total fertility rates, data on the total number of births expected may prove to have greater predictive validity and to be more useful in making population forecasts than data on short-term birth expectations. However, there has been very little research to determine how well actual fertility conforms with expected completed fertility. A very early study of a small group of engaged couples who were first interviewed in the mid-1930s showed that the average number of children wanted just before marriage (2.8 for women and 2.6 for men) was very close to the average number born (2.6) (Westoff, Mishler, and Kelly 1957). However, most of the research dealing with the predictive validity of birth expectations has concentrated on short-term expectations, as in several chapters of this book.

The greatest need is for research on the predictive validity of the birth expectations of young women, particularly those who are recently married or will soon be married. Obviously, it is necessary to wait at least twenty years before the birth expectations of these women can be evaluated definitively. However, it is also possible to make interim assessments of the expectations of birth cohorts as their numbers become older.

An initial effort to compare summary data on birth expectations within cohorts is presented in tables 15-1, 15-2, and 15-3. In table 15-1 the total numbers of births expected by white currently married women in the 1955 and 1960 GAF studies are compared with the numbers of children ever born to white ever-married members of the same cohorts, as reported in 1970 and 1975. In considering these comparisons, it must be kept in mind that the women for whom expectations are reported in 1955 and 1960 were only those who were currently married at that time. For example, in 1955 the members of the 1931–1935 cohorts were 20 to 24 years of age; the group interviewed represents only about two-thirds of all women in that age group. By 1975, twenty years later, 95 percent had married. Therefore, the comparisons are not between expected and actual fertility for representative samples of the same women, and some of the differences between expected and actual fertility must be ascribed to the changing composition of the group for which data are shown.

Despite these qualifications, the members of the 1926–1940 cohorts who were interviewed in 1955 and 1960 seem to have provided reasonably good indications of the eventual fertility of the ever-married portion of these cohorts in the 1970s. All the deviations of actual from expected fertil-

Table 15-1
Intracohort Comparisons of Number of Births Expected by White Currently Married Women in 1955 and 1960 with Number of Children Ever Born to White Ever-Married Women in 1979 and 1975, Cohorts of 1916–1920 to 1936–1940

Cohort	Number of Births Expected per 1,000 Women		Number of Children Ever Born per 1,000 Women			Percentage by Which Children Ever Born Differ from Births Expected	
	1955	1960	Age	Year	Number	1955	1960
1936–1940	—	3,018	35–39	1975	2,891	NA	−4.2
1931–1935	3,191	3,355	40–44	1975	3,224	+1.0	−3.9
1926–1930	3,096	3,237	45–49	1975	3,091	−0.2	−4.5
1921–1925	2,982	2,977	45–49	1970	2,777	−6.9	−6.7
1916–1920	2,898	—	50–54	1970	2,538	−12.4	NA

Sources (1955): Ronald Freedman, Pascal K. Whelpton, and Arthur A. Campbell, *Family Planning, Sterility and Population Growth* (New York: McGraw-Hill, 1959), pp. 486–487; (1960): unpublished tabulations from the 1960 Growth of American Families Study; (1970): U.S. Bureau of the Census, "Women by Number of Children Ever Born," Census of Population: 1970, *Subject Reports,* Final Report PC(2)-3A (Washington, D.C.: U.S. Government Printing Office, 1973), p. 1; (1975): ibid., "Fertility of American Women: June 1975," *Current Population Reports,* series P-20, no. 301 (1976), p. 34.
NA = data not available.

Table 15–2
Intracohort Comparisons of Number of Births Expected by Currently Married Women at Ages 20 to 24 and 25 to 29 in Surveys Conducted by the U.S. Bureau of the Census, 1967 and 1971–1979

Cohort	Year in Which Members Are:		Number of Births Expected per 1,000 Women at Ages		Percentage by Which Later Number Differs from Earlier
	20–24	25–29	20–24	25–29	
1943–1947	1967	1972	2,880	2,452	− 14.9
1947–1951	1971	1976	2,392	2,202	− 7.9
1948–1952	1972	1977	2,253	2,197	− 2.5
1949–1953	1973	1978	2,263	2,215	− 2.1
1950–1954	1974	1979	2,159	2,193	+ 1.6

Sources (1967, 1971, and 1972): U.S. Bureau of the Census, "Birth Expectations and Fertility: June 1972," *Current Population Reports,* series P-20, no. 248 (1973), p. 17; (1973): ibid., series P-20, no. 265, p. 17; (1974): ibid., series P-20, no. 277, p. 15; (1975): ibid., series P-20, no. 301, p. 13; (1976): ibid., series P-20, no. 308, p. 9; (1977): ibid., series P-20, no. 325, p. 8; (1978): ibid., series P-20, no. 341, p. 10; (1979): ibid., series P-20.

Table 15–3
Intracohort Comparisons of Number of Births Expected by Currently Married Women at Ages 25 to 29 and 30 to 34 in Surveys Conducted by the U.S. Bureau of the Census, 1967 and 1971–1979

Cohort	Year in Which Members Are:		Number of Births Expected per 1,000 Women at Ages:		Percentage by Which Later Number Differs from Earlier
	25–29	30–34	25–29	30–34	
1938–1942	1967	1972	3,037	2,915	− 4.0
1942–1946	1971	1976	2,619	2,536	− 3.2
1943–1947	1972	1977	2,452	2,468	+ 0.7
1944–1948	1973	1978	2,387	2,424	+ 1.6
1945–1949	1974	1979	2,335	2,282	− 2.3

Sources (1967, 1971, and 1972): U.S. Bureau of the Census, "Birth Expectations and Fertility: June 1972," *Current Population Reports,* series P-20, no. 248 (1973), p. 17; (1973): ibid., series P-20, no. 265, p. 17; (1974): ibid., series P-20, no. 277, p. 15; (1975): ibid., series P-20, no. 301, p. 13; (1976): ibid., series P-20, no. 308, p. 9; (1977): ibid., series P-20, no. 325, p. 8; (1978): ibid., series P-20, no. 341, p. 10; (1979): ibid..

ity for these cohorts are below 5 percent. Comparisons for the older cohorts (1925 and earlier) are less important for our purposes, since these women had already borne most of the children they would ever have by 1955 or 1960, but the results of the comparison are difficult to understand, particularly the fact that the 1916–1920 cohorts eventually had 12 percent fewer births than expected. The explanation probably lies in some sample bias in the 1955 study.

Tables 15–2 and 15–3 show how the total numbers of births expected have changed for various cohorts as they move from one age group to another. Again, it must be remembered that the comparisons do not relate to the same women or samples of the same women, but to the women who are currently married at the time of interview. A more thorough investigation of changes in expected completed fertility within cohorts would distinguish the changes among women who are represented at both times in the comparison from those who are represented only in the most recent survey. Nevertheless, the comparisons shown here are instructive. Table 15–2 shows that the cohorts of 1943–1947 reduced their expectations substantially between 1967 and 1972. Table 15–3 suggests that the expectations of these cohorts remained essentially unchanged between 1972 and 1977. Table 15–2 also shows a somewhat smaller reduction in total births expected for the cohorts of 1947–1951 between 1971 and 1976. These comparisons imply that the cohorts of the mid- and late 1940s were in the process of revising their childbearing plans to a substantial degree during the period around 1970. After birth expectations had fallen to the low levels reported by the cohorts of the late 1940s and early 1950s (around 2,200 births per 1,000 women) there is no evidence of any further change.

In summary, birth expectations of young married women appear to have served as valid indicators of completed fertility for the cohorts of 1931–1940 and as relatively poor indicators of completed fertility for the cohorts of the 1940s. Obviously, research is needed to document and study these intracohort changes in expected and actual childbearing in more detail, in a manner similar to that used by Ryder and Westoff (1967) in studying changes in total births expected in 1955, 1960, and 1965. Fortunately, the necessary basic data from the GAF studies, the NFS, the National Surveys of Family Growth (NSFG), the NNS, and the CPS are all readily available on computer tapes.

Such analyses should also be conducted on the basis of birth expectations collected in other countries. For example, the United Nations Economic Commission for Europe has published an excellent review of the results of fertility surveys, including birth expectations, conducted in the United States and certain European countries around 1970 (U.N. Economic Commission for Europe 1976). In addition, the World Fertility Survey

(WFS), conducted in a number of countries during the 1970s, is now providing much more of the basic data needed for analysis. However, none of the countries for which birth expectations are available have as long a record of data on this topic as does the United States.

It is difficult to evaluate the birth expectations of the cohorts of the 1950s because their members are still relatively young and have many reproductive years remaining. However, it is possible to compare their expectations with observed cumulative fertility rates and to form an opinion about the likelihood that they will have the number of births they expect. Since the total number of births expected by these cohorts is now on the order of 2,000 to 2,200 (reported by all women rather than married women only), it is clear that the vast majority of women are expecting no more than two births. For example, the 1954–1960 cohorts, who are represented without regard to marital status in the 1978 CPS, expect 878 first births per 1,000 women, 755 second births, and 400 third and higher-order births, which add to a total of 2,033 altogether. If these expectations prove to be valid predictors in the years ahead, 80 percent of all births will be first or second births. Therefore, it is useful to examine trends in the cumulative rate for first and second births separately and to compare them with the trend in total births expected. This has been done in figure 15–1 for first births. As this figure illustrates, the number of first births expected continues at a relatively high level (850 or more first births per 1,000 women, compared with 920 among the cohorts of the mid-1930s), but the trend in the cumulative rate for first births by age 25 is sharply downward. This means that women will have to bear unusually large numbers of first births at ages 25 and later if they are to achieve the level of fertility expected in 1978 (line A, figure 15–1). If they continue to have first births at ages 25 and over at the period rates observed at these ages in 1977, the cohorts of the early 1950s will complete their fertility with only 750 first births per 1,000 women. If, however, the cohorts of the 1940s and early 1950s have first births after age 25 at the rates observed for the 1916 cohort, which had the highest rates for first births at these ages among any cohorts in U.S. experience, they would complete their fertility with about 860 first births per 1,000 women, still below the expected level of 880 for the cohorts of the early 1950s.

Figure 15–2 shows the trend in the first-birth rate at ages 25 to 29 and 30 to 34 from 1917 to 1977 and indicates the approximate levels that the rates would have to attain if the cohorts of the late 1940s and the 1950s were to have the total number of first births expected in 1978. As this illustration shows, the rates would have to rise to a level close to the highest ever observed in the United States.

The same observations apply to recent trends in cumulative rates for second births and the numbers of second births expected by recent cohorts, as illustrated by figures 15–3 and 15–4. Again, the cohorts of the late 1940s

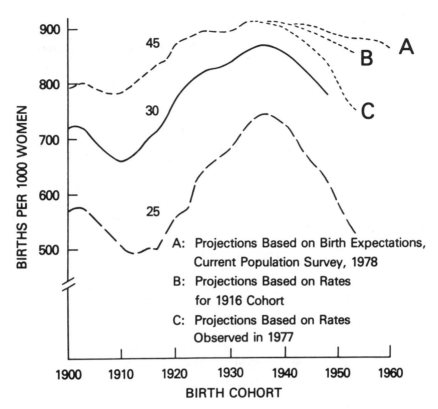

Figure 15-1. Cumulative Rate for First Births by Ages 25, 30, and 45: Birth
Cohorts of 1900-1960

and early 1950s would have to maintain rates close to the highest observed in U.S. experience after age 25 if they are to reach the numbers of second births expressed in the birth expectations collected in 1978. Also, as shown in figure 15-4, the rates for second births at ages 25 to 29 and 30 to 34 would have to be considerably higher than those observed in the 1960s and 1970s.

We may conclude from these considerations that the numbers of first and second births expected by the cohorts of the 1950s now appear to overstate the actual numbers of first and second births that these cohorts will ultimately have. In other words, it now seems that many of the presumably "postponed" first and second births will never occur. This conclusion should be regarded as an opinion subject to future verification, but the method of arriving at it illustrates the kind of analysis to which current birth expectations of young women should be subjected. In addition, similar analyses should be undertaken for third and higher-order births despite the

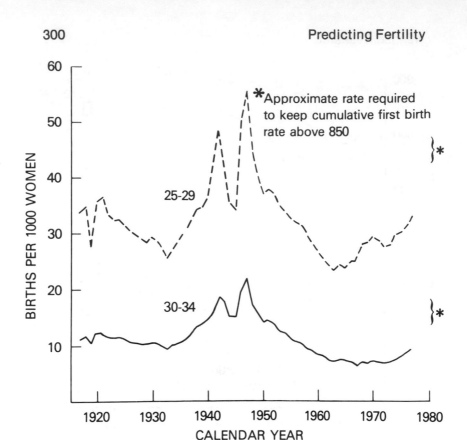

Figure 15–2. First Births per 1,000 Women at Ages 25 to 29 and 30 to 34: 1917–1977

low numbers currently expected, because some couples who have two children may revise their fertility intentions upward. So far, there has never been a cohort with as few as 400 third and higher-order births per 1,000 women, as expected by the cohorts of 1954–1960. It is possible that these expectations are unrealistically low.

The foregoing brief analysis recalls the desirability, noted in chapter 3 by Long and Wetrogan, of research on the stability of expectations for births of various orders. For example, it is possible that expectations for third and higher order births are less stable than those for first and second births. This is suggested by the experience of the 1940 cohorts, whose numbers reduced their expected numbers of third and higher-order births to a greater extent than those of first and second births. On the other hand, comparisons of the 1970 and 1975 NFS surveys showed that women who had zero, one, or two children by 1970 were less likely to have predicted

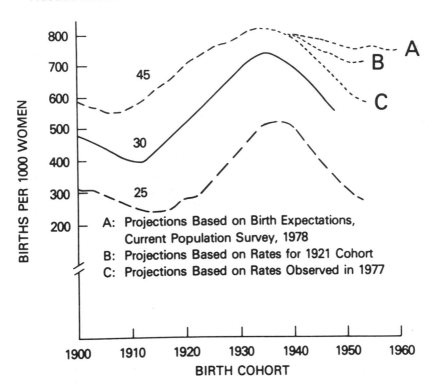

Figure 15-3. Cumulative Rate for Second Births by Ages 25, 30, and 45: Birth Cohorts of 1900–1960

their fertility accurately than women who had three or more children by 1970 (Westoff and Ryder 1977b). Obviously, the stability of birth expectations by parity and by total number of births expected needs much more attention than it has received.

A persistent difficulty involved in the use of data on birth expectations for making fertility forecasts arises from the fact that even if the long-term birth expectations of young women were to prove reasonably accurate, these women will have a major impact on fertility rates only for the ten years following data collection. Younger cohorts, not yet interviewed, will contribute the majority of births after that time. The question arises, then, as to whether data on birth expectations for young women can serve as reasonable guides to the birth expectations of still younger women for whom no information on birth expectations exists. Birth expectations have been used as such guides in the past, but insofar as we can verify expectations they have not always proved to be reliable. For example, the medium

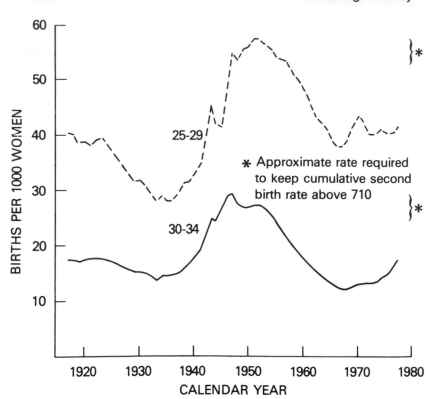

Figure 15–4. Second Births per 1,000 Women at Ages 25 to 29 and 30 to 34: 1917–1977

assumptions used in making population forecasts on the basis of the 1955 GAF study includes completed fertility rates of 2,867 for the cohorts of the 1950s, whose members are now expecting between 2,000 and 2,100 births per 1,000 women. There is no way around this problem other than to revise population projections fairly frequently (perhaps every five years), using the most recent data available at the time the projections are prepared.

In summary, research needed on long-term birth expectations includes the following elements:

1. Comparisons should be made between expected and actual completed fertility rates, with emphasis on verifying the expectations of young women. This research should separate observed fertility rates for women represented in the samples providing expectations from the fertility rates of women who were not represented in those samples.

2. More research should be directed toward the study of changes in birth expectations as cohorts grow older and the number of ever-married women rises. For this purpose, it would be useful for the census bureau to publish birth expectations for birth cohorts of women, rather than for standard age groups only.

3. The data resources needed to carry out the research proposed in this chapter are readily available for the United States. In addition, such research should be conducted with the use of data from other countries whenever possible.

4. Comparisons should continue to be made between the birth expectations of young women, their cumulative fertility rates up to the age at which they are interviewed, and the level of age-specific rates required to realize their birth expectations. This should help in assessing the validity of current birth expectations and in avoiding the temptation to take them at their face value.

5. The stability and validity of expected numbers of births of given orders should be studied. Emphasis should be given to first and second births, separately, because these orders of births will account for most births in the United States. Essentially, it has become very important to know whether the traditional preference for at least two children is surviving or whether more couples are choosing to have no children or one child only.

6. Finally, as was also recommended for research on short-term birth expectations, alternative methods of forecasting completed fertility rates, possibly on the basis of hypotheses relating fertility to social and economic changes, should be developed and the results compared with forecasts based on data on birth expectations. At the present time, there are no theories that link specific levels of completed fertility to changes in the social and economic variables affecting cohorts as they proceed through the reproductive years of life, and this absence of a predictive theory tends to place more reliance on birth expectations as predictors than may eventually be warranted. Nevertheless, unless better methods of forecasting fertility are developed, reliance will continue to be placed on birth expectations despite their many limitations.

References

Ryder, Norman B., and Westoff, Charles F. "The Trend of Expected Parity in the United States: 1955, 1960, 1965." *Population Index* 33 (1967): 153–168.

United Nations. Economic Commission for Europe. *Fertility and Family Planning in Europe around 1970: a Comparative Study of Twelve*

National Surveys. New York: United Nations Department of Economic and Social Affairs, Population Studies no. 58 (1976), pp. 97–147.

Westoff, Charles F.; Mishler, Elliot G.; and Kelly, E. Lowell. "Preferences in Size of Family and Eventual Fertility Twenty Years After." *American Journal of Sociology* 62 (1957): 491–497.

Westoff, Charles F.; Potter, Robert G., Jr.; and Sagi, Philip C. *The Third Child.* Princeton, N.J.: Princeton University Press, 1963.

Westoff, Charles F., and Ryder, Norman B. *The Contraceptive Revolution,* pp. 179–247. Princeton, N.J.: Princeton University Press, 1977a.

————. "The Predictive Validity of Reproductive Intentions." *Demography* 14 (1977b): 431–453.

16 Conclusions

Gerry E. Hendershot and
Paul J. Placek

Toward a Conceptual Framework

It may be useful to develop the tentative conceptual framework that seems to underlie much of the authors' thinking in the chapters of this book. This framework does not represent the thinking of any one author, or even of all the authors collectively, but contains, in the judgment of the editors, those elements that together constitute a synthetic whole.

In addition to birth expectations, the authors considered a variety of other fertility orientations. Perhaps the most systematic treatment of these different varieties of orientations was that of Ryder in chapter 7. He considered both the face validity and the empirical relationships among fertility ideals, desires, and intentions. On the face of it, these would appear to be progressively more specific measures in the order just listed: Fertility ideals are very general and set the conditions for more specific personal desires, which in turn have an important impact on fertility intentions. Despite that logic, Ryder concludes that intentions are more likely the cause of desires and ideals rather than their effects. Ryder also notes that he had concluded on the basis of previous research that there was no useful empirical distinction to be made between intentions and expectations. Other authors also recognize the difficulty of measuring fertility orientations unambiguously, but they are less pessimistic than Ryder about the outcome of the effort. In any case, most approach the problem as if there existed in the minds of most women an "expectation" about the number of children they would bear. This assumption underlies our framework.

Some Features of Birth Expectations

An expectation is a belief that a future event has a high probability of occurrence. A birth expectation is a belief that a given number of births is very likely to occur in the future. Expressing the concept in this way, we can highlight several features of birth expectations. First, birth expectations are beliefs or ideas, presumably subject to the same dynamics as all ideas and beliefs. Second, while birth expectations have a high probability and are very likely to occur, the degree of certainty required to raise a possible future event to the level of an expectation is not specified. Third, women

305

may have several different fertility expectations, that is, they may believe that several different numbers of future births are very likely. Fourth, relative satisfaction with individual achieved birth expectations may depend on birth outcome, such as the health or sex of the child.

Some of the implications of these features of birth expectations are important to their interpretation. For instance, since they are ideas, expectations may change in response to newly internalized beliefs, various psychic phenomena, and changing perceptions of external conditions. Such changes in expectations need not be regarded solely as evidence of unreliability or instability, but as a normal and understandable aspect of fertility orientations. This latter view is characteristic of Lee's approach in chapter 6 to expectations as "moving targets" that can be predicted.

The recognition that expectations entail some high but otherwise unspecified probability of occurrence also affects our interpretations of the data. For example, it is questionable that birth expectations exist at all if women do not think *any* number of future births very likely, that is, if they attach only low probabilities to every particular number (including zero) that they might consider. Also, women whose *subjective* probabilities of a given number of births are the same may have different *objective* probabilities. In other words, the level of objective probability considered high may vary from woman to woman; one woman might "expect" a given number of births if she assesses the odds as better than 50–50, while another women would not "expect" a given number until the odds reached, say, 90–10. We do know that among women who report an expected number of births, and who therefore presumably regard the event as likely, there is considerable variation in the level of certainty they express. In chapter 2 Oakley discussed data from the National Natality Surveys (NNS) indicating that roughly equal numbers of mothers expected more children "definitely" and "probably."

It may be that because women regard an objectively low probability as subjectively high, they may "expect" more than one number of future births. For instance, a woman might believe that at an objective probability of 0.4 the likelihood of no additional births was "high," and at the same time believe that at a probability of 0.5 there was also a "high" likelihood of one birth, and at a probability of 0.1 there was a "low" likelihood of two births. In such situations researchers would most often be interested in the *most* likely number—one birth—but they might also be interested in some weighted average of the several "expected" numbers. Not many women, however, would quantify their expectations as we have in this example. Instead, they would "sense" or "feel" some degree of certainty. Not being bound by the logic of mathematical probability, they might even "expect" at a high level of certainty two or more contradictory events.

Finally, women's satisfaction with precisely achieved birth expectations may be contingent on birth outcome. The birth of a retarded child or a child who dies early in life may serve as a stimulus to an additional expected birth. Similarly, sex composition of birth outcomes may affect future fertility. Women who wanted two births (say, a girl and a boy) may try again if the first two are girls. Several papers listed in appendix A deal with these types of contingencies.

The point here is not that birth expectations are illogical and their measurement hopeless, but that they may conform to a logic different from that familiar to the statistician. Ultimately, women's expectations must be transformed to a common statistical mode if they are to be useful for forecasting, but that transformation must be based on a better understanding of the original logic that produced them. Research of the kind reported by Hirsch, Seltzer, and Zelnik in chapter 12, and by Blake and del Pinal in chapter 13, both of which explore the reasons given by respondents for their fertility orientations, are helpful in understanding this logic.

Fertility Goals, Personal Resources, and Opportunity Structure

The model of expectation formation that predominates in the research reported in this book includes as immediate precursors of expectations both fertility goals and the means (opportunity structure and personal resources) for attaining those goals. Women are assumed to have some preferred ultimate family size that is formed early in life (prior to the teenage years, according to Hirsch, Seltzer, and Zelnik in chapter 12), and that is relatively stable thereafter. Also, they have some stock of resources to draw on in their efforts to achieve their fertility goals. There is a periodic or continuous assessment of fertility goals in relation to the means currently and prospectively available for their achievement, and this results in current expectations about future births. Since fertility desires generally are assumed to be rooted partly in personality, and therefore to be quite stable, variation in the *means* for achieving fertility goals becomes the principal proximate cause of change in expectations. Figure 16-1 depicts the model of expectation formation that we have just described.

However, Ryder (chapter 7) and Hirsch, Seltzer, and Zelnik (chapter 12) present evidence against the relative stability of fertility desires. Ryder shows that for the National Fertility Survey (NFS) sample, desires did change substantially between 1970 and 1975; and Hirsch, Seltzer, and Zelnik report a similar, though smaller, change in desires between their 1971 and 1976 samples of young women. Yet these authors do not so much deny the existence of a stable orientation toward fertility as suggest that stated first preferences may not be an adequate measure of them. As measured, fertility

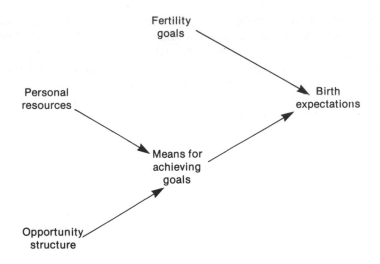

Figure 16-1. Model of Expectation Formation

desires are "rationalizations" of actual cumulative fertility and/or future expected fertility, much like those discussed by Pullum in chapter 8. In fact, Hirsch, Seltzer, and Zelnik advance that finding as an argument for regarding fertility desires, as measured by stated first preferences, as a surrogate for birth expectations. But none of these authors would necessarily disagree with the position described by Oakley in chapter 2 that the fertility goals relevant to a model of birth expectations lie deep within the person and are not retrieved by simple questions, although they may be retrieved by more detailed questions. In chapter 4 Westoff describes a technique developed by Lolagene Coombs that attempts (and in Westoff's view succeeds) in tapping underlying preferences for family size.

Given the assumptions of this model, the large and pervasive decline in birth expectations in the 1970s described by several of the authors (Long and Wetrogan, chapter 3; Ryder, chapter 7; Moore, chapter 9; Masnick, chapter 10; Hirsch, Seltzer, and Zelnik, chapter 12) must be accounted for in terms of changes in the *means* available to women for the achievement of their fertility desires. These means may be thought of as including both personal resources and a causal nexus or opportunity structure. Personal resources might include the money, time, effort, knowledge, or motivation needed to bear and rear children; the opportunity structure might include the institutional, legal, or organizational structures through which those personal resources could be applied. The distinction between personal resources and opportunity structure is made in order to emphasize that persons act (and anticipate action) within a social context, so that both personal resources and opportunity structure affect their expectations. Blake and del Pinal in chapter 13 give a good illustration of this point: They show that men's and women's perceptions of the personal costs and benefits of children depend on their perceptions of the probable division of labor between husband and wife in a marriage.

Explanation of changes in birth expectations, such as the decline in the 1970s, and forecasting of future trends in birth expectations, such as that called for by Lee (chapter 6), require consideration of both the personal resources and opportunity structures of women in, or soon to be in, the childbearing years. Personal resources might seem to have a greater potential for change than opportunity structures. Personal resources are known to change during the life cycle and in response to economic cycles; the laws and customs that define institutions, however, typically change more slowly. Thus, change in birth expectations might be expected in a cohort as it ages, and as its average personal resources change; also, the change might result from entry into the childbearing years of new cohorts whose personal resources differed, on the average, from those of earlier cohorts (see, for example, the discussion of Easterlin in chapter 1).

It is interesting to note in Ryder's study (chapter 7), which statistically sorted out the several sources of decline in birth expectations, that the aging and cohort effects were less than the period effects; that is, the decline resulted from some historical change that operated independently of cohort composition and aging of cohorts. That finding suggests either that the decline resulted from a change in personal resources experienced by most women, or that some institutional changes occurred in that period. Certainly there were institutional changes, such as the spread of publicly supported contraceptive services and the legalization of abortion; those changes enhanced means for limiting childbearing, and would therefore reduce expectations to the extent that those expectations exceeded fertility goals. But the evidence suggests that expectations were already below desires, so that personal resources must have been low and probably declining. Such an effect can also be read into the situation of the early 1970s: Inflation and recession were placing greater burdens on household budgets by increasing the direct costs of children; and increasing proportions of wives were in the labor force, thereby increasing the indirect or opportunity costs of childbearing.

It is not our purpose here to advocate a particular explanation of the decline in birth expectations in the 1970s. Nor does the fact that cohort and life-cycle changes were less important than historical changes in that period mean that the former are not important. The historical changes of that period may well be unusual, and we therefore need to understand the more predictable effects of cohort and life cycle, as Campbell recommends in chapter 15. We intend, rather, to illustrate the kind of considerations that must be made in attempts to explain and predict changes in expectations. The predominant factor in short-run trends in expectations will be the means available to couples to achieve their family-size goals; and those means, in turn, consist of their personal resources and their opportunity structures.

Prediction and Events: More on Fate and Control

Within the context of the model we have described, what are the conditions under which birth expectations will accurately predict future fertility? One source of inaccuracy is changing expectations; but since Lee has shown in chapter 6 that this problem is tractable, we will limit our consideration to situations in which expectations are stable. If we maintain the assumption made earlier that short-run fertility goals are relatively stable, we are left with this question: "How does variation in the means of achieving desired fertility affect the predictive accuracy of expectations?"

If the means for achieving fertility desires are fully adequate, women should expect and achieve their fertility goals. When they have the personal resources needed to bear and rear the children they want, and the institutional context makes it possible for them to apply those resources toward that end, most women should assess the probability as "high" that they will bear the number of children desired, and should then go ahead to realize their expectations. Such adequacy of means, both of personal resources and opportunity structure, may be referred to as a situation of *control* (see our discussion of fate and control in chapter 1). Where there is control, fertility expectations and actual future fertility will very often coincide. The predictability of individual fertility should therefore be very accurate.

As the adequacy of means declines, however, the average certainty of expectations will decline at first, and fertility will less often match expectations. With fewer personal resources and/or opportunities for applying them, subjective probabilities of bearing a desired number of children will decline, and unexpected outcomes will occur more often. Paradoxically, however, when the means of achieving desired fertility are very meager, the predictive accuracy of expectations may again turn upward, as shown in figure 16-2. The reason is that when personal resources afford so little control over fertility, the expectation is likely to be "whatever God sends" or its functional equivalent for the particular culture in question. The outcome of such uncontrolled fertility is known, on the average, from the

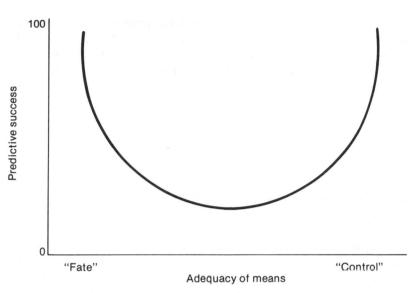

Figure 16–2. Predictive Success Given Varying Degrees of Control over Means

recent past experience of the population. Such a condition of deprived means for attaining fertility desires may be termed *fate*. It is questionable whether persons subject to fate actually have "birth expectations" in the sense of anticipating specific numbers of future births; however, their lack of control over their own situation makes it possible for demographers to predict their aggregate-level fertility correctly from their recent past experience.

The somewhat paradoxical conclusion, then, is that prediction of aggregate fertility is likely to be accurate when individual fertility is completely controlled (based on birth expectations within the "perfect-contraceptive population") as well as when it is completely uncontrolled (where fatalistic resignation to whatever the future brings determines future fertility). Of course, neither of these conditions is found in a pure form in the real world. However, conditions approximating those of "fate" are found in some in the populations described by Cho and Kantrow in chapter 14 and by Pullum in chapter 8. The conditions in the United States, the subject of most of the other chapters, are very far removed from fate, but probably also somewhat removed from perfect control. Despite institutional changes making it easier for couples to apply their resources to achieving their desired fertility, not all fertility-control services are available to all couples who may want to use them; furthermore, personal resources are often inadequate for bearing and rearing all the children desired. For countries in both situations, however, the movement is toward greater control; consequently, the usefulness of birth expectations for accurate predictions may increase in developed countries, while predictability using birth expectations may be reduced in less-developed countries. Thus, it is possible that in less-developed countries more reliance on social and demographic factors, and less reliance on birth expectations, would lead to more accurate predictions of aggregate future fertility.

A Final Word: What Should We Expect from Expectations?

The principal use for data about expectations of future births has been to forecast future fertility. A number of the chapters in this book have attempted to evaluate the success of that use by comparing reported expectations of future births with the births that actually occurred in that future period (Long and Wetrogan, chapter 3; Hendershot and Placek, chapter 5; Moore, chapter 9; and Campbell, chapter 15). Depending on the particular period considered and the judgment of the author, these comparisons were variously considered to validate or invalidate expectations as a predictive tool.

While we agree with Campbell (chapter 15) that such attempts should continue, we also suggest that the standard for evaluating expectations data be rethought. The business of predicting the future is notoriously risky. Even in fields with a long history of forecasting and a well-developed data base (such as agriculture and economics), prediction is far from perfect. The situation is even less favorable in the area of fertility forecasting, although the need is just as great. The field of predicting fertility has a modern history of only twenty-five years' duration, its data bases do not yet cover all of the population whose behavior it attempts to predict, and the data points are years apart and often not available until years after the fact. That expectations-based predictions have typically come within 10 to 15 percent of the fertility they predicted is commendable under those conditions.

A more reasonable standard of comparison than actual fertility are the forecasts made by other means. Forecasts based on simple tranformations of current period-fertility measures, for instance, may be compared with expectation-based forecasts, as Westoff and Ryder have done. Long and Wetrogan in chapter 3 recommend a similar approach, and in their own application of it arrive at a favorable conclusion about expectations data as predictors of fertility. Expectations-based forecasts should also be compared with those based on theoretical interpretations of social and economic trends. Campbell noted in chapter 15 that a theory relating those trends to predictions of fertility had not yet been developed. The beginning of such theories exist, however, in the cohort theory of Easterlin and the social-economic theory of Westoff, which we discussed briefly in chapter 1. The body of experience must be broadened and lengthened and forecasts based on all these ideas, including demographic studies of birth expectations, must be comparatively evaluated to improve the prediction of fertility.

Appendix A
Additional Selected References

The additional selected references that follow are references that have not been cited throughout the book. They are included here in order to provide a more complete representation of demographic studies of birth expectations.

Adamchak, Donald J. "Ideal Family Size and Family Background: An Examination of Mother's Employment and Daughter's Family Size Preferences." *Social Biology* 24 (1977): 170-172.

Anderson, Jeanne L. "Trends in Expected Family Size in the United States." *New York Statistician* 26 (1975): 1-2, 4, 6.

Beaujot, Roder P.; Krotki, Karol J.; and Krishnan, Parameswara. "Socio-cultural Variations in the Applicability of the Economic Model of Fertility." *Population Studies* 32 (1978): 319-325.

Blake, Judith. "Income and Reproductive Motivation." *Population Studies* 21 (1967): 185-206.

Bonham, Gordon, and Placek, Paul J. "The Relationships of Maternal Health, Infant Health, and Sociodemographic Factors to Fertility." *Public Health Reports* 93 (1978): 283-292.

Cartwright, Ann. "Mothers' Perceptions of Reasons for Family Size." In *How Many Children?* pp. 95-100. London: Routledge and Kegan Paul, 1976a.

———. "Nature of Intentions." In *How Many Children?* pp. 19-32. London: Routledge and Kegan Paul, 1976b.

———. "Family Size, Contraceptive Practice, and Fertility Intentions in England and Wales, 1967-1975." *Family Planning Perspectives* 11 (1979): 128-135.

Chatterjee, P.K. "Attitudes to Additional Children: A Study of Motivating Factors." *Journal of Family Welfare* 33 (1977): 76-84.

Coombs, Clyde H.; Coombs, Lolagene C.; and McClelland, Gary H. "Preference Scales for Number and Sex of Children." *Population Studies* 29 (1975): 273-298.

Coombs, Lolagene C. "Levels of Reliability in Fertility Survey Data." *Studies in Family Planning* 8 (1977): 218-232.

———. "Preferences for Sex of Children Among U.S. Couples." *Family Planning Perspectives* 9 (1977): 259-265.

———. "Underlying Family-Size Preferences and Reproductive Behavior in the United States." *Studies in Family Planning* 10 (1979): 25-36.

———— "Reproductive Goals and Achieved Fertility: A Fifteen-Year Perspective." *Demography* 16 (1979): 523–534.

Coombs, Lolagene C., and Fernandez, Dorothy. "Husband-Wife Agreement About Reproductive Goals." *Demography* 15 (1978): 57–73.

Coombs, Lolagene C., and Freedman, Ronald. "Some Roots of Preference: Roles, Activities and Familial Values." *Demography* 16 (1979): 359–376.

Coombs, Lolagene C., and Sun, Te-Hsiung; "Family Composition Preferences in a Developing Culture: The Case of Taiwan." *Population Studies* 32 (1978): 43–64.

Corsa, Leslie, and Oakley, Deborah. *Population Planning.* Ann Arbor: University of Michigan Press, 1979.

Davidson, Andrew R., and Jaccard, James J. "Social-psychological Determinants of Fertility Intentions." In *Population Psychology: Research and Educational Issues,* edited by Sidney H. Newman and Vaida D. Thompson, pp. 131–137. Washington, D.C.: U.S. Government Printing Office, 1976.

Dinkel, Robert M. "Number of Children Desired by U.S. Wives and Education of Wife, Husband, and Her Parents for Selected Religious, Residence, and Color Groups." Proceedings of the International Population Conference of the International Union for the Scientific Study of Population, Liege, 1971, pp. 1890–1902.

Fleisher, B.M., and Rhodes, G.F. "Fertility, Women's Wage Rates, and Labor Supply." *American Economic Review* 69 (1979): 14–24.

Foreit, K.G., and Suh, M.H. "The Effect of Reproductive Intentions on Subsequent Fertility among Low-Parity Korean Women, 1971–76." *Studies in Family Planning* 11 (1980): 105–113.

Freedman, Ronald; Coombs, Lolagene C.; and Bumpass, Larry. "Stability and Change in Expectations About Family Size: A Longitudinal Study." *Demography* 2 (1965): 250–275.

Freedman, Deborah S.; Freedman, Ronald; and Whelpton, Pascal K. "Size of Family and Preference for Children of Each Sex." *American Journal of Sociology* 66 (1960): 141–146.

Freedman, Ronald; Hermalin, Albert I.; and Chang, Ming-Cheng. "Do Statements About Desired Family Size Predict Fertility? The Case of Taiwan, 1967–1970." *Demography* 12 (1975): 407–416.

Freedman, Ronald, and Takeshita, John. "The Number of Children Wanted and the Number Born: Ideal and Reality." In *Family Planning in Taiwan: An Experiment in Social Change,* edited by Ronald Freedman and J.Y. Takeshita. Princeton, N.J.: Princeton University Press, 1969.

Frenkel, Izaslaw. "Attitudes Toward Family Size in Some East European Countries." *Population Studies* 30 (1976): 35–57.

Hermalin, Albert I., Freedman, Ronald; Sun, Te-Hsiung; and Chang, Ming-Cheng. "Do Intentions Predict Fertility? The Experience in Taiwan, 1967–74." *Studies in Family Planning* 10 (1979): 75–95.

Kiesler, Sara B. "Post Hoc Justification of Family Size." *Sociometry* 40 (1977): 59–67.

Kunofsky, Judith. "Population Projections: How They Are Made . . . and How They Make Themselves Come True." *Sierra,* January–February 1979, pp. 34–36.

Langford, Christopher M. "Women's Ideas About Family Size." In *Birth Control Practice and Marital Fertility in Great Britain: A Report on a Survey Carried Out in 1967–68,* pp. 16, 25, 95–103. London: London School of Economics, Population Investigation Committee, 1976.

Lawrence, Charles E., and Mundigo, Axel I. "Female Family Size Ideals as Population Policy Objectives for Latin America: Demographic and Methodological Considerations." *Policy Sciences* 8 (1977): 437–454.

Lee, Che-fu, and Khan, Mohammad M. "Factors Related to the Intention to Have Additional Children in the United States: A Reanalysis of Data from the 1965 and 1970 National Fertility Studies." *Demography* 15 (1978): 337–344.

Lee, Ronald Demos. "New Methods for Forecasting Fertility." *Population Bulletin of the United Nations* 11 (1978): 6–11.

McClelland, Gary H. "Determining the Impact of Sex Preferences on Fertility: A Consideration of Parity Progression Ratio, Dominance, and Stopping Rule Measures." *Demography* 16 (1979): 377–388.

Mendoza, Elvira. "Socio-economic Correlates of Attitude toward Family Size." In *Sociological Contributions to Family Planning Research,* edited by D.J. Bogue, pp. 36–70. Chicago: University of Chicago Press, 1967.

National Center for Health Statistics. "Expected Size of Completed Family Among Currently Married Women 15–44 Years of Age: United States, 1973." *Advance Data* 10 (1977). Prepared by Gordon Bonham.

Park, Chai Bin. "Lifetime Probability of Additional Births by Age and Parity for American Women, 1935–1968: A New Measurement of Period Fertility." *Demography* 13 (1976): 1–17.

Park, C.E., and Kim, M.I. "A Study on Wanted Number and Sex Composition of Children of Women in a Korean Rural Area, Based on Coombs Preference Scale." *Journal of Family Planning Studies* 3 (1976): 81–83.

Rao, S.L.N. "Recent Changes in Expected Family Size: Some Panel Results from Rhode Island." *Studies in Family Planning* 4 (1973): 70–72.

Ryder, Norman B. "The Predictability of Fertility Planning Status." *Studies in Family Planning* 7 (1976a): 294–307.

———. "The Specification of Fertility Planning Status." *Family Planning Perspectives* 8 (1976b) 283–290.

Schultz, T. Paul. *Fertility Determinants: A Theory, Evidence, and an Application to Policy Evaluation.* Santa Monica, California: Rand Corporation, 1974. Prepared for the Rockefeller Foundation and the Agency for International Development, R-1016-RF/AID.

Shah, Nasra M., and Palmore, James A. "Desired Family Size and Contraceptive Use in Pakistan." *International Family Planning Perspectives* 5 (1979): 143–150.

Stycos, J.M. "Haitian Attitudes Toward Family Size." In *Human Fertility in Latin America: Sociological Perspectives,* pp. 116–132. Ithaca, N.Y.: Cornell University Press, 1968a.

———. "Social Class and Preferred Family Size in Peru." In *Human Fertility in Latin America: Sociological Perspectives,* pp. 147–161. Ithaca, N.Y.: Cornell University Press, 1968b.

Terhune, Kenneth W. "Fertility Values: Why People Stop Having Children." Proceedings of the eighty-first annual convention of the American Psychological Association, Montreal. Washington, D.C.: American Psychological Association, 1973, pp. 351–352.

———. *A Review of the Actual and Expected Consequences of Family Size.* U.S. Dept. of Health, Education, and Welfare, Public Health Publication No. (NIH) 75-779. Calspan Report No. DP-5333-G-1, July 31, 1974.

Townes, Brenda D.; Beach, Lee Roy; Campbell, Frederick L.; and Martin, Donald C. "Birth-Planning Values and Decisions: The Prediction of Fertility." *Journal of Applied Psychology* 7 (1977): 73–88.

Townes, Brenda D.; Campbell, Frederick L.; Beach, Lee Roy; and Martin, Donald C. "Birth-planning Values and Decisions: Preliminary Findings." In *Population Psychology: Research and Educational Issues,* edited by Sidney H. Newman and Vaida D. Thompson, pp. 113–130. Washington, D.C.: U.S. Government Printing Office, 1976.

Van Keep, P.A. "Ideal Family Size in Five European Countries." *Family Planning Resumé* 1 (1977): 89–90.

Woolf, Myra. "Family Size." In *Family Intentions.* London: Her Majesty's Stationery Office, Office of Population Censuses and Surveys, Social Survey Division 55408, 1971, pp. 11–37.

Wynnyczuk, V. "Relations Between Socio-economic Characteristics and Desired Family Size: Findings on a Survey of 21-Year-Old Women." In Proceedings of the International Population Conference of the International Union for the Scientific Study of Population, Liege, 1971, pp. 1644–1652.

**Three Good Sources of Demographic Data on Birth
Expectations**

Division of Vital Statistics
National Center for Health Statistics
3700 East-West Highway
Hyattsville, Md. 20782

Population Division
Bureau of the Census
U.S. Department of Commerce
Washington, D.C. 20233

World Fertility Survey
International Statistical Institute
35-37 Grosvenor Gardens
London SW1W OBS
United Kingdom

Appendix B:
Survey Questions on
Birth Expectations

A wide variety of questions on birth expectations and other fertility orientations have been employed in the United States and World Fertility Surveys.
We have assembled questions used in recent major surveys and have shown
in parentheses the chapters of this book in which those survey questions
were the primary focus of attention.

Current Population Survey (chapters 2, 3, 6, 9, 10, 11, and 15)

1. Do you expect to have any (more) children?
2. How many (more) do you expect to have?
3. How many (more) do you expect to have in the next 5 years?
4. When do you expect your (next, first) child to be born?

National Natality Survey (chapters 2, 5)

1. Do you expect to have more children? (Check one box only)
   □ Definitely yes
   □ Probably yes
   □ Probably no ⎫
   □ Definitely no ⎭   Skip to _____
2. How many more children do you think you will probably have? (Please
   give your best estimate).

National Survey of Family Growth (chapter 5)

1. Do you and your husband intend to have a(nother) baby?
2. How many (more) do you intend to have?
3. Of course, sometimes things do not work out exactly as we intend them
   to, or something makes us change our minds. In your case, how sure
   are you that you will have (number) (more) babies? Would you say you
   are very sure or not very sure?
4. No one can be certain about the future, but you probably have some
   idea of how close you will come to the number you intend to have.
   What is the *largest* number of (additional) babies you expect to have?
   What is the *smallest* number of (additional) babies you expect to have?

5. When do you expect your (first/next) baby to be born?
6. When do you expect your last baby to be born—that is, about how many years from now?
7. If you do have (number) (more) babies, how many of these do you expect to have in the next five years?
8. The number of children people expect is not always the same as the number they would most like to have. Knowing how other things are for you and your husband, if you could choose exactly the number of children to have in your whole life, how many would you choose now?

National Fertility Study (chapters 4, 7)

1. Do you and your husband intend to have any children (another child)?
2. Do you intend to have your first (next) child within two years from now?
3. How many (more) children do you intend to have?
4. Given the circumstances of your life, how many children *in all* would you really consider the most desirable for you and your husband?
5. What do you think is the *ideal* size of a family—a husband, a wife, and how many children?

World Fertility Survey (chapters 8, 14)

1. I am going to ask you some questions about what you *want* to happen and what you *expect* to happen. First of all, do you *want* to have any children (another child) sometime?
2. Taking everything into consideration, do you *expect* you will have a (another) child sometime?
3. How many (more) children in all do you expect to have?
4. In what year would you prefer your next child to be born?
5. If you could choose exactly the number of children to have in your whole life, how many children would that be?

National Survey of Young Women (chapter 12)

1. Here are some questions on marriage and children. First, how many children would you like to have?
2. Why would you like to have (number) children?

Index

Index

About the Contributors

Judith Blake is the Fred H. Bixby Professor of Population Policy, School of Public Health and Department of Sociology, University of California, Los Angeles. Previously, she was a member of the faculty of the University of California at Berkeley. She received the Ph.D. from Columbia University. She is the author of many publications on population, mostly in the area of fertility. In 1980, she was elected president of the Population Association of America.

Arthur Campbell is deputy director, Center for Population Research, National Institute for Child Health and Human Development, National Institutes of Health. He is the author of many publications on fertility, and was president of the Population Association of America from 1973 to 1974.

Lee-Jay Cho is director of the East-West Population Institute at the University of Hawaii. He received the Ph.D. in sociology from the University of Chicago. He has done extensive research on fertility and other aspects of the demography of the United States and Asian nations.

Marilyn Hirsch is a research assistant and doctoral candidate in the Department of Population Dynamics, School of Hygiene and Public Health, The Johns Hopkins University. Currently she is studying choice of contraceptive methods and method-switching among teenaged women.

Louise Kantrow is a population-affairs officer in the Population Program and Projects Branch of the Department of Technical Cooperation for Development at the United Nations in New York. She received the Ph.D. in demography from the University of Pennsylvania and is the author of numerous articles on population.

Ronald Lee is a professor of demography and economics at the University of California at Berkeley. He was previously a member of the faculty of the University of Michigan. He received the Ph.D. in economics from the University of California at Berkeley. He has published numerous articles based on applications of the techniques of econometrics to the study of population, especially population history.

John F. Long is chief of the Populations Projections Branch of the Bureau of the Census. He received the Ph.D. in demography from the University of North Carolina.

George S. Masnick is associate professor in the Department of Behavioral Sciences of the Harvard School of Public Health; he is an associate of both the Harvard Center for Population Studies and the Joint Center for Urban Studies. He received the Ph.D. in sociology from Brown University. His publications include research on housing, fertility, the demography of higher education, the sociology of aging, and the demography of local population changes.

Maurice J. Moore, the author of many publications on fertility, received the Ph.D. in sociology from the University of Chicago. He was formerly chief of the Fertility Statistics Branch of the Population Division of the Bureau of the Census.

Deborah Oakley is an assistant professor at the University of Michigan. She is the author or coauthor of many publications on population, including, with Leslie Corsa, *Population Planning,* one of the few population books translated into Chinese. She received the Ph.D. from the University of Michigan. An activist as well as a scholar, Ms. Oakley has held leadership positions in a number of national and international population-related organizations.

Martin O'Connell is a statistical demographer in the Fertility Statistics Branch of the Population Division of the Bureau of the Census. Previously, he was a research associate at the Population Studies Center of the University of Pennsylvania, where he received the Ph.D. in demography. He is the author or coauthor of numerous articles on fertility.

Jorge H. del Pinal is a research associate in the School of Public Health at the University of California at Los Angeles. He received the Ph.D. in demography from the University of California at Berkeley. His previous positions have included work on the demography of developing nations at the Bureau of the Census and in Guatemala.

Thomas W. Pullum is an associate professor of sociology and director of the Center for Studies in Demography and Ecology at the University of Washington. Previously, he held positions with the World Fertility Survey in London, and at the University of California at Davis, the University of the Philippines, and the University of Chicago. His major areas of professional activity are mathematical demography and the fertility of developing nations.

Norman Ryder is a professor in the Office of Population Research at Princeton University. His contributions to the field of demography have earned him many honors, including election to the presidency of the Population Association of America in 1972. In recent years his work has focused on analysis of the National Fertility Studies of 1970 and 1975.

Judith Seltzer is a research assistant and doctoral candidate in the Department of Population Dynamics, School of Hygiene and Public Health, The Johns Hopkins University. She received the M.A. in demography from Georgetown University and has held several positions in the fields of population education and population information.

Charles F. Westoff is a professor of demographic studies and director of the Office of Population Research at Princeton University. He is the author or coauthor of numerous books and articles on fertility, many of them dealing with large-scale surveys, such as the National Fertility Studies of 1965, 1970, and 1975. In addition to directing those studies, he was executive director of the U.S. Commission on Population Growth and the American Future and served as the president of the Population Association of America in 1974–1975.

Signe I. Wetrogan is in the Populations Projections Branch of the Bureau of the Census. She received the M.A. in demography from Georgetown University.

Melvin Zelnik is a professor of population dynamics at The Johns Hopkins University, where he has collaborated with John Kantner in several pioneering national fertility surveys of young women and men. He has engaged in demographic research and teaching at several universities and has also served at the Bureau of the Census.

About the Editors

Gerry E. Hendershot studied sociology and demography at the University of Michigan (A.B. 1959) and the University of Chicago (M.A. 1964, Ph.D. 1970). He served on the faculties of the College of Wooster, Vanderbilt University, and Brown University before taking his present position as a demographic statistician in the Family Growth Survey Branch, Division of Vital Statistics, National Center for Health Statistics. On several occasions he has been a visiting research demographer at the University of the Philippines Population Institute in Manila. His research and publications have been in several areas of demography, including mortality, migration, and fertility. Since joining the staff of the National Survey of Family Growth, his research has focused on fertility, family planning, and the reproductive health of American women.

Paul J. Placek studied sociology at Florida State University (A.B. 1967, M.S. 1968) and demography, medical sociology, and biostatistics at Vanderbilt University (Ph.D. 1974). He has taught population and sociology at the University of Tennessee, Vanderbilt University, and the University of Maryland. He is a demographic statistician in the Natality Statistics Branch, Division of Vital Statistics, National Center for Health Statistics. His research and publications are in the areas of family-planning communications, maternal and infant health, and fertility. He is the project director of the 1980 National Natality Survey and the 1980 National Fetal Mortality Survey being conducted by the National Center for Health Statistics.

DATE DUE